# The Health Secrets Handbook

THIS IS A CARLTON BOOK

Published in 2010 by Carlton Books Limited
20 Mortimer Street
London W1T 3JW

10 9 8 7 6 5 4 3 2 1


The text in this book has previously appeared in *1001 Little Health Miracles* (2004), *1001 Little Healthy Eating Miracles* (2007) and *1001 Little Wellbeing Miracles* (2008).



A CIP catalogue record for this book is available from the British Library.

ISBN 978 1 84732 660 7

Senior Executive Editor: Lisa Dyer
Managing Art Director: Lucy Coley
Designers: Anna Pow and Barbara Zuñiga
Production: Kate Pimm

Printed in China

# The Health Secrets Handbook

# Contents

# Introduction

Did you know that you'll eat less if you're blindfolded or that wrapping presents could help you burn 100 calories an hour?

On the following pages we've gathered together over 2000 little health gems, based on current scientific evidence, to help you stay healthy and happy in every area of your life. Whether you want a natural remedy to beat stress, an easy way to drop calories or hayfever and headache cures, this book is packed with easy-to-follow tips to help make your life brighter and better.

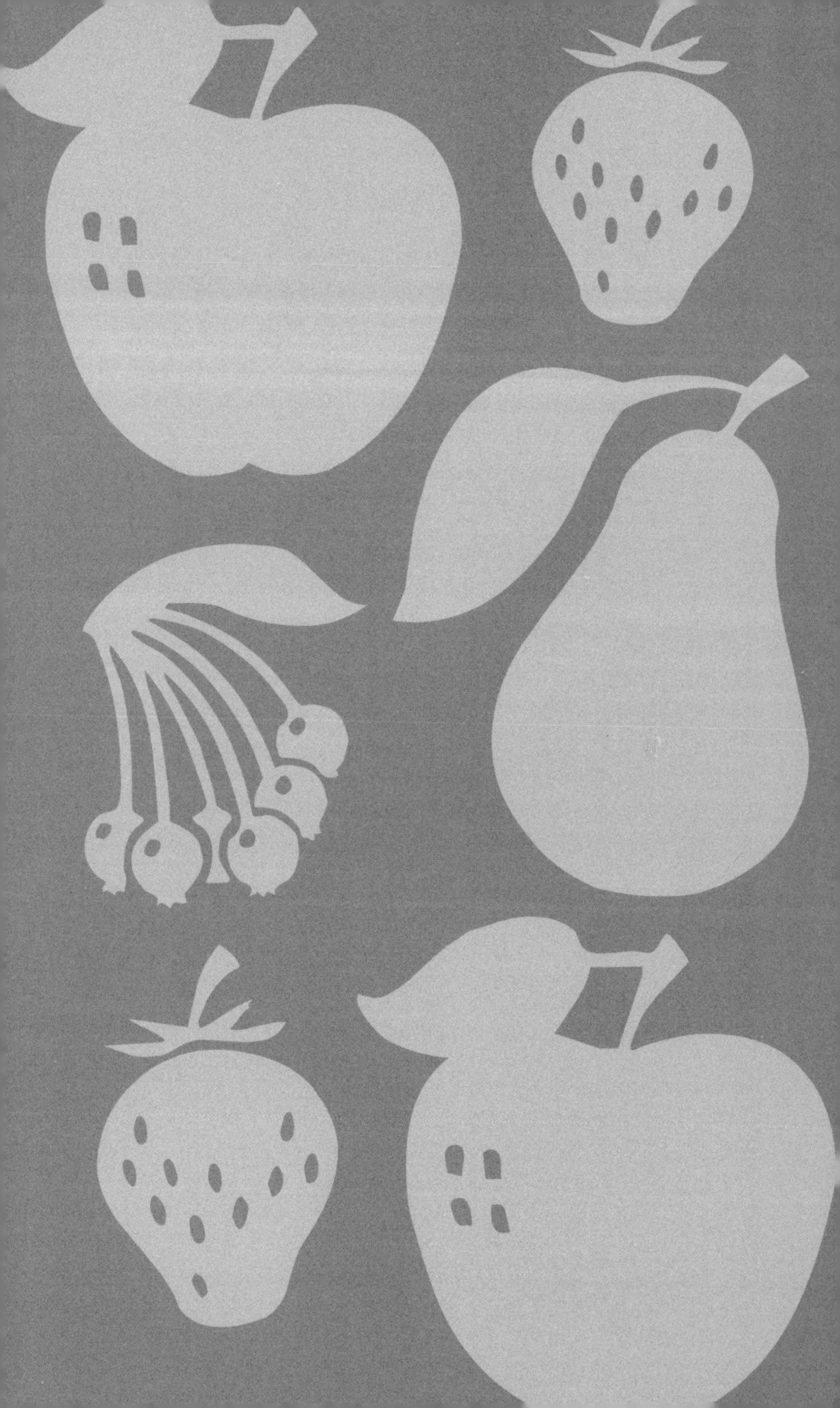

# Healthy Lifestyle

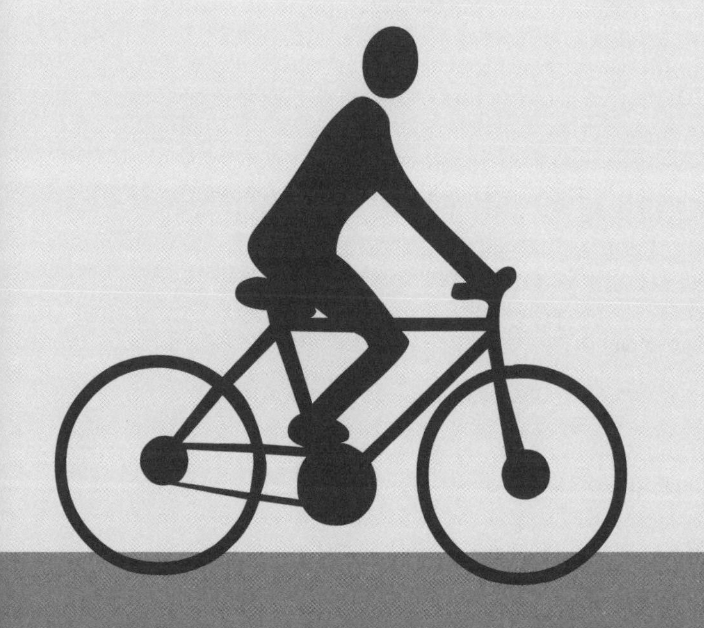

From easy ways to increase your mental fitness to giving up bad habits, here you will find a huge range of tips for healthier living. Along with tactics for changing poor attitudes toward food in the "food philosophy" section, there is advice on weight maintenance and calorie counting, eating habits and anti-ageing and how to choose healthy foods for family dinners, snacks and eating out.

# climate changes

## COTTON ON

During periods of high-heat and high-humidity, it's easier to develop the yeast infection candida. Opting for cotton underwear can help prevent problems arising, as can loose trousers and skirts.

## STAY WET IN WINTER

Water is important all year round but in winter, because of central heating and lots of stress on the body as temperatures change suddenly from cold outside to hot inside, it's even more important to drink eight glasses a day.

## RING THE WINTER CHANGES

Rings that get tighter in the winter could be a sign of fluid retention caused by too much salt, along with tighter shoes and socks that leave lines on ankles that aren't there in warmer weather. If this happens, drink more water.

## BANISH BODY ODOUR FASHIONABLY

Sweat and underarm odour are worse in the summer because it's harder for sweat to evaporate, leaving it in contact with the body for longer. Wear loose clothes in natural materials like cotton or linen, and avoid nylon.

## STEAM AHEAD TO BEAT WINTER COUGHS

People are more prone to developing coughs and lung problems in dry weather, which can dry out the inner membranes of the lungs and cause trauma to them. To alleviate seasonal coughs, have regular hot baths or steam inhalations.

## CHOOSE SEASONAL FOODS

In winter, root vegetables are more nutritious because the plants push their energy reserves into the roots to avoid the cold. In summer, flowering fruits like tomatoes contain more goodness. So follow nature for the healthiest diet.

## DON'T GET SORE, GET SCREENED

Cold sores are more common in the summer, when sudden exposure to sunlight puts the skin under stress. To avoid them, acclimatize slowly and use a sunscreen.

## WALK YOURSELF HAPPY

Just 15 minutes of daylight a day can help prevent the winter blues by giving your body a good dose of vitamin D, so get out in the fresh air.

## DON'T HAVE A FAT WINTER

Many people put on weight during the winter because their activity levels drop and food cravings increase with colder weather. Try indoor exercises like yoga to help you spring into spring.

## COOL AS A CUCUMBER

Cucumbers, mung beans and watermelon are particularly good foods to eat in the summer because they help keep your body cool and aid salt balance.

## TURN OFF WHEN YOU TURN IN

Sleep quality and quantity are both better when the bedroom temperature is on the low side, so turning off the central heating or turning down the thermostat on winter nights could help you get a better night's sleep.

## HIBERNATE FOR BETTER IMMUNITY

Studies have shown that in winter people need more sleep than in summer to reboot their immune systems, so let yourself have an extra half an hour in bed for that all-important extra winter resistance.

## PUT A HAT ON INFECTIONS

We lose a lot of our body heat through the skin on our head and neck, so covering up with a hat and scarf can help your body fight off infections by keeping you snug.

## SEE THE LIGHT

If you find yourself craving more starchy and sugary foods during the winter months, you may be suffering from seasonal affective disorder (SAD), which can be helped by daily exposure to natural sunlight or by light-box treatment.

### ESCAPE GERMS WITH ECHINACEA

Sudden, abrupt changes in the ambient temperature can take a toll on the body's energy levels, making it more prone to succumb to infections. If you're faced with hotter or colder climates, take echinacea, which has been shown to strengthen the immune system.

### BREATHE EASY ALL YEAR ROUND

Spring is called the allergy season but air quality is, in fact, worse in winter than at any other time. Fight allergies by upping your intake of free-radical fighters in fresh fruit and vegetables.

## ageing

### BE A HONEY IF YOU WANT TO STAY SHARP

Too much sugar in the diet has been found to leave damaging beta amyloid deposits in the brain, which can contribute to brain degeneration and Alzheimer's disease. Swap sugar for healthier alternatives like honey or maple syrup.

### COP YOURSELF A FEW EXTRA YEARS

Recent studies have shown that copper is essential for reducing age-related disintegration of body tissues. Get your doses from oysters, crab, nuts, soya beans, wholegrains, peas and lentils.

### WORK OUT TO WARD OFF DISEASE

Studies have shown that regular exercise boosts the levels of white blood cells in the blood. These white cells are responsible for fighting illnesses from flu to cancer and preventing tissue degeneration, so regular exercise really could help you fight ageing.

### DON'T BE FAZED, TAKE EFAS

Essential fatty acids (EFAs), found in oily fish, walnuts and oils such as olive, sunflower, linseed (flaxseed) and evening primrose, reduce inflammatory chemicals in the body and lead to better mental health and clarity. To keep your wits about you as you grow old, make sure you have some every day.

## BONE UP ON CHEESE

The calcium in cheese, particularly full-fat cheese, is essential for preventing the bone-thinning disease osteoporosis. Experts say that having three small portions of dairy products a day can help maintain strong bones.

## REMEMBER YOUR GLASSES

As we get older our sensitivity to thirst decreases, leading to dehydration and possible health problems. So it's even more important for older people to make sure they drink at least eight caffeine-free, non-alcoholic drinks a day.

## MUNCH DOWN YOUR BLOOD PRESSURE

Eggs, wheat, kidney, soya, alfalfa and rice bran all contain high levels of the vitamin-like substance coenzyme Q10, which is thought to boost immunity, lower blood pressure, prevent heart attacks and reduce the symptoms of ageing.

## POWER UP YOUR MEMORY

Gingko biloba, a tree extract that has been used by the Chinese for about 2,800 years, improves mental function by soaking up harmful free radicals and improving neurotransmission within the brain, promoting good blood circulation and enhancing memory.

## WORK AWAY JOINT PAIN

Strengthening your muscles with regular exercise could help prevent or end pain from joints and bone degeneration in later life. A tiny increase in thigh strength could reduce risk of knee osteoarthritis by up to a third.

## MAKE EVERY DAY A D-DAY

Experts say vitamin D is essential for the body to absorb enough calcium to keep bones healthy and strong. The vitamin is converted in the body on contact with sunlight, so make sure you get outside for some fresh air every day as you get older.

## WALK THE WALK

Walking improves circulation, bone strength and immune functions and can help people look between five and eight years younger in middle and later life. Half an hour a day is ideal.

### BE A SUPERBRAN

Fibre has been shown to be important in preventing constipation and helping lower cholesterol. It also protects against colon cancer and helps regulate blood sugar.

### FOLLOW THE RULER

The falling ruler test measures reaction time, which deteriorates with age. Ask someone to hold a wooden ruler by the top, large numbers – 45cm (18in) – down, suspended centred above your thumb and middle finger. Have them drop the ruler without warning three times, while you try to catch it, then average your score. The 28cm (11in) mark is normal for a 20-year-old and 15cm (6in) for a 60-year-old.

### KEEP LIGHT TO STAY BRIGHT

After the age of 65, overweight people have a higher chance of a decrease in mental function than people of normal or lower weight, so it's important to stay slender.

## bad habits

### UNEARTH HIDDEN DIET HORRORS

Write down everything you eat for three days. Do you add a lot of butter, sauces or salad dressings? Rather than eliminating these foods, cut back your portions.

### JUMP FOR BETTER JOINTS

Get into the high-impact habit. Studies have shown that to keep muscles and bones strong, resistance training that involves impact, such as running, walking, skipping rope and weight training, can be more beneficial than smooth, slow movements like swimming and cycling.

### FENG SHUI YOUR BAD HABITS AWAY

According to feng shui practitioners, bad habits could be due to problems in the bedroom health area. Draw a plan of your room with the main entrance at the bottom and divide it into nine roughly equal squares. Your health area is the middle square on the left. Make sure it is clutter free or fill it with round-leaved plants.

## GIVE IN TO CHOCOLATE

Chocolate – especially dark chocolate – can boost your mood by increasing levels of the amino acid L-tryptophan, which encourages feel-good serotonin to be released, so don't feel guilty about tucking in.

## WRITE IT DOWN

Size up your bad habits by listing all the pros and cons. Having a clear list of good and bad points to compare makes it far easier to measure up the benefits of giving up a bad habit. Look at the list every time you feel your motivation slipping.

## STOP LATE-NIGHT SNACKING

Eating a big meal at night, or snacking through the evening, impairs sleep quality by sending your body mixed messages and giving it heavy work to do, making it more difficult for you to get to sleep. Instead, eat earlier in the evening.

## DO IT TODAY

Procrastinating – putting everything off until tomorrow – not only reduces your efficiency but also causes stress. The longer you hold "to do" lists in your head, the more stressful they become. Vow to do one chore every day.

## DON'T BE PICKY

Rather than eliminating the problem, picking spots can introduce dirt and bacteria onto the skin surface, increasing chances of infection, not to mention the effects of redness and scarring. So, for healthier skin, don't pick – cover up blemishes instead.

## CULL YOUR CRAVINGS CULPRITS

Foods you crave and eat the most may be causing a lot of your health problems, say researchers who are worried about people becoming dependent on sugar highs from snack foods. Chief culprits to cut are pastry, cakes, biscuits (cookies) and doughnuts.

## WALK OFF THE WEIGHT

If you're a couch potato and don't spend much time outside, make yourself walk in the fresh air for at least ten minutes a day. Not only will it boost your metabolism and help stretch out muscles, the natural light will raise vitamin D levels.

## CUT CAFFEINE TO STOP STRESS

Coffee drinkers can have up to a third more stress hormones circulating in their system than non-coffee drinkers, making them more prone to stress. Aim for no more than three cups a day, swapping the rest for water or herbal teas.

## SET AN ALARM TO CRACK THE CRAVING

If you get a craving for a bad habit – like smoking or filling up on cakes or ice cream – set a timer for five minutes, then see if you still have the craving when it goes off. Experts believe this time lapse can cure cravings.

## TAKE A BREAK AT WORK

Far from being efficient, workaholics who don't take breaks during the day are up to a quarter less efficient than those with healthier working practices. Working through breaks is a false economy, so make yourself have at least three breaks – when you DON'T think about work at all.

## KEEP HUNGER IN THE CAN

Downing a carbonated drink at breakfast is likely to make you more hungry at lunchtime, even if it's one of the sugar-free varieties. Don't start your day with the fizz.

## EAT EARLY TO STAY SLIM

Recent research studies have shown that people who regularly eat breakfast consume more vitamins and minerals throughout the day than those who skip breakfast, and they are also less likely to be overweight.

## BE A HUNGER MONGER

Instead of scoffing food whenever you get the opportunity, think about eating moderately and according to your natural appetite instead. To do this, rate your hunger on a scale from one (absolutely starving) to ten (completely stuffed). Then, only start eating at two or three and finish at seven.

## SWITCH SWEETS FOR FRUIT

If you find yourself munching on high-sugar, high-calorie sweets and snacks for a treat, try switching to chopped fruit or no-sugar yogurt instead. Both of these are sweet, but healthy, natural alternatives.

# hangovers

## PALE IS BEAUTIFUL

Recent research suggests that dark, sweet drinks like brandy, rum and whisky contain more "congeners", which produce the effects of hangovers, than paler drinks like white wine and vodka.

## THINK QUALITY NOT QUANTITY

Cheaper brands of drinks often contain more toxins and are therefore harder for the liver to cope with, causing worse hangovers. Go for quality rather than quantity – the expense might motivate you to limit your drinking, too.

## BE A WATERBABY

The dehydration that alcohol causes often plays a major role in the hangover scenario. Matching alcoholic drinks, glass for glass with water, and then slugging back another glass or two of water before going to bed, will help combat this.

## DETOX WITH A BEET DRINK

For a detoxifying antidote to all that partying, try beetroot juice mixed with the juices of carrot, apple, celery and ginger. The celery contains various antioxidant compounds that will help neutralize the effects of cigarette smoke, while the ginger will help relieve any nausea, stomachache or diarrhoea.

## HAVE HONEY TO BURN OFF ALCOHOL

Before or while you're drinking, have a large glass of grapefruit juice, and eat some honey. The grapefruit is a liver tonic, and the honey helps your body burn off alcohol in your system.

## ALTERNATE DRINKS TO AVOID A HANGOVER

Alternate alcoholic drinks with water if you want to keep yourself hangover free the next day by keeping your body hydrated and giving your liver a chance to work on excess alcohol.

## BOOST YOUR B INTAKE FOR BETTER MORNINGS

Take a combination of B-complex vitamins, vitamin C and zinc before a night of drinking, and then again in the morning, to help your system replace what you have lost with your overindulgence. Research shows that your system turns to B vitamins when it is under stress, and alcohol depletes levels further.

## BARK BACK AT PAIN

Willowbark tablets are a natural alternative to over-the-counter headache pills because they contain a form of salicylate, which is the active ingredient in aspirin.

## DON'T SOBER UP WITH A COFFEE

Drinking caffeine, which is in its highest concentrations in filter coffee, is a diuretic and will rob your body of even more water and nutrients. Try water or a sports drink instead, to replace electrolytes and give you an energy boost.

## CALM WITH CAMOMILE

Camomile and peppermint tea are good stomach settlers if you've overindulged, while aloe vera can neutralize excess stomach acid and soothe an irritated gastrointestinal tract.

## SPICE UP YOUR LIFE

Ginger is one of the most effective natural remedies for nausea and indigestion, stimulating metabolism to encourage the elimination of toxins.

## FEEL FINE AND DANDELION

The herb dandelion is a traditional liver tonic that has been shown to reduce the severity and duration of headaches.

## PRESS YOUR LUCK

Try the ancient Chinese art of acupressure to relieve morning nausea. With your thumb, apply continuous pressure to the soft area between your thumb and index finger on either hand for several minutes.

## MILK A CURE

Milk thistle is renowned for its ability to support and stimulate the working of the liver, which is the organ primarily responsible for detoxifying alcohol within the body. Take a dose of milk thistle before you go out and one when you get back for the best results.

## DON'T GET A RUM DEAL

Drinking rum, brandy and whisky is more likely to cause a hangover than drinking white wine, gin or vodka because they contain methanol, formaldehyde and formic acid, which are the chemicals chiefly responsible for a hangover's headache and accompanying rapid heart rate.

## BECOME AN ICE MAIDEN

Soothe a throbbing hangover headache the natural way with an ice pack. Soak cotton wool pads in cold camomile tea and then place them on your eyelids to reduce the swelling.

## CROSS OUT CROISSANTS

Eating a breakfast of croissants, buttery brioches or high-sugar cereals can send your blood sugar level on a roller coaster ride of ups and downs, while fatty foods can make you feel sick. Rather than endure this, stick to healthy options like fruit and wholegrain foods.

## REFRESH YOURSELF WITH A SEA BREEZE

Bloody Marys and Sea Breezes are two of the least toxic alcoholic drinks because the vodka they are made with doesn't contain any congeners and they contain health-giving fruit juices, too.

## FILL UP WITH FOOD

Taking alcoholic drinks on an empty stomach brings about a drop in blood sugar that makes you feel light-headed and drunk, then keeps it low throughout the night and into the following day, resulting in a major hangover.

# live long & healthy

## BE PART OF THE CROWD

Death rates are twice as high for the most socially isolated people compared with those with strong social ties, so your friends really can help you live longer.

## THE PEEL-GOOD FACTOR

Adding more potassium to the diet can lower blood pressure, while a diet deprived of potassium can actually raise blood pressure. Eating one banana per day provides the extra 400mg of potassium needed to slash the odds of suffering a fatal stroke by 40%.

## GIVE YOURSELF A RAW DEAL

According to studies, if you don't consume fruit daily, your risk of stomach cancer doubles or even triples, and raw is best. Munch on raw fruit and vegetables.

## WEAR A COPPER

Copper is an essential supplement for reducing age-related disintegration of body tissues and it is an a nonallergenic material. Many people, particularly arthritis sufferers, wear copper bracelets for the absorption of the mineral into the skin.

## HAVE A HEARTY DOSE OF ONION

Consuming half an onion a day, or the equivalent in juice, raises HDL (good) cholesterol by an average of 30% in most people with heart disease or cholesterol problems, extending life expectancy and boosting health.

## CURIOSITY KEEPS THE CAT ALIVE

The more curious you are, the more likely you are to live longer, say scientists who found that curious people were 30% less likely to die than people who weren't.

## OH FOR OKINAWA

Okinawans live longer than any other race on earth. Their secrets include eating lots of soya products, stopping eating before they are completely full and daily exercise.

## BE OPTIMISTIC

Optimists live about 20% longer than pessimists, so making yourself believe that the glass is half full rather than half empty really could enhance your health.

## REST ASSURED

Rest is as important as exercise in helping your body stay healthy for longer. Regular exercise along with daily relaxation and at least one rest day a week may add years to the life span.

## MAKE EACH MEAL SMALLER

People may be able to extend the length of their lives by cutting calorific intake by just 10%, as long as they aren't depriving themselves of essential nutrients as well.

## GET SPIRITUAL

People who attend religious ceremonies regularly are likely to live significantly longer than their non-religious friends, so maybe it's time to rediscover old beliefs.

## GO BACK TO YOUR ROOTS

People who behave as if they're younger live longer and age less quickly. You don't need to dress in the clothes you wore as a teenager, just revive a few of the things you liked doing when young.

## PINE FOR YOUR YOUTH

Pine bark extract (pycnogenol) and grape-seed extract contain powerful antioxidants that can help your body counteract the damaging signs of ageing.

## SAY OM TO BEAT AGEING

Meditation reduces stress, which is one of the major causes of the ageing process, and taking up yoga and other meditative techniques in old age has been shown to enhance quality of life.

# love

## GET IN THE MED FOR LOVE

In the Mediterranean, pistachios and pine nuts are considered aphrodisiacs and certain spices, like cinnamon and nutmeg, are said to arouse both men and women.

## TIE THE KNOT TO STAY ALIVE

Being married encourages healthy behaviour. Married people are apparently more likely to wear seat belts, be active, eat breakfast and not smoke, so tying the knot could help your health.

## CHOC FULL OF DESIRE

Chocolate releases endorphins into the body that make us feel happier and more relaxed, which is why it's considered such an effective aphrodisiac. Enjoy!

## KISS AND MAKE UP

Arguments between couples weaken their immune system, making them more susceptible to illness. People who feel loved and supported are less likely to suffer blockages in their heart arteries than unhappy people.

# sex

## SEX IS GOOD FOR YOU

Working the muscles around your sex organs regularly keeps them strong and healthy. For men, this can help reduce the chance of suffering prostrate cancer and for women it helps prevent incontinence problems. You can safely consider your lovemaking to be a health-giving activity.

## LIVE LONGER WITH THE BIG-O

Orgasms could help you live longer. People with an active sex life who regularly reach orgasm are half as likely to die at an earlier age than those who don't. So the older you get, the more important sex is!

## GET SOME SATISFACTION

Sexual dissatisfaction is potentially a serious risk factor when it comes to heart attacks in women, with women who are satisfied in bed being much less likely to suffer from heart problems.

## ZINC INTO THE MOOD

A natural aphrodisiac and fertility booster, zinc is found in pumpkin and sesame seeds, cheese, chicken and turkey, wholegrains, pine nuts, brown rice, fish and seafood. Not forgetting (surprise, surprise) oysters!

## SAFEGUARD HIM WITH REGULAR SEX

Men who have sex every other day are significantly less likely to develop life-threatening prostate cancer than those who sow their oats less often, so upping your sexual antics could aid his health as well as yours.

## MORNING GLORY

The male's testosterone levels have been found to drop by nearly a quarter in the mid- to late evening, so don't take it personally if he doesn't desire you before going to bed. Testosterone levels and, therefore, sex drive, are usually highest first thing in the morning.

## TAKE TO THE FLOOR

Make your orgasms more powerful and work your pelvic floor muscles at the same time by contracting and relaxing them.

## ENJOY SEX THROUGH THE BIG CHANGE

Women going through menopause who eat about 100g (3½oz) of tofu daily or drink one cup of soya milk receive an oestrogen boost that makes sex more satisfying and pleasurable.

## TAKE IODINE FOR LOW SEX DRIVE

In some people, low sex drive could be due to an underactive thyroid gland, so if you seldom feel in the mood, visit your doctor to have your thyroid checked; increased iodine could be the answer.

## THYME FOR BED

Chromium, found in thyme, and also wholegrains, meat, cheese and brewer's yeast, is thought to increase sperm count in men and sex drive in both sexes.

## GET LIVELY WITH LIVER

Vitamins A and E are vital for the production of sex hormones, which boost sex drive. They can be found in liver, dairy produce, oily fish, dark green leafy vegetables and yellow-orange fruits.

## TRYP THE SEX FANTASTIC

Foods containing tryptophan, such as bananas, milk, cottage cheese and turkey, not only encourage sleep but can also boost sex drive by increasing comfort sensations and reducing stress. Milk chocolate contains tryptophan, too, plus phenylethylamine, a chemical thought to be released at times of arousal.

## BE A DOMESTIC GODDESS

Bizarre as it may sound, the smell of cinnamon buns has been shown to boost male sexual arousal. Pumpkin-pie scent was also found to be very erotic, so spending a few hours in the kitchen could pay exciting sex dividends.

## GET HOT TO LOSE WEIGHT

Having sex burns approximately 150 calories every 30 minutes, so if you have vigorous sex for an hour you could burn about 300 calories – which is roughly equivalent to what you would burn if you went for a brisk one-hour walk. Why not try for a marathon?

## DON'T LET STRESS SPOIL SEX

Vitamin C and magnesium, essential for the proper functioning of sex organs, are used up in times of stress, so it's important to replenish them with foods such as citrus fruits, red berries, potatoes, kiwi, chicken, tuna and green leafy vegetables.

## GLOW WITH THE FLOW

Sex helps increase blood flow to your organs. As a fresh blood supply arrives, the body's cells, organs and muscles are filled with fresh oxygen and hormones; and as the used blood is removed, it takes away the waste products that are responsible for feelings of fatigue.

## GET HEART HEALTHY IN BED

Sex helps lower cholesterol levels. More importantly, it tips the HDL/LDL (good/bad) cholesterol balance towards the healthier HDL side by promoting blood flow and increasing feelings of wellbeing.

## USE SEX AS A STRESS BUSTER

Research studies reveal that people who have frequent, pleasurable sex handle stress better. The profound relaxation that typically follows sex, when the hormone rush causes the body to relax, may be one of the few times when people allow themselves to let go completely.

## NATURE'S FAVOURITE PAINKILLER

Endorphins are released from the brain during lovemaking. These natural opiates act as powerful analgesics in the body, easing aches and pains.

## MAKE HAY WITH DHEA

The natural hormone DHEA, which is produced in response to sexual excitement, helps strengthen the immune system, improves cognition, promotes bone growth, and maintains and repairs tissues in the body. It may also contribute to cardiovascular health and even function as a mild antidepressant.

## BUILD UP BONES IN THE BOUDOIR

Regular sexual activity appears to lift levels of testosterone and oestrogen hormones, which act in the body to strengthen bones and muscles.

## BE A HONEY IN BED

Honey contains high levels of boron, which helps the body metabolize and utilize oestrogen and enhances levels of testosterone, the hormone responsible for revving up sex drive.

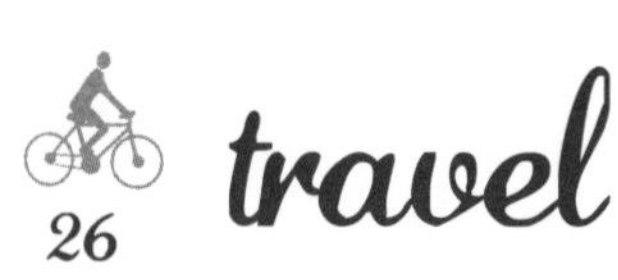

# travel

## TRAVEL A LITTLE AT A TIME
Jetlag tends to be a problem if four or more time zones are crossed, and the effects are generally worse travelling eastwards rather than westwards because the body copes better with a lengthening day than with a shortening day.

## DO IT BY DEGREES
Normally, brain temperature fluctuates by about 1.5°C (2.7°F) every day. The brain is at its minimum temperature at daybreak, and its maximum at midday. Mimicking these fluctuations could combat jetlag by reducing tiredness and tricking the brain into thinking it's a different time of day.

## PLAN OUT TIME-ZONE PROBLEMS
Save important activities for when you have most energy – in the morning after flying west; in the evening after flying east.

## MOVE TO PREVENT MOTION SICKNESS
On a ship or plane, move to the centre where it tends to be more stable. On a ship, go to the top deck and look out at the water to put your eyes and inner ear in sync.

## DRINK WATER, NOT ALCOHOL
Jetlag effects are generally made worse by dehydration, caffeine and alcohol, which put stress on the body and increases fatigue.

## TREAT TRAVEL SICKNESS WITH GINGER
Ginger is a traditional herbal remedy and is available in chewable ginger root and as sweets. Side effects seem to be minimal but it's always wise to check with your doctor since it has been shown to have some blood-thinning effects.

## BE WARY OF LOCAL WATER
Local water can cause digestive upsets. Drink bottled water when abroad and be careful of fruit and salad that's washed in local water, as well as hazards like ice cubes.

# treats

## CURL UP WITH AN OLD FAVOURITE

Take ten minutes to shut yourself away with a good book or poem, or let your creative juices flow and write something yourself. Concentrating on one thing and forgetting worries will help reduce stress.

## BOOK YOURSELF SOME SCENT TIME

Book an aromatherapy massage to relax yourself, stimulate circulation and lower stress and tension. Don't feel guilty about the time you're giving to yourself – you'll cope with life better if set aside time to enjoy the things you like to do.

## BUY YOURSELF A FOODY TREAT

The next time you visit the supermarket, treat yourself to one thing that wouldn't normally be on your shopping list and, some time during the week, take time to enjoy it. Keep it healthy – such as yogurt-coated raisins, carrot cake or plain popcorn – and your treat will be guilt free!

## BEAT YOUR TROUBLES WITH BUBBLES

Whenever time permits, indulge in a 30-minute "home spa" session in your own bathroom. Soak your troubles away in your favourite bubble bath; lie back, close your eyes and let pleasant thoughts flood in.

## RENT A LAUGH TO FEEL HAPPY

Give yourself a break from emotionally charged news broadcasts and mind-numbing television, or from the usual list of evening chores. Instead, rent a favourite comedy programme tape or DVD that you know will put a smile on your face.

## SURROUND YOURSELF WITH FLOWERS

Research studies have shown that flowers provide an emotional lift. You don't need to spend a fortune to spread flowers throughout your house – buy one bouquet and split it up, putting a flower or two in several different vases.

# weight maintenance

## TAKE AN EVENING OFF

Even people who are dieting can have a night off once in a while! Decide what you're going to have and allow yourself to indulge for the evening, but make it one night only – it's back to healthy eating the next day!

## WATER FILLER

Your body can often confuse hunger with thirst, so next time you think you're hungry try first drinking a glass of water before you reach for the snacks. That way, you'll start to read your body's signs better and only snack when you're genuinely hungry.

## DON'T SKIP TO BE SLIM

Many people think skipping a meal makes it easier to cut calories, but you will actually be more likely to overeat later. Instead, aim to have three balanced meals per day plus two or three small healthy snacks.

## DOUBLE UP ON WEIGHT LOSS

Take a two-pronged approach to losing weight to make it sustainable – instead of trying to cut, say, 500 calories a day from your diet, cut out half the amount and make up the rest with exercise. This would mean cutting out 250 calories and burning off a further 250 by, for example, walking briskly for around 3 km (2 miles).

## EAT SMALL TO EAT LESS

A lot of food satisfaction comes from how food looks on the plate, so to trick yourself into feeling satisfied with smaller portions, simply use smaller plates. It might sound silly, but studies have shown that people feel fuller if they think they've eaten a plateful, no matter what size!

## FULL STOP

Stop eating when you're full. It sounds simple, but many of us are conditioned to finish what's on our plates regardless of whether we've had enough. After every mouthful, pause and think about whether you really want the next one.

## QUALITY NOT QUANTITY

The sight of a buffet table is enough to send most dieters running for cover, but don't despair – a good trick for keeping buffets healthy is to eat larger portions of fewer things, instead of lots of little nibbles. Pile up on protein, fruit and vegetables, and foods high in fibre.

## LEAVE A NOTE

Many people snack on high-calorie foods without realising they're doing it. Train yourself out of it by leaving a note on the outside of your fridge to remind you that if you're going to have a snack you should a) want it and b) enjoy it.

## CUT TO THE CHASE

If you're serving bread with a meal or in a sandwich, make sure you cut thin slices rather than doorsteps (thick slices). Most people will eat the same number of slices no matter how thick, so reduce calories by making slices thinner.

## KEEP YOUR BALANCE

As a general guide for someone who does moderate exercise and isn't greatly over- or underweight, one pound of body fat equals 4000 calories. This means that in order to shed a pound a week, you would need to reduce your total number of calories by just over 500 calories a day.

## EQUAL REWARDS

If you find overeating a problem, find a non-food alternative which you also find rewarding. This could include exercise, prayer, yoga, listening to music, browsing the internet, phoning a friend, reading a magazine, or many other alternatives.

## DIP YOUR NUTS

For a healthy after-dinner snack that won't pile on the pounds, choose nuts or dried fruits dipped in dark chocolate – at least 70% cocoa solids is best.

## SAVE YOURSELF FOR THE BEST

One useful guideline in cutting calories is that if it seems too good to be true, it probably is! Often, people who choose "low fat" versions of their normal desserts or treats are disappointed when they just don't taste the same. Why not "save up" your calories and have the occasional indulgent treat instead.

## DITCH THE PASTRY

Quiche is often seen as a healthy choice, but the problem is the pastry. A standard 23-cm (9-inch) pastry case contains 41 g of fat, 63 g of carbohydrates and 818 mg of sodium. Choose a pastry-free omelette instead.

## DIET WITH DAIRY

Calcium actually helps your body to expel fat, helping you to lose weight and maintain healthy cholesterol, but only if the calcium comes from dairy products. Lower-fat dairy products have the most absorbable minerals, so try to choose them wherever possible.

## TRUST AN ANGEL

Instead of your usual afternoon cake or biscuits, try angel layer cake (or angel cake), which is much lower in fat. To make an even healthier snack, serve it with fruit purée.

## A NEW COAT

If you're on a low-carb diet but want to make fish or chicken in breadcrumbs, try using crushed pork rinds instead, mixed with a few herbs or spices. That way, you'll get the crispy outer shell and stay carb-free.

## SEE THROUGH SOUP

Instead of soups containing cream, choose those with tomato or clear broth as their base. For example, instead of leek and potato or cream of mushroom, try tomato and herb or carrot and coriander.

## CHEESE MELT

If you're a toasted cheese sandwich fan, but don't want the extra calories, make yourself a low-fat version by grilling the toast and adding a small amount of cheese which has been melted in the microwave. That way you can cut down on non-essential fat.

## MIX YOUR OWN YOGURTS

Replace fruit yogurts, which can contain quite high levels of sugar and fat, with your own fruit purée. Add it to low-fat natural yogurt and top with a sprinkling of seeds for an extra health boost.

## CUT A QUARTER

When butter or oil is needed in recipes, try reducing the amount by a quarter. For instance, if your recipe calls for 50 g (2 oz) butter, try cutting it down to 25 g (1.5 oz). If you can't taste the difference, reduce it by another quarter next time. You will be surprised just how little fat is really necessary.

## GO FOR COTTAGE

Try puréeing low-fat cottage cheese into a smooth paste and using it instead of full-fat cream cheese in recipes and as a spread. Alternatively, combine half and half.

## ROLL UP A TREAT

If you simply can't live without biscuits or cakes with your afternoon tea, choose healthier options. Fig rolls contain less saturated fat and more fruit content than chocolate biscuits or those with cream fillings. Mixed berry or fruit and spice oat biscuits have a low GI, too.

## REAP THE REWARDS

Set yourself realistic goals and reward yourself (not with chocolate!) for achieving them. Try something like "for one week I will eat one additional fruit or vegetable portion a day and avoid second helpings".

## MIST YOUR PAN

Instead of sloshing butter or margarine into the pan to prevent sticking while you're frying, invest in a plant mister and fill it with olive oil, which is a healthy cooking oil. Then, you can be sure you're only using as much as you really need.

### SMOOTH OPERATOR

Thick smoothies can actually fill you up for longer than a solid meal because their volume causes the stomach to expand more. This makes them a great choice for breakfast or lunch, when you may have to wait some time before your next meal.

### GRATE, FINE

It's the fat in cheese that helps it melt uniformly – low-fat varieties often melt in patches or take much longer. To make sure your low-fat cheese melts properly, grate it first using the fine side of your grater.

### NO YOLKS PLEASE

An easy way to lower the calorie content of your egg sandwiches is to hard boil eggs and use only the egg whites for the filling. That way, you cut out on the calorific yolks but keep the eggy taste.

### PICK LOW FAT

Instead of ice cream on desserts, choose low fat soya versions or simply use frozen yogurt for a yummy pudding without all the saturated fat or calories

## counting calories

### GO NAKED

If you're used to eating roast chicken with the skin on, removing the skin will reduce the calorie count from 220 to 155 for an average portion, as most of the fat is in the skin. Trim the calories further by removing any excess fat before cooking.

### SWAP SHOP

Swap a bowl of normal ice cream (at 310 calories and 20 g fat) for low-fat frozen yogurt (at 200 calories and 2.5 g fat) – that's a saving of 110 calories and an astounding 17.5 g fat per serving! It tastes wonderful, too.

### HALVE YOUR SANDWICH

Try opting for a half a sandwich at lunchtime, rather than your usual whole one – it's an easy way to halve your calories and you might find you feel just as full but less sluggish as a result.

## DRINK LIGHT

Choose light beer, which has an average of 95 calories per bottle, rather than the usual kind, which has around 150 calories. It might sound like a small saving, but if you're having it two or three times a week it could soon add up into a meaningful cut in the calorie count.

## DILUTE YOUR DRINK

Alcohol adds many hidden calories – why not spread out your daily dose of wine into one or two spritzers and opt for low-calorie mixers where possible? You can save around 50 calories in a gin and tonic merely by switching to light tonic.

## STAY LOW WITH $H_2O$

Liquid calories are digested much more quickly than solid, and provide a lot of extra calories without filling you up, which means it's likely you'll eat just as much food as you would without them. Two cups of fizzy drink each day is 220 calories, which is 10 kg (23 lb) in weight over a year. Water is the best option.

## SKIM ON THE MILK

Each time you swap 1 cup of skimmed milk for one of whole milk, you'll save 70 calories. Based on one serving a day, at the end of the year you will save more than 25,000 calories and potentially lose 3 kg (7 lb).

## SAY CHEESE

If you swap 30 g (1 oz) reduced-fat cheese (90 calories) for 30 g (1 oz) regular cheese (115 calories), you'll save 25 calories. And if you swap it for fat-free cheese you'll save 75 calories per ounce – perfect for sauces or pizza where the taste of the cheese isn't paramount.

## PICK OF THE PIZZAS

If you want to add a serving of ice cream to your pizza meal, save the calories by choosing a vegetarian pizza over one with meat, which will reduce the calorie content from around 1000 to 700, leaving you an extra 300 to finish your meal off in style!

## THINK DRINKS

If you're trying to cut down on your calories, don't forget to count what you drink as well as what you eat. There are at least as many calories in the average can of fizzy drink as in a slice of cake.

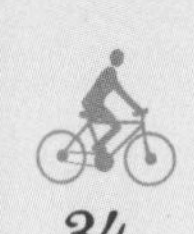



### A HOT DATE

Instead of reaching for the chocolates after a meal, pop a date into your mouth. They contain much less sugar than chocolates and a range of health-giving vitamins and minerals, but still have a rich, sweet taste.

## eating habits

### SEE A PROFESSIONAL

If you're having trouble cutting sugary and fatty foods out of your diet, or you're trying to stick to a plan but the weight just isn't coming off, consider consulting a dietician. Most offer a one-off consultation that might help kick-start you into making some basic practical changes.

### STICK TO YOUR SIZE

One of the most dangerous temptations in dieting is the tendency to add a little bit more food. If you're on a calorie-restricted diet plan, make sure you stick strictly to portion sizes or weigh food carefully to avoid this common pitfall.

### EAT TOGETHER

Try to get your whole family to sit down together for a meal at the table. It's thought that children from families who regularly eat together have healthier attitudes to food and are less likely to be obese than those who don't. Studies have shown that people who eat while watching TV eat more and enjoy their food less than those who sit at a table to eat.

### STOP BEFORE STUFFED

Try to eat until you are sufficiently satiated, rather than completely stuffed! In other words, try stopping when you feel 75–80% full and only eat more if you feel you really need to. To do this, you will have to learn to get "in touch" with your feelings of hunger and fullness.

## BE PREPARED TO WORK

One of the most common reasons people reach for biscuits and other unhealthy snacks is that they're simply less work. Get ahead of yourself and spend 15 minutes or so peeling and chopping vegetables like carrots, fennel, cucumber, peppers and celery, or fruit such as apples and pears. Bag it all up and keep it in the fridge so you can reach for it whenever you want.

## STICK TO THE SAME TIMES

If you often resort to snacking between meals, take a proactive step towards eliminating your bad habits by eating meals at regular times for a week. This will help keep calories more balanced and reduce hunger pangs and cravings.

## EAT MORE OFTEN

If you find it hard not to snack between meals, eat more often – three meals a day doesn't suit everyone so try changing your routine to five or six smaller meals a day. For some people it's a way of eating that can help to keep blood sugar levels stable and keep you mentally alert and physically energetic all day long.

## THE CHINESE WAY

Trick yourself into eating smaller portions of rice and noodle dishes by using chopsticks instead of a fork. The longer you take to eat, the more chance you give yourself to fill up before you've finished your plateful.

## IN THE KITCHEN AT PARTIES

Many people find it difficult to control their eating at parties. As you arrive, take a look at the food and choose what you will eat. Fill up a plate rather than grazing at will, when you are much more likely to overeat.

## KNOW YOUR WEAKNESS

If you know you have certain times of the day when you reach for snacks, try to pre-empt the problem by preparing a light meal or healthy snack ahead of time so you can reach for it when the craving strikes. Keep a bowl of fruit near your desk or on your kitchen table so you can pick from the bowl at any time during the day.

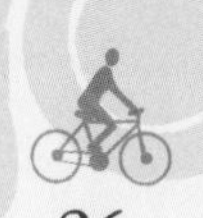



## MORE THAN FOOD

To a lot of people, food isn't just food. Make a list of how you feel when you feel tempted to snack and what alternatives there might be. If you're bored, try changing what you're doing rather than reaching for a snack.

## LEAVE SOMETHING BEHIND

For a week, make it a rule never to finish everything on your plate. At the end of the week, think back to whether you really noticed the difference. If you didn't, you can happily make your portions a little bit smaller.

## COOK FROM SCRATCH

If you rely on fast foods or microwave meals, which are often high in saturated fat and added salt or sugar, try to make an effort to cook from scratch at least two or three nights a week instead. Switch one day at a time so you end up with only one or two processed-food days.

## BECOME A COLLECTOR

Cooking for yourself, using fresh ingredients from scratch, doesn't have to be a long-winded affair. Collect a folder of ten-minute recipes and stock your cupboard accordingly so you're always prepared for those "need-food-now" moments.

## DO IT THE SLOW WAY

Calorie-controlled diets often work for a short time, but many people put on weight again after they stop, and they return to their old eating habits. Instead of dieting, cut calories every day in small ways, such as having fewer snacks and smaller portions. You'll lose weight more slowly but it's more likely to stay off.

## WALK IT OFF

Make a point of going for a gentle walk after a meal, especially if you're eating out in the evening. Walking home instead of getting a taxi will help your meal "settle" and can aid the digestive process.

## START WITH JUICE

If you're used to knocking back a glass of wine as you cook, pour yourself a tomato juice instead, or even a glass of water, and drink that before you start on the alcohol. That way, you'll drink less and regulate your calorie intake.

## SAVOUR THE FLAVOUR

Take a more Buddhist attitude to food by savouring every mouthful. Make yourself mindful of what you eat, what the flavours really taste like and how the food feels in your mouth. Pause after each mouthful and think about whether you really want more. Slowing down will make you feel fuller.

## GET REGULAR

Eat regular meals – skipping meals can lead to hunger, often resulting in overeating. When you're very hungry your blood sugar levels plummet and it's tempting to forget about good nutrition. Snacking between meals can help curb hunger, but make sure the snack is healthy rather than high in fat or sugar – and don't eat so much that your snack becomes an entire meal.

## FRUIT TEST

Some people find that eating fruit after a meal can cause bloating and gas problems – if you think fruit affects you in this way, try eating it an hour or two before or after a meal and see if it feels any different.

## DRINK AWAY HUNGER

Are you really hungry – or dehydrated? Lack of water can make you think you're hungry, leading to overeating and weight gain. Cravings for salty foods are also a telltale sign of dehydration. Drink 2 litres (4 pints) of water daily at regular intervals.

## THE ORIENTAL WAY

A great food to choose for working lunches is sushi, especially if you add a healthy salad or vegetable serving which will add some fibre to the meal. The fish will give you a boost of omega-3 oils to help brainpower, but make sure it's really fresh.

## KEEP THE TREATS

Diets that cut out all "treat" foods have been shown to be ineffective at keeping weight off in the long term. Instead, choose a healthy-eating style where you minimize (but don't cut out completely) unhealthy foods, replacing them with better choices. If nothing's forbidden, you won't be so tempted by it.

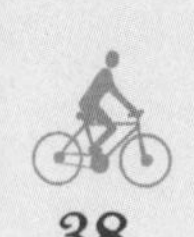


## TIDY UP YOUR LEFTOVERS

Leaving food lying around is just too tempting – you might reach for a second helping – so put everything away as soon as you've served it.

## STRESS FACTORS

Stress is often a trigger for eating – when we're stressed, not only are we likely to eat more, but we're more likely to go for the fast option as our bodies speed up. Our bodies can also crave certain types of food, such as those high in fats and sugars. Think about how this relates to your eating habits, and make changes in your life to reduce stress if necessary.

## STOCK UP AT THE OFFICE

If you have a microwave in your office, stack your desk with some diet staples like individual packs of oatmeal and dried fruit – that way, you'll always be able to make yourself an energy-boosting, low-fat snack.

## TAKE THE LONG VIEW

There will be times when you'll slip up and overeat or pick less healthy foods because they sound good, you're stressed or you just feel like it. Healthy eating is a lifelong goal and one slip up won't make any difference in the long run. If you overdo it one day, eat less the following day to redress the balance.

## AGE BEFORE APPETITE

As you age, your metabolic rate changes as well as your lifestyle, so even active older people need fewer calories than when they were young. Alter your diet as you grow older by cutting down on fatty foods and making carbohydrate portions smaller.

## TOTAL YOUR DAY

Try and balance up your eating every day so that when you go to bed, you do it with a clean slate. For instance, if you have an unhealthy lunch or snack in the afternoon, make your evening meal a super-healthy salad with fish and fresh fruit. If the evening's been unhealthy, resolve to start afresh the next morning.

## TUNE IN

Eat when you're hungry, not just out of habit. Getting more in tune with your body's requirements will help you maintain healthy eating habits – by listening to what your body really needs instead of simply reaching for the biscuit tin every time you're bored, upset or angry.

## DAY BY DAY

Make changes gradually and don't expect to totally revamp your eating habits overnight. Start to remedy excesses or deficiencies with modest changes, which will add up to create positive lifelong eating habits. For instance, if you don't like the taste of skimmed milk, try semi-skimmed; replace white rice with brown basmati, and so on.

## MOVE ON

Be realistic about your target weight. It's likely to be unhealthy to aim to maintain your teenage weight as you get older, as your natural body weight increases with age as well as being affected by factors such as pregnancy. If you eat a healthy, balanced diet, the chances are your weight is fine.

## LOOK AT YOUR FRAME

Don't be fooled by the media into thinking you should be thinner than is healthy – set yourself a sensible target weight which isn't hard to maintain with a healthy diet and normal levels of activity. If you often feel genuinely hungry or exercise too much, your target weight is probably too low.

## DON'T DO A DIET

The word diet has negative connotations and can reduce body image – it's a sad fact that most people who admit to dieting don't manage to keep the weight off. Instead of concentrating on losing weight, make good health your aim.

## KEEP A DIARY

If you've been trying to diet and not succeeding, try keeping a food diary for a week or two – write down everything you eat and drink. Seeing it in black and white can help you to identify vulnerable times of day, unhealthy eating patterns and areas you might not be aware of.

## EXERCISE YOURSELF HAPPY

Studies have shown that one of the best ways to prevent overeating is to take regular exercise. This is because exercise releases feel-good endorphins in the body, and people who feel happier and more fulfilled are less likely to overeat.

## ACTIVATE YOURSELF

Metabolism varies among individuals but only by up to 100 calories daily, so claiming a slow metabolism isn't an excuse for weight gain. Instead, look to the details of how you eat and how active you are, counting up hidden calories and making practical changes.

## GET SOME THERAPY

If you feel your eating is out of control, or you struggle to implement changes for more than a few weeks at a time, perhaps it's time to consider some kind of behaviour therapy, which aims for gradual but permanent changes in behaviour alongside a sensible eating plan? Ask your doctor for advice on what kind of therapy or counselling to try.

## SUMMER STRETCH

Throughout the summer, eat in line with the longer daylight hours so that your food intake is spread more evenly throughout the day. This usually means smaller, more frequent meals, which will make sense if it's hotter, too.

## KNOW YOUR PITFALLS

To improve your eating habits, you first have to know what's wrong with them. Do you add a lot of butter, creamy sauces or salad dressings to your meals? Rather than eliminating them completely, just cut back your portions instead.

## YOUR OWN JUDGE

Don't let other people determine how much you eat. Ask to serve yourself if you're out, and don't listen to friends or colleagues who say you should eat more or less. Be your own judge of what's a healthy portion for you.

## EAT WHEN ALERT

Don't eat first thing in the morning, before you are fully awake, or last thing at night because your mind is not alert at these times and you might overeat without meaning to.

# food philosophy

## PORTION PICKER

Studies have shown that people given larger portions eat more no matter how hungry they feel. Instead of serving dinner on to plates, which means one person is deciding the portion sizes, serve foods in bowls on the table and allow everyone to take as little or as much as they want.

## DIET DETOURS

A cake here and missed workout there – it happens! Don't starve or punish yourself in any other way to try to compensate if you slip up. It's far healthier for your brain and body – and you're much more likely to continue the diet successfully – if you let it go rather than prolonging the guilt.

## COLOUR COORDINATE

The way food looks can be as important as how it tastes in the satisfaction ratings. Help yourself enjoy your food more by taking a few minutes to make sure it's well presented on the plate.

## LONG-TERM COMMITMENT

Dedicate some time to making long-term changes in the way you and your family eat. Every time you go to the supermarket, swap one of your usual unhealthy food choices – like a packet of biscuits – for a healthy choice such as dried fruit or oatcakes. That way, you're more likely to keep up the healthy changes.

## GIVE TASTE A CHANCE

Because processed foods often have stronger tastes than freshly cooked meals, your tastebuds can become used to them. If you cut them out, flavours that used to seem appetizing may well lose their appeal as your palate regains its sensitivity and you start to appreciate tastes more.

## FOCUS ON FLAVOUR

Don't forget to taste your food. It may sound ridiculous, but many people – especially those prone to overeating or comfort snacking – get satisfaction from eating rather than actual food. Engage the senses in the pleasure of eating.

## STAY STABLE

Excess body fat increases your chances of high blood pressure, heart disease, stroke, diabetes, some types of cancer and other illnesses. But being too thin can increase your risk of osteoporosis, menstrual irregularities and other health problems. The worst from a health point of view, however, is to fluctuate between the two. Aim to find a stable weight and stay there.

## GET SOME SATISFACTION

Foods that fill you up best and reduce hunger pangs are those that are high in protein. Fish and skinless chicken are good examples, and to feel most satisfied you should aim to include a serving of these foods in each meal.

## SLOWLY DOES IT

If you feel you've lost touch with the enjoyment of eating, consider joining the Slow Food organization, a global movement that's dedicated to encouraging people to reconnect with the pleasure of eating healthy, wholesome foods.

## EAT BLINDFOLDED

If you worry about overeating and can't seem to tell when you're full, try eating blindfolded! Studies have shown that people eat 25% less food when blindfolded and feel fuller more quickly. Just make sure your plate is to hand and not the cat's dinner!

## ADJUST YOUR ATTITUDE

Understanding your food psychology can help you gain control over your eating. Every few months, make time to sit down and think about your attitudes to food. Include things like how you ate as a child and how you feel when you overeat, and use these insights to help you change your eating habits. Many unhealthy eating behaviours are simply bad habits.

## LIMIT THE CHOICE

We tend to eat more when our eyes tell our brains that there's lots of variety to choose from. Cut back on the choice available and serve food on one large platter instead of several small ones; studies have shown that you will eat less overall.

## DON'T PULL THE TRIGGER

Appetite can be affected by certain foods, which trigger good memories and cause the release of chemical messages to the brain – which in turn trigger the stomach to feel hungry. If you understand your trigger foods, it might be possible to intercept this process before hunger strikes, and to avoid them.

## GIVE YOURSELF A MINI-BREAK

Psychologically, you're more likely to stop snacking if you have to keep opening new packets. If overeating is a problem for you, consider buying mini-portions of your favourite snacks – opening each one as you eat it and collecting a pile of wrappers will help you limit intake.

## CHOOSE A BOWL

If you're eating a stackable food like pasta, rice or noodles, eat from a bowl rather than a plate to help you feel fuller quicker. Eating a pile of food rather than one spread out on a plate tricks the body into thinking it's eaten more.

## MAKE IT A TALL ONE

Our brain tends to recognize height quicker than width. If you drink from a tall thin glass as opposed to a short fat one, your brain will think you're having more even if you drink the same amount.

## BE REALISTIC

Sometimes you'll still have a take-away, a burger, a ready-meal, or simply not be able to resist the allure of deep fried crisps, chips or creamy desserts. Relax and enjoy it – healthy eating is all about balance and as long as you're eating well most of the time, it's fine to give in occasionally.

### TAKE STEPS

If you've recognized that your eating has emotional cues, put in place some steps to allow you to take control – Stop, Breathe, Reflect (on why you're about to eat) and Choose (to eat the food, not eat it, eat half of it, eat an alternative, and so on). Get into the habit of doing this whenever you feel the impulse to reach for food outside mealtimes.

### DARE TO BE DIFFERENT

Eat differently, not less. Instead of your next serving of pasta, bread or rice, try a large portion of mixed salad. A full plate of salad is physically and psychologically filling, but contains few calories and plenty of vitamins and minerals.

### ASK YOURSELF A QUESTION

Before you reach for that sugary snack, ask yourself, "If I eat this food now, is it worth it?" These questions bring mindfulness to eating rather than just doing it on impulse or obeying urges. It doesn't guarantee the eating won't happen – it just gives you a chance to make a better decision.

### LOOK AT THE LABEL

Use food labels to create balance and diversity in your diet (see Understanding Labels, page 8). By looking at the labels and learning to understand them, you can include less healthy foods in your diet as long as they are balanced with foods that are healthier. This will help you to keep to your recommended daily amounts.

## healthy snacking

### AU NATURAL

If you're a fan of peanut butter, but not of the high levels of unhealthy trans fats – which can't be properly digested by the body – it contains, switch to a natural product. While no lower in calories, these are free of hydrogenated oils. Great spread on crackers or oatcakes and eaten with an apple as a mid-morning snack.

## CARE FOR CAROB

If you want an alternative to caffeine-rich chocolate that is cocoa and dairy free, try chocolate substitutes made with the tree bark of the carob tree. These taste naturally sweet and so will contain quite a lot less sugar than many chocolate bars.

## CUT THE CHEESE CONTENT

Instead of smothering your pizza or salad with lots of high-fat low-flavour cheese, switch to a highly flavoured cheese like Parmesan, extra mature Cheddar or a blue cheese such as Stilton or Gorgonzola, and use a smaller amount. A tablespoon of Parmesan contains only 2 g of fat (one of which is saturates).

## SERVICE-STATION TRAP

Car journeys can be long and you might find yourself eating to keep awake. And, of course, service stations are waiting for you with a tempting array of super-sized snacks. To avoid the temptation, set off on your journey with a good choice of healthy snacks to see you through.

## STAY WELL STOCKED

Lots of people get hungry for sugary snacks in the evening, and if you're at home watching TV it can be difficult to resist that bar of chocolate. Keep healthy snacks to hand – low-fat yogurt, dried or fresh dates, figs or mango, oatcakes – and only have the chocolate if you still want it after you've had two healthy snacks.

## KEEP IT FRESH

All fruit is healthy but dried fruit is significantly higher in calories than fresh fruit. This is because the moisture is taken out, leaving more sugar per serving. If you're trying to lose weight, it's best to stick to fresh fruit, which you can eat more of for the same number of calories.

## ON THE MOVE

Next time you reach for a snack when you're out shopping or in the car, stop and think whether you're really hungry. Are you bored, tired? Does it just happen to be there? Carry a healthy snack such as nuts or oatcakes in your bag for times like this.

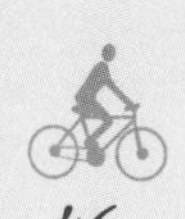



## LOOK BELOW THE SURFACE

Don't be fooled into thinking yogurt-coated nuts and raisins are healthy foods. They are filled with calories, sugar and fat without any of the active cultures of fresh yogurt. In fact, the yogurt taste is often just flavouring. Just 20 yogurt-covered nuts provide around 460 calories, 32 g fat and 8 tsp sugar. Instead, choose nuts in the shell – they will take longer to eat, giving your brain more time to recognize you are full.

## AIR-POPPED CORN

Popcorn is a great filler and fibre provider and has only 100 calories and 3.5 g fibre per regular serving – much less than nuts and dried fruit. But choose air-popped corn rather than fried, and don't add lashings of salty or sweet toppings.

## CUT THE COFFEE

There might be a coffee bar on every street corner, but that doesn't mean you need to stop for a top-up at every one! Coffee drinks can be really high in fat and calories because of the milk and syrup – mocha coffee has 11 g fat, cappuccino 6 g and regular white coffee 1 g fat, so choose carefully – and don't dip in a sweet snack.

## IT HAD BETTER BE CELERY

Celery is a super snack food – not only is it crunchy and refreshing, it genuinely does take your body the same amount of calories to eat and digest it as it gives you. Avoid smothering it with creamy dips and go for healthy versions instead, such as hummus made with olive oil or low-fat yogurt mixed with garlic and fresh herbs.

## SERVE YOURSELF A SALAD

So that you've always got a healthy option when you open the fridge door, make up a large bowl of salad a couple of times a week and get into the habit of serving it with every meal, adding extra vegetables to your diet.

## CHOOSE DECAF

Many people swear by the caffeine in tea, coffee, chocolate and many soft drinks to give them a boost whenever they're flagging, but caffeine addiction can lead to fatigue and lack of concentration. Give yourself a break for a few days or switch to decaffeinated drinks – even if just a cup or two a day.

## FISHY PATE

To help you get your extra portions of fish, make your own fish pâté using canned fish with your favourite sauce – think horseradish with salmon and mackerel, or tomato with tuna – to use as a sandwich spread during the week.

## KEEP IT INDIVIDUAL

Never take a whole box or packet of snacks or food to eat in front of the computer, television or while reading, because you might absentmindedly eat more than you intend. Serve yourself an individual portion in a bowl instead, and get yourself a refill only if you really want more.

## DANGER ZONES

Most people have "danger times" for snacking during the day (for a lot of women it's around 4 pm). Make an effort not to be around fatty snacks at this time, or take along a healthier alternative such as nuts and seeds.

## GRAB A GRAPE

Keep a bunch of grapes in your fridge and grab a handful when you fancy something sweet. They release sugar quickly, so are great for satisfying cravings – wait ten minutes and only reach for the chocolate if the grapes really don't hit the spot.

## CAN YOU BURN IF OFF?

For each pound of body weight you want to burn off, you need to use up roughly 3500 calories, so unless you're about to become a marathon runner, think carefully about which snacks you choose.

## UP WATER LEVELS

Drinking water is essential for keeping your system healthy – not only does it keep your cells hydrated and help your organs function optimally, it also keeps food flowing through the digestive system, which means you'll derive more benefits from your healthy foods.

## SUGAR-FREE YOUR IMMUNITY

Cutting down on snack foods containing refined sugar can limit your susceptibility to fatigue, colds and winter bugs. High levels of sugar affect immunity by reducing the efficiency of white blood cells.

## LOW-CAL YOUR HOT DRINKS

Try using skimmed, or fat-free milk instead of your usual whole or semi-skimmed version in hot drinks where calories can add up without you realizing. This could save you 30 calories per cup of tea or filter coffee, even more if you drink cappuccino or latte. And ditch the syrups and flavourings.

## GO BANANAS

For an energy boost to help you through a late-afternoon dip in energy, choose a banana. They're packed with potassium for extra energy.

## PACK UP THE CAR

If car journeys are a time you find it difficult not to snack, pre-empt your cravings by packing fruit and vegetables in snack-sized portions, or healthy rice cakes or dried fruits. Pack enough for the family, so you won't be tempted by their snacks.

# eating out

## STICK TO THE RULES

Keep to the ground rules wherever you are. Whether you're eating at home or eating out, make a concerted effort to apply the principles of healthy nutrition by eating a variety of healthy foods, limiting fat, sugar and salt, and keeping portion sizes in check.

## SIZE MATTERS

Be aware of portion size when eating out – if the restaurant offers meals in several sizes, choose the smallest. Or get creative and order two starters or a child-sized meal. You can also share meals or ask the restaurant to put half the meal in a take-away container before it's served.

## DON'T BE SHY

Never feel like you're stepping out of line or putting anyone out if you request healthier options or substitutions in a restaurant, pub or bar. You're not being difficult, so don't be swayed – you're simply doing what it takes to stay committed to your healthy-eating plan.

## NO SKIPPING

Don't be sucked into the false economy of starving yourself at lunchtime if you know you're going out in the evening. Being hungry will just make you eat more, and you'll be more likely to reach for unhealthy snacks. Choose healthy, filling foods such as vegetable soup with lentils or beans, or a baked sweet potato.

## STICK TO THE ROUTINE

Try to keep to regular mealtimes, even if you're eating out, to help you ward off food cravings and keep your blood-sugar levels regular. If you're booking a table for lunch or dinner, book it for your usual eating time rather than forcing your body to wait until later.

## TWO FORKS ARE BETTER THAN NONE

Next time you're tempted by a calorie-packed pudding at a restaurant, why not share instead of having a whole one to yourself. It will give you the benefit of all the taste with half the calories. You just need to find a willing partner!

## SALAD DAYS

Don't be fooled into thinking all salads are healthy. For instance, thanks to excessive dressing, croutons and added cheese, a standard chicken Caesar salad can total 1130 calories and add more than 90 g of fat to your diet! Make it healthier by cutting out the croutons and dressing with a small amount of vinaigrette.

## ASK FOR ADVICE

Don't be afraid to ask for advice in a restaurant. If you're worried about which dishes contain more fat or calories, ask the waiting staff. Or tell them you're cutting calories and ask the chef to recommend the best option.

## NO NEED TO VEGETATE

Don't use your dietary limitations as an excuse not to venture out to eat – even restaurants that don't offer vegan options can usually whip up a meatless pasta or vegetable plate if you ask. Ask the waiting staff or phone ahead and speak to the manager or chef directly.

## DON'T BLOW IT

Having a light snack, such as wholemeal toast, a banana or a low-calorie yogurt before you go out to dinner will take the edge off hunger and stop you gorging on the bread basket the minute you sit down. Make it a low-sugar wholegrain snack, or have a glass of skimmed milk.

## SWAP FAT FOR FIBRE

Try to swap high fat foods for low fat, high fibre wherever you can. For instance, instead of roast or fried potatoes with your meal, ask for extra vegetables or salad instead. Most restaurants are used to catering for a range of dietary requirements so these types of request aren't rare.

## HALF AND HALF

Make your food choice healthier by swapping half the meat for low-fat vegetarian options such as thick slices of marinated tomato, courgette or aubergine. Serve with buns instead of meat or with burgers as a cheese alternative.

## A FORK FULL

If you want the taste of salad dressing without the extra calories, try the fork method – order dressing on the side and dip your fork into it before each mouthful. It might sound silly, but most restaurant salads are overdressed, and this is a way of making sure you only get as much as you want and consume fewer calories.

## BREAD WARNING

In restaurants, filling up on bread before your meal starts is a hidden danger, especially as you're likely to be eating more than normal anyway. Choose grain breads wherever you can, share with someone else and eat without butter to minimize health costs.

## WORLD-WISE

Trying different world foods is a great way to make changes to your diet – experiment with different flavours and amalgamate those you like into your diet.

## FRUIT DESSERTS

If you're eating out, try to choose desserts containing fruit whenever possible. Even higher-fat options such as apple crumble and fruit tarts usually contain fewer calories than non-fruit cakes and creamy puddings.

## BE CORDIAL

Instead of fizzy drinks, which can contain lots of additives and sugar, and therefore be high in calories, try mixing sparkling mineral water with a fruit juice or cordial for a much healthier flavoursome drink.

## THINK THIN

If you're out at a pizza restaurant, steer clear of thick and stuffed crusts, which contain hidden calories. Instead, go for the traditional Italian thin-crust version, which contains less fat and carbohydrate.

## END WITH A SALAD

If you want pudding but you don't want to ruin your healthy eating plan, choose a healthy fruit salad or a sorbet, which are lower in calories than other puddings.

## CHOOSE SASHIMI

A great food to choose for working lunches is sashimi, especially if you add a healthy salad or vegetable serving to add some fibre to the meal. The fish will give you a boost of omega-3 oils to help brainpower when you get back to work, but make sure it's really fresh.

## PLAN AHEAD

If you have to entertain or eat out a lot for your work, organize your week in advance and try to have only one function a day where you'll allow yourself to be tempted by unhealthy food, and don't have too much of it. Give yourself one or two occasions a week to relax and blow out and stick to healthy options for the rest.

## OIL-LESS

When ordering grilled fish or vegetables in restaurants, ask for the food to either be grilled without butter or oil or prepared "light", which means it is cooked with less oil or butter than would normally be used.

## GET REAL

It's time to make some changes to your attitude towards eating out – with today's modern lifestyles, eating out is more a part of life than a special occasion for many, which means you can't always use it as an excuse to let go. Be realistic about how often you eat out and think about how to include it in your lifestyle changes.

## PLUMP FOR TOMATO

When ordering pasta and rice dishes, look for tomato-based sauces rather than cream-based ones because they are much lower in fat and calories. And the tomato in the sauce counts as one of your five-a-day, so you can tuck in guilt-free!

## A HEALTHY CHOICE

Many restaurants indicate healthy choices on their menus, and most sit-down places will modify menu items on your request. Additionally, fast-food restaurants now offer a wider range of healthy choices and most will provide nutritional information if asked, or you can check on their websites in advance.

## START WITH A SOUP

Soups are a great starter choice because most are lower in calories than the other menu options and will fill you up more, so you eat less. Choose a clear soup and bear in mind that cream-based soups are higher in fat and calories than most other soups.

## BRING ON A SUBSTITUTE

If you're eating out late and you don't want to eat too many carbohydrates, ask if your starch serving can be replaced with extra steamed vegetables.

## PEER PRESSURE

If you're out with friends and it looks like everyone's having a starter, don't feel pressured into it unless you want to. You could always ask if anyone wants to share one with you to limit your intake.

## MASH UP A SIDE DISH

If you have a choice of side dishes, opt for baked or mashed potato rather than chips. Even if these choices are not listed, you can ask if there are other options or request vegetables instead.

## HOLD BACK

Try not to eat out in "eat as much as you like" restaurants, or those with buffet-only choices. You are more likely to overfill your plate and overeat in these places than when ordering from a menu.

## LOSE THE FAT (BUT KEEP THE TOYS)

Children love the kid's meal offered in restaurants – more for the fun box and toys than for the food. Let them order the kid's meal, but ask for substitutions for the unhealthy fizzy drinks and chips (fries).

## ON THE SIDE

Often, restaurants smother salad in dressing, giving you far more oil that you would choose at home. Order the dressing in a jug on the side and you can be sure you only use as much as you need.

## NO MORE FRY-UPS

Look for items on the menu that are baked, grilled, dry-sautéed, broiled, poached or steamed as these cooking techniques use less fat in the food preparation and are generally lower in calories. Steer clear of deep-fried foods.

## GO LIGHT ON CHEESE

When you're ordering a meal containing cheese in a restaurant, ask the chef to make it light on the cheese – you'll still get the cheesy taste without all the added calories.

## SEE THE WHOLE

Think of eating out in the context of your whole healthy-eating plan. If it's a special occasion that simply won't be the same without your favourite foods, go for it. Moderation is the general rule but as long as it doesn't become a habit, a bit of excess now and again is fine. Remember not to starve yourself in advance as it leads to bingeing and overeating.

## LEAVE A THIRD

Portion sizes in restaurants are usually at least double what a person would normally eat, especially as you usually have more than one course, so it is important to keep that in mind when ordering and eating. If your portion is too large, a good rule of thumb is to leave a third of each serving.

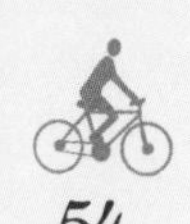



## BEFORE-DESSERT COFFEE

Try ordering your tea or coffee before dessert rather than at the end of your meal. After you've drunk it, the rest of your meal will have had 20 minutes or so to settle and make you feel full, and you're less likely to want to order dessert.

## AN EYE ON THE ALCOHOL

One of the ways extra calories slip in to meals is with high-calorie alcohol – don't allow yourself to lose track of how much you're drinking. Empty your glass before you accept a top up and try to stick to one or two glasses per meal, alternating with a glass of water. Look out for low-calorie mixers and drink spritzers.

## ENJOY YOUR EATING

Whatever you do, don't let healthy eating ruin your meal out – if you're in danger of letting calorie-reduction tips overwhelm you, stick to one or two tips, and if you do it often enough they will become habits.

## MAKE A RULE OF TWO

Make a rule of eating only two courses – choose either a starter or a pudding, but don't have all three courses. Check the menu and see what really takes your fancy, then choose your tastiest meal.

## LET YOURSELF FILL UP

It takes 20 minutes for our stomach to send the message to our brain that we're full, so make sure you take the time to chew and taste your food to avoid overeating.

## LIMIT YOUR OUTINGS

Limit the amount of times you and your family eat out each week. Studies have shown that children and teenagers consume nearly twice as many calories and more fat when they eat out than at home.

## A LA CARTE

It's usually a good idea to stick to the à la carte menu rather than fixed menus. The portion sizes are usually slightly smaller – and the chef will be more receptive to you asking for changes.

# fast food & take-aways

## SIZE UP THE PORTION

If you're ordering fast food, make sure your portion hasn't been supersized without you realizing. Many restaurants will assume you want more food for the same price. If unsure, ask for a regular or medium size.

## HALF AT A TIME

Pre-made sandwiches in supermarkets are often designed for the hungriest people. Be aware of how much you eat by serving yourself one half at a time and only starting the second half if you are hungry.

## AVOID UNREFINED

Subjecting foods to processing and refining, often at high temperatures, is a very effective way of robbing them of any nutritional value they might have originally possessed. Some processed foods have added vitamins and minerals but others have none at all. It's best to avoid them.

## TAKE IT AWAY

Order food to take away rather than eating in fast-food restaurants, as studies show that people tend to consume more food when they are not eating at their own table. Plus, you also have the option of providing a healthier side dish such as fruit or vegetables.

## DELI-BELLY

If you're heading out for fast food, choose the deli-style shops and counters rather than pre-made options. Staff are more likely to take into account your requests to make your choice healthier, such as reducing butter or mayonnaise, and they're usually made with fresher ingredients.

## BUN OFF

If you're eating out at a burger joint, reduce the amount of refined carbohydrates and calories in your meal by removing the top half of your burger bun and eating it with a knife and fork. Ask for a salad rather than fries, but keep the cheese and tomato.

## CHOP THE CHINESE

Next time you reach for the phone to order that Chinese takeaway meal, be aware that the average take-away contains a whopping 1000 calories, which means it's likely to be around half of your daily intake. And that's before pudding!

## A SHAKY CHOICE

Milk shakes might sound like a healthy option, and they are if you make them at home with skimmed or semi-skimmed milk and fresh fruit. However, in restaurants they are usually made with full fat milk, sugary fruit syrup and flavourings – in which case they're not a good choice. Far better to have water or a smoothie if they're on offer.

## A LIGHTER OPTION

Most fast-food establishments now offer healthier menu options such as soups, salads, sushi, chicken sandwiches and non-meat hamburgers. Choose these lighter options if you're in a rush and need to buy something to eat on the go.

## VEGGIE BURGER SUBSTITUTE

Next time you're tempted by a burger – which is high in saturated fat as well as salt, and may not be made from good-quality meat – order a vegetarian version instead. With the same sauces it's often hard to taste the difference, and it's much better for you.

## WHAT'S NOT THERE

It's not just what's in fast foods that's alarming. What they leave out – vitamins, minerals and fibre, to name a few – has just as bad an impact on your health and your digestive system, slowing it down and causing ill health and fatigue.

## DON'T CUT THE MUSTARD

Choose mustard instead of mayonnaise on restaurant or fast food meals to cut calories by reducing fat. If your fast food option is pre-made with lots of mayonnaise, get the same effect by scraping off the excess.

## GRILL YOUR BIRD

Chicken is a great source of protein but it's not always the healthiest menu choice – make sure you choose grilled chicken pieces rather than those which are fried or breaded, and don't go for food like nuggets unless you are sure they're made with real chicken meat.

## BEWARE OF BIG

In recent years, the portion size of salty snacks like crisps has increased by 93 calories, soft drinks by 49 calories and chips by 68 calories, so you're getting more than you used to even if you order the same thing. Check the labels when you're choosing unhealthy snacks.

## CURRY'S FINE

Don't think you can't have a curry on your healthy eating plan – curries can be fattening but there are ways around it. Simply choose plain boiled rice over fried and opt for dry meats (like tandoori) instead of those with creamy sauces. Add a vegetable dish like dahl instead of oily bread.

## FISHY FRIDAYS

One of the UK's favourite take-away meals is fish and chips – far from being banned from healthy-eating lists, it's much better news than many Chinese or Indian alternatives. To make it healthy, go small on chips, or remove them altogether, and replace with a salad at home.

## LOOK FOR REPLACEMENTS

Don't settle for what comes with your sandwich or meal without considering a healthy option. Instead of chips, choose a healthy side salad or fruit bowl, and ask for salsa or tomato-based sauces instead of cheese and mayonnaise.

# family food

## INVOLVE THE KIDS

Do encourage your children to be involved in choosing and preparing food from an early age – that way, they're more likely to develop a healthy attitude to food that will last them a lifetime.

## LET THEM EAT OATCAKE

Oatcakes are great fibre-filled additions to healthy lunchboxes, as are rice cakes, especially the wholegrain ones, and corn cakes. These foods also make great travelling snacks as they are easily transported and children like them. Avoid those that are flavoured as they're usually coated with salty flavourings, and choose low-salt varieties where you can.

## SUGAR HIT

Many parents worry that their children's behaviour will be adversely affected by foods containing lots of sugar at parties, but some studies have shown that hyperactivity is more likely to be caused by overstimulation. Either way, let them blow out once in a while.

## VEG SUBSTITUTE

Rice salads made with brown rice or pasta salads of wholewheat pasta are great choices for healthy lunches for kids. If you struggle to get your kids to eat brown rice, don't despair – simply cut down on the white rice and add extra chopped vegetables for fibre instead.

## LEAD BY EXAMPLE

The best way to help your family adopt healthy eating habits is to have them yourself. It's hard for children to eat healthily if they see you snacking on high fat, sugar or salt foods. Try new fruits and vegetables and set a routine for your meals and snacks that they can follow.

## CUT OUT THE WHITE

Buy seed- or oat-topped wholemeal rolls, wholemeal breads with poppy seeds or nuts (if allowed – some schools don't allow nuts because of allergies) or wholemeal pittas for your children's lunchbox instead of overprocessed white bread.

## SUGAR TRAP

Yogurts and fromage frais are popular with most kids but many – especially the tubed varieties which are so easy to eat – are sugar-laden, with even a mini-pot containing more than 1 tsp of sugar and little or no real fruit. Limit the amount your children eat, or give them sugar-free or natural yogurt, with fresh fruit on the side.

## JOBS FOR TEENS

Give your teenagers some autonomy in the kitchen by taking a night off and allocating them one night a week to make the family meal. That way, they'll learn to cook for themselves before they leave home, and hopefully they'll enjoy planning and preparing a healthy meal.

## A BALANCED LUNCHBOX

In a recent UK government survey, the contents of 74% of lunchboxes for kids were below the nutritional standards set for school meals. For a child aged 9–12 lunch should provide 585 kcal of energy, 23.7 g of fat (of which 7.5 g saturates), 81.3 g of carbohydrate and no more than 1.83 g of salt.

## TEETHING PROBLEMS

Many baby biscuits and toddler's teething rusks contain sugar, which can damage baby's teeth before they've even emerged properly! Check labels carefully and choose biscuits that are sweetened with natural fruit juices – such as apple or grape – instead.

## VITAL VITAMINS

Children need certain vitamins to keep their concentration levels high at school, and some – such as B-vitamins, vitamin C and particularly vitamin E, have been shown to help correct some behavioural problems. Supplements are useful, but vitamins from food are always best.

## BREAK OUT THE BROWN

Sandwiches are a great lunchbox favourite but kids often prefer white bread, which isn't as good for them as wholemeal varieties. Try making their sandwiches with one slice of wholemeal and one of white, but remember to put the white slice on top so it's the one they see first.

## CHOOSE CHEESE FOR SNACKS

Cheese is an excellent snack food for children, but beware of the snack-size individually wrapped versions, which can contain more salt than if they're cut from a bigger block. Check the label and if in doubt, pack a wrapped finger of ordinary cheese instead.

## CAN'T BEAT A BANANA

Bananas are a great snack food and perfect for lunchboxes but they can often get bruised by vigorous movement! Invest in a Banana Guard for your child, a plastic housing which will keep the banana bruise-free until lunchtime!

## GREEN UP YOUR SARNIES

Make yourself a rule for your children's sandwiches – never let a sandwich leave your home unless it's got some greenery in it. Spinach, lettuce, spring greens and watercress are all good sandwich fillers, and if you cut it up small, they'll probably get bored before they can pick it all out!

## DRINK UP

Water is always by far the best drink for kids. Your children should always have access to water, and should have more water than any other drink during the day. If they're not keen on plain water, try sparkling mineral water for special occasions, or add a slice of lemon or lime or a dash of pure fruit juice for flavour.

## STIR UP A SOUP

Soup is lovely in winter, and you can use just about any combination of vegetables to make it. Heat to just below boiling, pour it into a small, warmed flask and it'll be just the right temperature by the time you get to lunch. It's also a great choice for children's lunchboxes.

## MILK THE HEALTH BENEFITS

Plain milk is a great choice for kids, because it contains essential vitamins and minerals and doesn't cause tooth decay. Children up to the age of two years should drink whole milk for the extra calories. After that they can move on to semi-skimmed, but don't give skimmed milk until children are at least five years old.

## A GOOD CHEESE

"Lite" versions of cheese may be lower in fat than the original but, unbelievably, they sometimes contain sugar, so it's important you check labels carefully. Spreads do too. You're probably better off with half the amount of your normal cheese.

## OFFER AN OLIVE

Olives are a great snack for children as they are healthy snacks – filling and without sugar or fat. They can be salty, though, if stored in brine, so wash before eating or offer water alongside them.

## TAKE A DIP

Children love the process of dipping into sauces, so give them a sauce or dip they love, then slip some raw vegetables – sugar snap peas, carrot sticks, celery or peppers – into their hand and they'll (hopefully) eat them without fuss.

## SMUGGLE SOME VEG

Sandwiches, rolls, pizzas and pitta breads are a great place to hide vegetables to help your kids get their five a day. Try grated carrots, finely chopped peppers, sliced cucumber and shredded greens.

## EAT, DRINK AND BE HEALTHY

Try to limit your children's intake of drinks that may contain sugar – like fizzy drinks, fruit squashes and cordials – to mealtimes only as they often contain high amounts of sugar, which is healthier for teeth if taken with food and in one go rather than in little bits. Opt for low sugar or high juice varieties if you can.

## A REAL SMOOTHIE

If you're struggling to get your children to eat their five portions of fruit and vegetables a day, remember smoothies! Homemade, they are a great way of tricking your kids into eating healthily, especially if made with live yogurt. If you buy them, make sure you choose those made with real fruit rather than concentrate.

## DRIED UP

For healthy family or kid's snacks, try dried fruits like raisins, apricots or prunes, which are sweet in taste because of the natural fructose sugars they contain but which also provide a healthy vitamin and mineral boost.

## DRINK TIMES

Juices are best drunk at mealtimes, and not sipped throughout the day, when they're more likely to damage teeth. Limit children to the one glass of pure fruit juice a day that counts towards their five portions of fruit and veg.

## SEASONAL SHOPPING

Whenever you can, buy fresh fruits that are in season like apples, cherries, strawberries or peaches to use for snacks for your children. Cut them up into bite-sized pieces and put in small Ziploc bags or plastic pots for easy snacking.

## SAFE SALT LEVELS

As a general rule, the maximum amounts of salt children should have at different ages are 2 g a day (0.8 g sodium) aged 1–3; 3 g a day (1.2 g sodium) aged 4–6; 5 g a day (2 g sodium) aged 7-10; and 6 g a day (2.5 g sodium) aged 11 and over.

## CUT SOME FAT

Cut the amounts of saturated fat in your children's sandwiches by using less butter, spread or mayonnaise and choosing low-fat fillings such as lean ham, turkey, chicken, tuna in brine, or cottage cheese.

## PLAY A HEALTH TRICK

Don't feel guilty about tricking your kids into eating and drinking more healthily – it's for their own good. If they make a fuss about drinking light drinks, for example, decant sugar-free versions of their favourite fruit squashes into the usual bottles when they're not looking!

## A CHOCOLATE DIP

Make your children a healthy but "naughty" dessert by dipping bits of fresh fruit in melted dark chocolate and allowing it to cool, or even invest in a chocolate fondue set and get the whole family dipping. Try tropical fruits like mango and pineapple.

## GROWING UP

As kids approach school age, they should gradually move towards a diet that's lower in fat and higher in fibre than when they were calorie-hungry youngsters. And by the age of five, their diet should mirror an adult's – low in fat, sugar and salt and high in fibre, with five portions of fruit and veg a day (see www.5aday.nhs.uk).

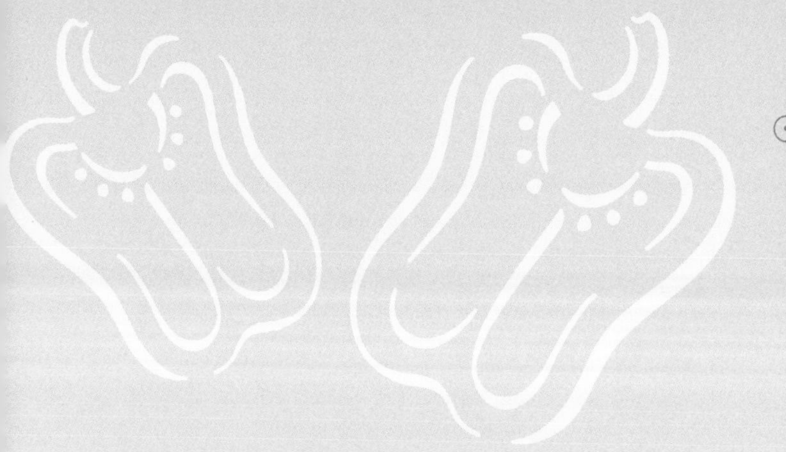



## SECRET INGREDIENTS

To get your family eating more vegetables without them noticing, slip them into favourite dishes – for example, add finely sliced mushrooms to bolognese, chopped red pepper to tomato sauces and steamed leeks or celeriac to mashed potato.

## PACK A HEALTHY PUNCH

In the UK, around half of all children take packed lunches to school, totalling 5.5 billion lunches a year, but it's estimated that less than half contain fruit and nine out of ten contain foods that are high in sugar, salt and saturated fat. Children are choosy, but try making just one healthy change a day, and offer lots of variety.

## KEEP KIDS SALT FREE

It's important to ensure children don't have too much salt. While adults should have no more than 6 g of salt a day, children need even less as they have smaller bodies and less-developed organs. Check processed foods such as crisps, ready meals and sauces, even breakfast cereals, including those aimed at children. Opt for those with the least sodium.

## DON'T DEPRIVE THEM

Encourage your child to eat healthily 90% of the time and let them choose and plan what they would like to eat for their "fun foods" for the other 10% (1 or 2 snacks each day). This removes the feeling of being deprived of certain foods and wanting them even more. And because you're allowing everything in moderation, it teaches responsible food planning and fosters a sense of independence.

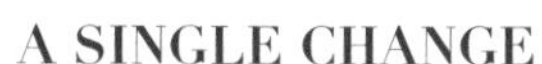

## A SINGLE CHANGE

Many people go into auto-pilot mode when cooking their usual family recipes because they cook them so often. Before you start to cook, think of one change you could implement to make it healthier – frying mushrooms in olive oil instead of butter, for example, or swapping half the meat for beans or lentils.

## TREAT YOUR KIDS DIFFERENTLY

Remember that nutrition guidelines for adults are inappropriate for most children under the age of five. Children have small stomachs so it's important to maximize the calories in their food by, for instance, using whole milk and carbohydrate-heavy meals. They require small but frequent meals to meet their energy needs.

## USE YOUR LOAF

Instead of biscuits and cakes, give your children healthier versions with less refined sugar like banana bread, cheese scones or fruit loaf, which have a "cakey" taste without being too high in sugar or fat.

## STICK TO WHAT THEY LIKE

If your children love one or two types of vegetable but won't eat the rest, don't worry. Feed them two portions of the one they like – although a varied diet is best, getting enough portions is more important. Introduce new kinds gradually.

## STAY AT 150

If you want to let your kids have snacks but don't know how much is too much, watch the portions and keep each item around 150 calories each. In fact, make your life easier and go for pre-portioned snacks like 100-calorie packs, fun-size chocolate bars, or 25 g (1 oz) bags of crisps (potato chips).

## THE BEST START

Children who eat a healthy diet balanced between the four main food groups – meat and fish, dairy products, fruit and vegetables, and bread, potatoes and other carbs – are much less likely to be obese or overweight as adults or to suffer from health problems such as heart disease.

## SNACKS ON THE GO

Great ideas for kids travel snacks are chopped or sliced raw vegetables such as carrots and celery, and crackers, oat biscuits or wholewheat breads, which are full of wholegrains and low in fat and sugar.

## DON'T FORBID FOODS

Studies have shown that forbidding foods will only make your children want them more. Help them to maintain a healthy attitude to food by allowing everything in moderation and offering healthy snacks.

## PACK IN THE FRUIT

Try to make it a rule to put two pieces of fruit into every packed lunch you make. You don't have to stick to apples and bananas – try grapes, fruit salad, a slice of melon or a mix of dried fruit.

## CHUNKY CHIPS

Why not swap chips (fries) for healthy homemade potato wedges? Simply cut potatoes (in their skins for added fibre) into wedges, brush with a little olive oil and bake in the oven until they are soft in the middle and crispy on the outside.

## ORANGE LOVER

Oranges are high in vitamin C and they're a really good portable fruit because they don't bruise easily. Slip one into your child's lunchbox or satchel for a healthy snack.

## BE PREPARED

If you find cooking on weekdays a struggle, prepare in advance by spending an evening or afternoon at the weekend cooking up in bulk and freezing meals to ensure your family have fresh-cooked food every night.

## FATTEN THEM UP

Children under five years old need more fat than older children and adults, but steer clear of cakes, biscuit and chocolate in favour of foods that contain plenty of other nutrients like meat, oily fish and whole dairy produce.

## FEED LITTLE MINDS

Blood-sugar levels are linked to concentration, so allowing your children to skip meals or snack on high-sugar snacks rather than low-GI alternatives (like oats and fruit) could have an effect on how well they do at school.

## LIMIT THEIR FIBRE

Although vegetables and fruit are healthy for adults, young children shouldn't eat too many fibre-rich foods. They may fill them up so much that they can't eat enough fat and protein with them to provide adequate calories and nutrients.

## A GOURMET BABY

Give your baby a head start in the taste stakes by puréeing and freezing unusual combinations of fruit and vegetables in ice cube trays. If you aren't sure which flavours to combine, scour the baby aisles at your local supermarket for ideas. Carrots and apples are a good starting point.

## FRUITS OF THEIR LABOUR

Cook meals with your children and make it fun. They're more likely to eat what they've helped prepare, especially if you've given them some choice about flavours. They'll also take great pride in watching you eat what they've prepared. Also, encourage them to enjoy their food and take time to eat rather than wolfing it down.

## TEENS IN A FIZZ

Fizzy cans of drink are unhealthy for everyone but they're particularly bad for teenage girls as they have been linked to low bone density (because they rob bones of strengthening calcium), which can cause osteoporosis. Try sparkling water instead.





## BE PREPARED

Always have kid-friendly veggies prepared – such as baby carrots, sugar snap peas, red peppers, cherry tomatoes and washed, chopped cucumber. When your child complains he's starving between meals, you can offer him a healthy snack. If he's really hungry, he'll eat it.

## HIDE THE TREATS

Keep chocolate, crisps (potato chips) and other unhealthy snacks in a high cupboard away from other foods. Your kids will be much more likely to demand snack foods if they can see them or they're in accessible cupboards or drawers. It's good for you too, as you may reconsider going to the trouble of reaching for the snacks.

# Eating for Health

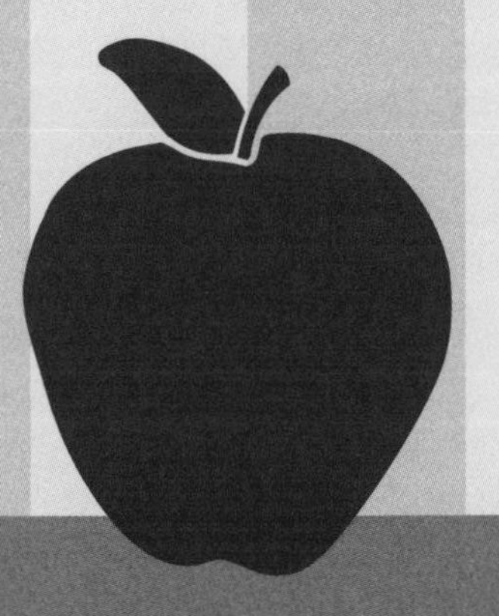

Whether you want the lowdown on food labels, additives, pesticides and GM foods or want to improve your health through the foods you eat, there are many simple ideas here to help you make changes that have a positive effect on your health. In addition to information on nutritional guidelines and food groups, there are tips on reducing fat, sugar and salt in your diet as well as food remedies to counter a range of health ailments.

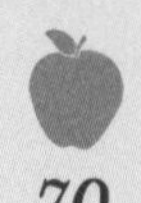



# understanding labels

## STARCH WATCH

The term "modified starch" describes starch that has been physically or chemically treated for food product preparation, often for use as a thickener. It doesn't mean it has definitely been genetically modified. Check with the supplier to be sure.

## JUST ONE DATE

You will see "use by" dates on food that goes off quickly such as smoked fish or ready prepared salads, so don't use it after this date. "Best before" dates are more about quality. When the date expires, the food might begin to lose its taste or texture.

## COUNT THE FAT CALS

Make use of the "calories from fat" label on your food. No more than 30% of your daily calories should be from fat – if you're eating 1500 calories a day, this is 500.

## TRAFFIC LIGHT LABELS

Some supermarkets are adopting a labelling system of traffic lights. This signals whether nutrients we should be cutting down on – fats, sugars, salts and carbohydrates – are at high (red), medium (amber) or low (green) amounts per 100 g (4 oz) food, and enables the shopper to see at a glance if the item is relatively healthy or not.

## FIBRE FILLER

Fibre not only helps keep your digestive system healthy but it can also reduce cholesterol levels. Best of all, it has no calories and it can help you feel full. Try to pick foods that have at least 3 g of fibre per serving, such as all-bran breakfast cereals.

## PORTION DISTORTION

Take note of how much a recommended serving is (100 g, 4 oz, 1 cup, and so on) and try to stick to that amount, only having more if you're still hungry afterwards. Often a serving size will be much less than you're used to eating – restaurant and take-away meals have super-sized over the years.

## DON'T BE AVERAGE

Remember that recommended daily allowances are based on averages, so if a food claims to give 25% of the RDA of vitamin C, that's for someone consuming 2000 calories a day (depending on age, the daily average required by women). If you're consuming fewer than 2000 calories, one portion will give you more than 25%.

## BACTERIAL BENEFITS

Check the sell-by dates on the yogurt tubs in the supermarket, and buy those that are most fresh. Yogurt lasts for about 10 days beyond the sell-by date, but the sooner you eat it the better in terms of reaping the maximum bacterial health benefits.

## INTERNATIONAL DATES

When you're looking at use by and best before dates, be aware that different countries use different date formats. For instance, in the USA 07/03/07 means July 3, 2007 where as the same date in the EU/UK refers to 7 March, 2007.

## GET YOUR DAILY ALLOWANCE

Each day your diet should balance out to give you 100% of your daily amounts for each nutrient. If a food has a daily value of 5% or less, it is considered to be low. Between 10% and 19% is a good source, and 20% or more is excellent. Choose your foods accordingly.

## KNOW YOUR EGGS

Eggs labelled as "Barn eggs" come from birds that live in a shed but are able to move around and often have access to perches, nest-boxes and litter, allowing them to forage and roost. These are not Free Range, which offers birds a similar interior to barn eggs, but also gives continuous access to open-air runs.

## FORBIDDEN FRUIT

Choose foods labelled with the name of the fruit rather than "fruit flavoured". For example, strawberry yogurt must contain strawberries, but strawberry-flavoured yogurt probably doesn't contain any fruit and usually includes additives to create the flavour. Also, if there's an image of real strawberries on the packaging, the product's flavour must, by law, come wholly or mainly from strawberries.

## FOOD WITH FREEDOM

In the UK, the RSPCA has developed a farm and animal welfare labelling scheme that gives consumers the opportunity to purchase meat, poultry, eggs and dairy products from monitored farms. Look out for products labelled Freedom Food. Some campaigners say the scheme doesn't go far enough and it's still best to choose organic. Organizations in other countries, such as the ASPCA in the USA and the RSPCA in Canada and Australia, have similar food-monitoring systems.

## SEEK OUT ORGANIC LABELS

The Soil Association in the UK has developed a certification scheme for foods that have been produced to their stringent organic guidelines. It is a recognized logo that, if it appears on a label, should reassure you that the food you're buying is as free of nasties as it can be. The equivalent in Australia is the Organic Federation of Australia, or in the USA choose food labelled USDA (United States Department of Agriculture) Organic.

## GO VEGGIE

If you're looking for foods without animal products in them, look for those labelled "vegetarian", which guarantees it contains no ingredients derived from animal sources.

## CHECK YOUR FATS

"Cholesterol Free" or "Low Cholesterol" means that the product does not contain any or only small amounts of animal fat or saturated fat, but it does not necessarily mean the product is low fat. Vegetable oils are cholesterol-free but made entirely of fat.

## PLACE OF ORIGIN

Thirty per cent of consumers are concerned about country-of-origin food labels in the EU, which can be vague and misleading. For example, Welsh lamb can be sent to France, slaughtered there, and sold as French lamb – you would naturally assume that the lamb spent its entire life in France. Some labels read "produce of the EU or South America" or "produce of EU, Brazil or Thailand". Ask the supermarket staff or your butcher to provide exact details as you have a right to know.

## NOT THE WHOLE STORY

Remember that companies are not obliged to give detailed nutrition information about their food products unless they make a claim about their food, such as "low fat" or "high fibre". In other words, something labelled "90% fat free" could contain 10% fat, which is a lot higher than the 3% it needs to be to be labelled "low fat". Check before you buy.

## KEEP AN EYE ON SATURATES

Don't just look for total fat content on labels. The proportion of saturated fat – the really bad stuff – is important too. Products with 5 g of saturated fat per 100 g are classed as high-fat products, whereas those with 1 g are healthy low-fat options.

## TOP UP YOUR FIBRE

Foods that are labelled "more fibre" or "added fibre" contain at least 2.5 g more fibre per serving than the original food, which means they are usually better choices. Do check labels, though, to make sure sugar, salt and fat haven't also been added.

## SUGAR HIGHS

People with diabetes or who are worried about their blood sugar levels should avoid all food products where sugar is listed first under the ingredients list and keep to a minimum products where sugar is listed in second place. These foods are likely to cause blood sugar peaks.

## BEWARE OF HIDDEN SUGAR

If the label on your food says "low cholesterol", what that means in practice is that it contains less than 20 mg of cholesterol and a maximum of 2 g saturated fat per serving. Be careful of hidden sugar in these products, which manufacturers use as an alternative to fat.

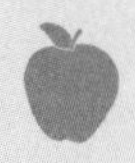



## NON-LABELLED PRODUCTS

In the UK, shops are required to give basic nutritional information. For non-labelled items such as fresh breads and other bakery produce, check the price labels on the products in the supermarket – they should contain basic information and a list of ingredients to help you plan your diet.

## PRESERVE YOUR HEALTH

Food which is labelled "no preservatives" means exactly what it says, but don't confuse it with the label "no preservatives added" – this is used to label food that could contain natural preservatives such as salt and essential oils.

## A LIGHT TOUCH

Although some light products have certain guidelines to which they must adhere, sometimes the word refers to the taste or colour. For instance, "light" olive oil has no fewer calories or less fat than regular olive oil – it simply tastes more delicate.

## LEAN TOWARDS LEAN

A great way to get your protein without the added fat that often accompanies it is to choose food that is labelled "lean", which means that per serving it contains 10 g or less of fat, of which 4.5 g or less are saturated, and less than 95 mg cholesterol. Remember that this is for an 85 g (3 oz) portion, though. Larger portions will contain more fat.

## SEDUCED BY REDUCED

"Reduced" on a food label can be a little misleading. What it actually means is that the product contains 25% less of the specified ingredient (for instance, reduced fat or reduced sugar) than the usual product. Check the label to see exactly how much there is per serving.

## LOW-SALT IS BEST

Products high in salt contain 0.5 g of sodium (1.25 g of salt) per 100 g of produce, whereas those low in salt contain around 0.1 g, and medium is 0.2–0.4 g. Try to choose low-salt products whenever you can.

## STAY BELOW THREE

Fat is usually measured in grams. A good rule of thumb for keeping to the right amount per day is to choose foods that have less than 3 g of fat for every 100 calories in a serving.

## SEARCH FOR THE SALT

Foods that are labelled as "low sodium" or "low salt" contain a maximum of 140 mg of salt per serving. This is a good label to look out for on foods that may contain hidden salt, such as soups and sauces.

## THE LOW-DOWN ON SUGAR

In general, products are high in sugar if they contain 10 g of sugar per 100 g of the product. They are low in sugar if they contain 2 g per 100 g of product. Use this information on labels to help you choose. No added sugar means just that, and nothing more – it doesn't mean the product is necessarily low in sugar. Many foods (such as fruit) contain natural sugars, so no added sugar really means that no extra refined sugar has been added.

## DON'T BE FOOLED

Foods labelled "healthy" might not actually be terribly healthy. They have to have decreased fat, saturated fat, sodium, and cholesterol, as well as some added vitamins, but there isn't a specific amount by which they have to be reduced to carry this label. Check the label carefully.

## WATCH OUT FOR PERCENTAGES

Beware of percentage labels on foods saying things like "20% more chicken" in a pie. This only means something if the product had a decent amount to start with. For example, if it's a 200 g pie that used to contain 20 g of chicken, that's only 4 g more meat, which isn't much at all.

## BE GLUTEN FREE

For coeliacs (those allergic to wheat) claims about gluten in foods are very important. However, manufacturers are not obliged to state how much gluten is in a food item. As it is impossible to remove all the gluten from wheat, the gluten content may not be clear. Look carefully at the ingredients list to see how much the food contains, or choose one that carries the Food Standards Agency's Gluten-free label.

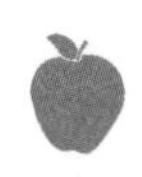



## FAT FREE, SUGAR HIGH?

Products labelled as "fat free" or "sugar free" are guaranteed to contain less than half a gram of fat or sugar per serving, but remember that usually products are only one or the other. Check that the reduced fat or sugar hasn't been replaced with a higher dose of the other to enhance taste.

## CHECK THE LIST

If you're looking at ingredients lists, remember they are given in descending order, so the ingredient there is most of will be listed first and the one there is least of, last. This is important in, for instance, products where you would expect meat to be the main ingredient.

## SALT OR SODIUM

Some manufacturers make trying to work out salt in products difficult by giving sodium levels instead. Work it out yourself by multiplying the sodium content by 2.5 to get the salt content and try to keep salt below 1.25 g per 100 g.

## BEHIND THE BIG SELL

Items labelled "traditional" often contain a number of non-traditional ingredients, including E-numbers, and there's no law against using the word on foods. Check the ingredients lists carefully to make sure it's not just a marketing ploy. Other words that fall into this category are "farmhouse", "wholesome" and "original".

## LARGE DOSE

If a food is labelled "High in…", it will contain at least 20% of the recommended daily amount of that particular nutrient. Check the label carefully to find out exactly how much each serving provides.

## A FRESH FEEL FOR EGGS

"Country-fresh" eggs, accompanied by a nice picture of hens running around in the sunshine, could come from caged battery-farmed hens that have never seen natural daylight. The same applies to eggs labelled "farmhouse", "farm fresh", "selected" and "traditional". The only way you can be sure is to choose free range and/or organic.

## LAY OFF THE JUICE

Fruit juice contains 100% pure fruit juice (although it may be made from concentrate), but a "juice drink" only has to contain 5% pure fruit juice to get its name. That's a tiny dribble in every bottle and the remainder can be water, artificial sweeteners, sugar, colours, flavourings and even thickeners.

## THE LIGHT TRAP

Versions of food that are labelled "light" can contain up to two thirds of the amount of fat or calories of the usual version, so although they are good alternatives to fatty foods they're not necessarily healthy choices.

## HIGH FIBRE FOR HEALTH

High-fibre foods are good healthy choices because they fill you up without adding extra calories. Foods that are labelled "high fibre" must contain 5 or more grams of fibre per serving, so you know that if you choose them you're getting a really high dose.

## FAIR DEAL

Buying Fairtrade doesn't just help local workers all over the world to get a better deal out of farming and producing foods. Because of the guidelines on how many chemicals are used to protect human health, it also means that fair-trade food usually contains far fewer toxins, too.

## BEWARE TEMPTING OFFERS

You might be tempted to pick up foods that are labelled "a good source of..." but beware – all this label means is that it provides at least 10% of the daily recommended value of a nutrient, which for some vitamins can be fairly small amounts.

## SERVE YOU RIGHT

If you choose foods that are labelled "calorie free", you can be sure that the food you're eating contains fewer than five calories per serving. Beware of serving size, though, as some manufacturers may specify small servings to get their product under the barrier.

## LOW-CAL DOESN'T MEAN HEALTHY

If a food is labelled "low calorie", it means there are less than 40 calories per serving. It doesn't, however, give any guidance on how healthy the ingredients are, how many additives it contains, or how processed the food is, so do have a look at the label.

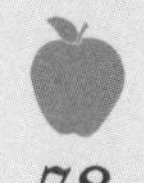



# genetically modified foods

## HAVE YOUR SAY

Take a stand against GM foods by avoiding foods which contain GM ingredients and writing to the manufacturer to let them know about your decision. If only a small percentage of the population did this, it could lead to manufacturers losing sales and possible changes in policy.

## CHOOSE ORGANIC

If you want to avoid GM foods, buy organic. Although there are a percentage of non-organic ingredients allowed in foods labelled organic, none of the ingredients are allowed to contain GM material.

## MODIFY YOUR CHOICE

About 80% of processed foods contain maize or soya – or their derivatives – and so could potentially contain GM ingredients. Any label saying "modified maize starch" or "modified soya protein" is almost certainly GM.

## HALF TRUTHS

There could be more genetic modification in your food than you think. Genetically modified bacteria and fungi are used in the production of enzymes, vitamins, food additives, flavourings and processing agents in thousands of foods as well as health supplements. Check with the manufacturer if you're unsure.

## AVOID PROCESSED THE MOST-EST

The best way to make sure you avoid GM food is to avoid heavily processed foods, which are more likely to contain modified soya or crops. In fact, 75% of processed foods are thought to contain GM ingredients. The worst culprits are ready meals, followed by foods such as bread, biscuits, sausages, pies and chips.

## SWEETENING YOU UP

Aspartame, the diet sweetener, is a product of genetic engineering. By buying low-fat or "diet" alternative drinks or foods, which may contain this substance, you could inadvertently be giving your support to genetic modification.

## NO GUARANTEE

Did you know there is a threshold of 0.9% GM ingredients that foods can contain and still be labelled as GM free in Europe? This means that even foods that aren't labelled as GM could contain nearly 1% GM foods. Recognized organic foods, however, are guaranteed to contain none.

## THE HONEY TRAP

The most difficult areas to control
GM in foods are items like honey, where free-roaming bees may have visited GM-crop fields, inadvertently contaminating the honey. This is why Canadian honey is not on sale in Europe. Check labels carefully to be sure.

## BUY ORGANIC DAIRY

Dairy products like milk, meat, cheese and eggs that come from animals fed on a GM diet do not have to be labelled as GM, so it is impossible to tell if the animals have been produced using GM or not. Buying organic will assure that they are GM free.

## BACK YOUR LOCAL

It can be difficult for those catering for high numbers – in schools, old people's homes and other mass-catering events – to be sure their food is GM free because of the large suppliers they have to use, but it's not impossible. Encouraging people to use locally sourced ingredients helps.

## CORNY BUSINESS

In the western world, many crops are now routinely grown using GM seeds or processes. This includes 45% of corn and 54% of canola, which show up on ingredients lists as corn meal, corn syrup, dextrose, maltodextrin, fructose, citric acid, lactic acid and of course, corn oil.

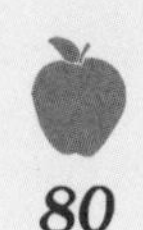



## THE BUTCHER'S BUSINESS

Many animals are now fed a GM diet. Visiting a local butcher will help you to remove these products from your diet because they work on a smaller basis than supermarkets and therefore should be able to tell you what diet the animals consumed, helping you avoid GM if you want to.

## SOY SORRY

Most packaged foods contain soy in some form, which can show up on ingredients lists as soy flour, soy protein, soy lecithin and textured vegetable protein. A staggering 85% of these will be GM. Check the ingredients list, then scour the shelves for non-GM alternatives.

## STAY OFF THE HORMONES

About 22% of cows in the USA are injected with genetically modified bovine growth hormone (rbGH), so if a dairy product is not labelled organic, non-GMO or hormone-free, it is likely that some of it came from cows injected with rbGH, which is thought in Europe and Canada (where it is banned) to have adverse effects on health.

## LOG ON TO BE SURE

If you live in the USA and aren't sure about whether your usual food items contain GM ingredients, you can check them by logging on to www.truefoodnow.org, a site which offers an extensive list of foods by brand and category, indicating whether or not they contain GM ingredients.

## GET POLITICAL

If you're worried about GM foods, it's a bit of a geographic lottery. In the USA, many foods contain GM ingredients whereas in Europe it's a much lower number. Visit your government's health advice pages to find out more about the area you live in.

## CHECK YOUR OIL

Most generic vegetable oils and margarines used in restaurants and processed foods are made from soy, corn, canola or cottonseed – the four major GM crops in the USA. Unless these oils specifically say "Non-GMO" or "Organic" they are probably genetically modified. Non-GM substitutes to try include olive, sunflower, flaxseed and hemp oils.

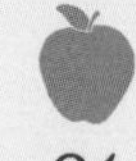



### WORDLY WISE

More than 50% of papaya (paw paw) from Hawaii is genetically modified to resist a virus so choose papayas grown in Brazil, Mexico, or the Caribbean, where there are currently no GM varieties.

### THE FACTS

There is currently no real evidence that any GM crop or ingredient has a negative effect on human health or on the environment. But as there's no evidence to the contrary either, many pressure groups advocate avoiding GM until we can be sure.

### LOOK OUT FOR HVP

Watch out for the ingredient "hydrolyzed vegetable protein" (HVP) on ingredients lists, particularly for processed foods such as cakes, biscuits and other sweet snacks. This is a commonly used flavour enhancer, which is derived from corn and soy, so could therefore be GM.

## pesticides & chemicals

### FISHY BUSINESS

In the past couple of years, the EU has significantly reduced the level of dyes that can safely be fed to farmed salmon, because of concerns that the dyes, at high levels, can affect people's eyesight. If you have to eat farmed salmon, European-produced salmon is the safest.

### FISH FOR PURITY

Oily fish show fairly high levels of pesticide and chemical residue. However, many of the fish tested are probably farmed and if you buy organic farmed or wild-caught versions, the residues are much lower.

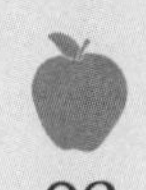



## REMEMBER TO WASH

In recent studies, the foods most contaminated with pesticides were found to be apples, peppers, celery, cherries and grapes. You should make sure you wash these items thoroughly, immersing them in water and drying carefully.

## AND THE GOOD NEWS...

Not all food preservatives are bad news – the antioxidant food preservative BHT, which is used to prevent fat from going rancid in packaged foods, is currently being researched as a cure for cold sores. As with all preservatives, however, there are still so many gaps in the knowledge it's best to avoid them where possible.

## CHEMICAL COCKTAIL

An astounding 447 chemicals are available to non-organic farmers, and around 31,000 tonnes are used every year. The most dangerous have been linked with a range of problems including cancer, decreasing male fertility, foetal abnormalities, chronic fatigue syndrome in children and Parkinson's disease, so choosing organic is safest.

## WATER RETENTION

Chemicals, such as pesticides and fertilizers, sprayed on foods during the growing process are thought to be held for longer in watery fruit and vegetables, such as cucumbers and watermelons.

## WHAT'S YOUR POISON?

Most people think fruit and vegetables are higher in pesticide residues than other foods but according to a report by the FDA in the USA, the highest residues are actually found in bread, flour and potatoes. Buying organic versions of these foods will dramatically reduce residues, although there may still be some traces.

## ORGANIC IS BEST

While non-organic farmers have hundreds of pesticides at their disposal, only four substances are used on UK Soil Association organic farms – sulphur, soft soap, copper and rotenone. The latter two are "restricted", which means that organic farmers must prove there is no alternative before they can be used.

## A PLUM DEAL

The five fruits shown to be least contaminated with residues in the UK are star fruit, plums, peaches, kiwi fruit and hard-skinned exotic fruits like passion fruit and pomegranate.

## PEEL AWAY PESTICIDES

An apple a day is supposed to keep the doctor away, but the average eating apple – the most pesticide-heavy fruit – has been sprayed 18 times with many different chemicals. Most of the residues of chemical fertilizers and pesticides stay on the skin. If you buy non-organic apples, make sure you peel them or at least wash them thoroughly. This will also remove dirt and bacteria.

## PILL POPPING

Total farm antibiotic use has increased by 11% in three years in the UK – many intensively reared farm animals in the UK are still given antibiotics in their feed on a daily basis. The resistance that is built up by the animals as a result is thought, in turn, to contribute to antibiotic resistance in humans. The only way to be sure you're not getting a dose is to eat organic meat.

## CRACK THE CONSPIRACY

Many people think eggs are safe from pesticide residues and dangerous chemicals because they're covered with a hard shell, but in fact they are just as susceptible as poultry meat. Choosing organic will help you be sure your eggs are pure.

## TRY TO RESIST

The USA has already banned enrofloxacin, a drug that causes resistance to the important medical antibiotic ciprofloxacin, which is added to the drinking water of chickens and turkeys. However, it's still used in the UK on many non-organic farms.

## BEST OF THE BUNCH

Among the foods found to be least contaminated with pesticide residues worldwide are asparagus, avocados, bananas and broccoli, so you can generally eat these without worrying, although it's still safest to wash before use. Other good choices are corn on the cob, cauliflower, marrow, squash and swede.

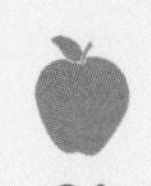



### PICK YOUR PORK

The drug tylosin is routinely added to intensively farmed pig feed to control disease. It is also thought to increase levels of the hospital superbug VRE and to cause resistance to antibiotics used to treat food poisoning. Become an informed consumer.

### LIVER YOUR TIMBERS

Be extra careful to choose organic when you're buying animal products where toxins may be concentrated, like offal. The chemical nicarbazin, which has been shown to cause birth defects and hormonal problems in animals, has been found in amounts up to 20 times the legal limit in chicken livers.

### CAN YOU STOMACH IT?

In the past, the enzyme chymosin, used in hard cheeses, was taken from the stomach linings of calves. Since the GM variety was introduced in 1990, it is used in more than 70% of US cheeses. Its use is not allowed in organic cheese. In the UK, chymosin is used in the production of vegetarian cheeses, and does not require labelling.

### WASH ORGANICS TOO

Don't assume that just because your foods are organic they'll be pesticide free. Most of the residues found in organic foods are probably the unavoidable results of environmental contamination in the past, or by drift when sprays are blown in from non-organic farms. Be sure to wash ALL fruit and vegetables.

## nutritional guidelines

### VARIETY IS KEY

Eat a variety of nutrient-rich foods. You need more than 40 different nutrients for good health, and no single food supplies them all. Your daily food selection should include wholegrain products (wholegrain cereals, brown rice, wholemeal bread, etc), fruits and vegetables, dairy products, and meat, poultry, fish and other protein foods.

## BALANCE YOUR PLATE

Nutritionists used to suggest meals should be one-third each of carbs, protein and veg, but the most recent advice is that your plate should be half full of vegetables, a quarter carbs and a quarter protein. Make sure you balance every meal to ensure a healthy intake.

## BULK UP ON PROTEIN

Meals containing higher levels of protein and a lower amount of carbohydrate keep you fuller for longer than those that are low in protein and high in carbohydrates. Try altering the balance of foods on your plate to help maintain fullness, particulary at lunchtime.

## AGE-RELATED ALTERATIONS

Remember that as you grow older, your calorie requirements will change even if you maintain the same levels of activity. Make time to think about your life-eating balance a few times a year to see if you need to alter your intake.

## GROWING-UP DIETS

Teenagers and older children who are growing fast often have higher requirements for nutrients. For example 15 to 18-year-old boys need more thiamin (vitamin B1), niacin (vitamin B3), vitamin B6, calcium, phosphorus and iron than adult men. Similarly, 15 to 18-year-old girls need more niacin, calcium, phosphorus and magnesium than adult women.

## CALORIE COUNT

For an adult man who is moderately active the daily guidelines are around 2500 a day. For women, who usually have less muscle bulk and therefore a lower metabolism, it's 2000 a day. Dropping 500 calories a day is a calorie-controlled diet.

## SPOT THE DIFFERENCE

The main point of difference between US and EU/UK nutritional labels is that the EU/UK requires nutrients to be shown per 100 g or 100 ml. The nutrient amounts may, in addition, be given per quantified serving or portion (if the number of portions in a pack is stated on the packaging).

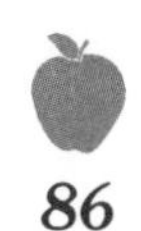



## BOOST THEIR BRAINS

For children aged between four and six, growth has slowed down but general development is ongoing and rapid, so getting enough calories is really important. Studies have shown that children with healthy diets perform better in school, so aim to give boys of this age 1700 and girls 1500 calories a day.

## GOLDEN OLDIES

Scientists have found that consuming a diet rich in wholegrain foods may lower the risk for cardiovascular disease and reduce the onset of metabolic syndrome, especially in older people so it's even more important to eat them as you age.

## ALLOW FOR DIFFERENCES

Remember that US Recommended Daily Allowances (RDAs) differ from UK RDAs, therefore figures and statements of percentage contribution of nutrients could be misleading on imported products. Check where your products originated to be sure.

## COUNT KIDS' CALORIES

Aged between seven and ten, children need around 2000 calories (for a boy) or 1800 calories (for a girl) to keep their bodies functioning optimally. Eleven to 14-year-old boys need an average of 2200 calories a day and girls a slightly lower 1900, but bear in mind that these amounts are calculated for average activity, so if your child is sporty, he or she will probably need more.

## THUMBS UP TO CHEESE

Did you know that a portion size of cheese is just the size of a thumb? Or that one muffin or bagel portion is the size of a ping-pong ball? This means you're more than likely getting more than one portion with each serving, so take this into account when planning menus.

## TODDLERS DON'T RUN ON EMPTY

If you have children aged one to three, try to make sure they get around 1200 calories a day from all the major food groups to meet their growth and energy needs. Try to keep down the amount of "empty" calories – in processed foods – and to include as many different foods as possible.

### TEEN SPIRIT

The recommended daily amount of calories for a teenager over 14 years old is actually around 300 calories a day higher than that for an adult because their body is using up lots of calories in growth and development. Aim for around 2800 calories for boys and 2200 for girls and avoid skipping meals.

### CLIMB THE FOOD PYRAMID

Many organizations use the food pyramid to help you understand how to eat better. At the base of the plan are plenty of breads, cereals, rice and pasta, vegetables and fruits. Add 2–3 servings a day from dairy and 2–3 servings from meat, and go easy on fats, oils and sweets, which are at the top of the pyramid.

### DAY-TO-DAY NEEDS

Per day, the average 40-year-old woman should be eating 175 g (6 oz) of wholegrains, three handfuls of vegetables and two of fruit, 500 ml (18 fl oz) of milk or dairy products, and around 175 g (6 oz) of protein from meat, fish or beans.

### EAT LESS EMPTIES

As a general rule, try and keep your intake of "empty" calories (from sugary snacks, processed foods, alcohol, biscuits and cakes) to around 200–250 a day. These high-energy/low nutritional value foods should make up less than 10% of your total daily intake.

## food planning

### WEIGH UP THE WEEK

It's important to get a good balance of food every day, but it can be confusing and easy to lose track. To check, think about what you eat and drink over the course of a week – jot it down if it helps. If it balances out overall, even if you have the odd bad day, you're on the right track.

### THREE OF YOUR FIVE A DAY

Most people know they should eat five portions of fruit and vegetables a day, but did you know that three of these, ideally, should be vegetables because they are lower in sugar and higher in fibre?

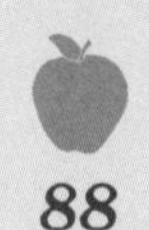



## PUT IN WHAT YOU GIVE OUT

Start thinking about your balance of calories in and calories out. So, if you've had a really active day you might need a larger dose of carbohydrates to refuel your body's lost energy, but if you've been relatively inactive, you could probably make do with a smaller portion.

## EAT ONE CARB PER MEAL

The best way to moderate your carbohydrate input is to limit it to one portion per meal. This would be equivalent to 1–2 slices of wholemeal bread, a cup of cereal, rice or oats, or a baked sweet or regular potato.

## GO LIGHT ON THE CARBS

Watch the amount of starchy carbohydrates you're serving at each meal. Carb-heavy meals tend to be calorie-heavy meals. Don't be tempted to base an entire meal around noodles, rice or bread even though it's sometimes easier. Replace with more vegetables or a salad instead.

## BE AN EARLY RISER

Get up five minutes earlier in the morning and use the time to sit down and plan your daily intake of food and drink. Knowing ahead of time what you're going to eat will make you less likely to binge and more likely to eat in moderation. If you're eating to weekly plans, use this morning time to revise your day's diet.

## BAKE A CAKE

Instead of buying cakes or biscuits in the supermarket, make your own at home and substitute wholemeal flour for the usual white variety – it will make your homemade cakes nutritious as well as tasty.

## FRUIT IN THE FRIDGE

Try fresh fruit salad for dessert instead of calorie-packed puddings. To make it easier, make a large bowl at the beginning of the week and keep it in your fridge so it's easy to dip into every night.

## STICK TO A SERVING

It's difficult to know what's meant by "one serving", especially if you're trying to count calories. Generally, the recommended serving of cooked meat is 85 g (3 oz), which is roughly the size of a pack of cards.

## JUST SAY NO

Did you know that 500 ml (18 fl oz) of ice cream is the equivalent of four portions of your daily dairy and fat intake? Think about that next time you're offered an extra scoop.

## TAKE A HANDFUL

How do you know what a serving of fruit or vegetables is? In general, it's about a handful of most types, or a medium apple, pear or orange. Bear in mind that for vegetables the amounts are measured cooked rather than raw. This is especially important for "shrinking" foods like spinach.

## SENSIBLY DOES IT

Always remember that effective weight-loss programmes should include healthy-eating plans that reduce calories but do not rule out specific foods or food groups, together with physical activity. This should give a slow and steady weight loss of 0.5–1.5 kg (1–3 lb) per week.

## SERVE YOURSELF WELL

According to advice from the USDA (mypyramid.gov), for a balanced daily diet, you should aim for 6–11 servings from the bread, rice, cereal and pasta group (around 100 g or 4 oz), 3 of which should be whole grains. Then add 2–4 servings of fruit, 3–5 servings of vegetables and 1–2 of protein.

## GROW YOUR OWN

If you're tired of not being able to find cheap organic vegetables, why not grow your own? Vegetable patches and allotments are becoming increasingly popular and they're a great way to ensure good quality produce. If you're short of space, tomatoes, lettuce and fresh herbs also grow well on windowsills and in window boxes.

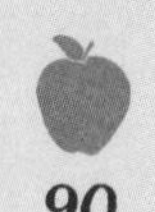





# food groups

## AN EVEN KEEL

Foods rich in soluble fibre have the ability to slow down the absorption of glucose into your bloodstream and to stabilize blood-sugar levels, helping prevent feelings of hunger. Choose oats, brown rice, barley, apples, pears, peas, strawberries, sweet potatoes, carrots and beans.

## FEEL THE PULSE

For extra fibre smuggle lentils into soups and sauces. They are great if used as a thickening agent instead of flour, and give winter soups heartiness and flavour.

## FAT BALANCE

Eat more "good" fats than "bad" (saturated) throughout the course of a week to get a balance. Good fats are the naturally occurring fats that haven't been damaged by high heat, refining, processing or other tampering such as "partial hydrogenation". The best of these are found in olive oil, oily fish, nuts, avocados and seeds.

## EAT UP THE SKIN

If you want to give yourself a fibre boost, eat up the peel and skin of your fruit and vegetables rather than peeling and throwing it away. The skin is often the most fibrous part, especially in root vegetables. Wash or scrub them first to remove any lingering pesticides.

## WATCH YOUR JUICE LEVELS

Although vegetable juice seems a really healthy choice, it isn't very high in fibre and actually contains quite high levels of sodium, which is the damaging element in salt. Choose low-sodium varieties if you can, and limit your intake to one portion (as stated on the pack) a day.

## BE PRO-PROTEIN

If you're a vegetarian, it's important to make sure you get enough protein – you should aim for 2–3 portions of milk or dairy products and two portions of other protein (such as nuts, tofu or fish) per day.

## PUT ON THE PROTEIN

The addition of protein to a meal helps to slow down the absorption of carbohydrate into the bloodstream and makes you feel fuller, so you'll eat less. This means protein can help leave you feeling satisfied and productive for longer after eating, even if you've only eaten a small portion.

## GET A FEEL FOR FIBRE

Insoluble fibre takes a longer time to chew and provides volume to food without adding lots of calories. It keeps your digestive system in good working order. Soluble fibre helps stabilize blood-sugar levels, warding off hunger cravings. There's some of both in fruit and vegetables.

## BEANS ARE BEST

Beans – particularly kidney beans, black beans and chickpeas – are great carbohydrate choices if you're trying to regulate blood sugar because they provide plenty of fibre, while being low in calories.

## PROTEIN POWER

Recent studies have found that adding more protein (found in fish, meat, eggs and beans) to meals also has a "thermic" effect on digesting your food, meaning it can increase your metabolism and help to burn off fat. Your body requires more energy (calories) to burn protein off than it does carbohydrates and fats.

## DRINK FROM FOOD

Fruit and veg that have a higher water content – such as puréed vegetable soup and watery fruit like melon, celery and watermelon – can help fill you up, so you'll eat less throughout the day. Just drinking water does not have the same effect since it exits the stomach more rapidly.

## PALM YOUR PROTEIN

The average woman needs approximately 85 g (3 oz) of protein per serving, and the average man needs just 25 g (1 oz) more (110 g or 4 oz). A serving should fit into the palm of your hand – a good way of measuring it if you're out and about.

## EAT AWAY FAT

Put yourself together a fat-burning meal by combining green leafy vegetables with a lean protein source such as fish or turkey to form the bulk of the meal. Then add a small portion of natural starchy carbohydrates like oats, sweet potato, wholewheat pasta or brown rice.

## GO FOR GOOD FAT

Fats can be heavily disguised in foods, even with labelling systems, and it's often difficult to know how to get the right balance. To add good fat to your diet, cook with olive oil, add flax oil to a morning shake and try to include nuts, seeds or avocados in your meals.

## FIGHT FATIGUE

Foods that combat tiredness include complex carbohydrates, potassium and magnesium-rich foods, and foods high in iron and vitamins B and C. Good meal choices to beat fatigue would therefore be meat or fish served with steamed vegetables and fresh fruits.

## DON'T SEE RED

Try eating fish, chicken or turkey instead of red meat a few times a week. Red meat is a good constituent of a balanced diet, especially the leaner cuts, but in a healthy diet it's not necessary to eat it more than two or three times a week.

## MAKE THE SWITCH

To help your heart stay healthy and give your digestive system a flush through, swap pulses or grains, which contain the same nutrients, for your usual meat or fish a couple of nights a week.

## MAX YOUR MONOS

Try to maximize your intake of monounsaturated fats (like olive oil, avocados, walnuts, almonds and sesame seeds) and omega-3 fatty acids (from cold water fish, hemp and flax seeds), which have health benefits for all the organs of the body, including the brain and heart.

## SATURATION POINT

Minimize your intake of saturated fats from red meat and full-fat dairy products, trans fatty acids from processed foods, and omega-6 fatty acids like safflower and sunflower oil, all of which can create problems in your body if eaten in excess.

## BUILD MILKY BONES

Not only is skimmed milk lower in fat than semi-skimmed and whole milk, the bone-building calcium it contains is actually easier for your body to access because fat can interfere with calcium absorption.

## GET THE WHOLE PICTURE

To increase your fibre intake, which helps regulate the digestive system and boosts health, it's a great idea to include wholegrains in your diet. You can do this by using wholemeal pasta, oats and wholemeal flour in cooking.

## KEEP FUEL LEVELS UP

Carbohydrates provide the body's preferred fuel: glucose. A diet rich in complex carbohydrates such as grains, cereals and starchy vegetables provides the best staying power because these foods are digested slowly and continue releasing energy for many hours after eating.

## DRINK IN YOUR FIBRE

Soluble fibre is a really important part of any healthy diet because its soft texture helps your muscles to move food through the digestive system, for efficient digestion. It also boosts water absorption in the body. Drink water when you eat fibre for optimum nutritional benefits and avoid processed foods as they are low in fibre.

## HALF AND HALF IT

If your family love the taste and lightness of white bread but you want to make sure they have their daily dose of healthy wholegrains, try using half wholemeal flour and half white flour in bread and other baked goods like muffins and pizza bases. You could also make sandwiches using one slice of white with one slice of brown, which looks attractive, is tastier and offers a healthy alternative to an all-white bread sandwich.

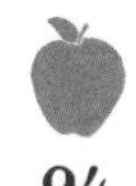



# health-giving substances

## HELP THEM TO GROW

For children and teenagers, it's important to ensure high levels of the amino acid L-arginine, which works with lysine and ornithine to stimulate the production of growth hormones and enhance infection-fighting antibodies. Good sources are nuts, sunflower seeds, chocolate, raisins and brown rice.

## BE A GOOD EGG

Vegetarians who don't eat meat or fish should try to include eggs in their diet as a regular feature as these are the only other source of the amino acid L-Lysine, which has been shown to work with vitamin C to reduce damage to arteries.

## TOP UP THE TYROSINE

Tyrosine is an amino acid that is a component of thyroid hormone, reported to aid in the treatment of depression, anxiety, fatigue and Parkinson's disease. It is found in meat, fish, eggs and dairy products and is better taken naturally because high-dosage supplementation has been linked to cancer development.

## THE HARD TRUTH

Raw food is often richer in nutrients and enzymes and requires more chewing than cooked foods. This extra work is beneficial because it mixes the food with enzymes in the saliva to kick start the digestive process and ensure that you absorb as many nutrients as possible.

## BRIGHT IS RIGHT

When choosing fruits and veggies, look for a bright hue – as a general rule, the brighter the colour, the more nutrients the food contains. Blueberries, kale and red peppers are especially full of antioxidants, which help to counteract the negative effects of pollution and the sun on our bodies.

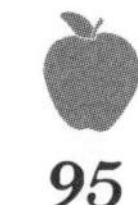



## SUP SOME SULPHUR

It's not only calcium and magnesium you need for healthy bones, skin, hair, nails and connective tissues in the body – sulphur is essential for the production of collagen. Find it in lean beef, dried beans, eggs, fish and cabbage, which are even more important to include in the diet as you age.

## PRESSURE POINT

Vanadium is a required trace element that has been beneficial in treating some forms of high blood pressure and for reducing the body's production of cholesterol. It is also reported to reduce insulin requirements in type I diabetes, and is found in black pepper, mushrooms, shellfish and parsley.

## DON'T BIN THE GARLIC

Don't worry if you're not sure whether to use that old head of garlic you've found at the back of the cupboard – aged garlic has been shown to have high levels of sallylmercaptocystein (SAMC), a sulphur compound that has been shown to slow the growth of prostate cancer cells. Fresh garlic doesn't have this effect.

## THUMBS UP TO FRY-UP

Next time you have a hangover, cook yourself a protein-rich meal such as bacon and eggs. It's high in the amino acid taurine, thought to help heart health and repair the brain, nervous system and skeletal muscles as well as improving the body's utilization of sugar and insulin.

## MOP UP YOUR TOXINS

Foods high in sulphadryl groups are an important part of a healthy diet because these chemical compounds have been shown to mop up poisons and toxins, including metals like aluminium. Onions, garlic, chives, red pepper and egg yolks are all great sources.

## CUT UP A CABBAGE

In order to protect yourself against cancers, it's important to increase your intake of plant phytochemicals, which contain tumour-busting enzymes. They are present in all fruit and vegetables, but cabbage, broccoli, cauliflower, Brussels sprouts and tomatoes contain the highest quantities.

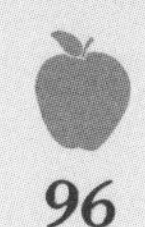



## MAKE AN ALPHA BET

Alpha carotene has been reported in some studies to be ten times more effective against cancer than the better-known beta carotene. Natural sources include carrots, squash, pumpkin, peaches, dried apricots and Swiss chard, which contain good amounts of both types of carotene.

## ADAPT FOR HEALTH

To ensure you're as healthy as you can be, make sure your diet contains adequate levels of natural medicinal adaptogens such as garlic, echinacea, ginseng, liquorice, ginger, schisandra root and ginkgo biloba, which offer a health makeover in the way they adapt their beneficial qualities to individual needs.

## BETTER CHOOSE BETA

Beta carotene is an essential substance in the body – it works with vitamin E against cancer, and with other vitamins against ageing and other damage, boosts immunity and promotes eye health. It's found in many foods but the best sources are broccoli, kale, cabbage, carrots, pumpkin, spinach, squash, sweet potatoes and apricots.

## WHAT A HEADACHE

If you suffer from headaches a lot or your eyes feel sore and tired, make sure you're getting enough riboflavin, especially if you're taking hormone replacement drugs, which can deplete natural levels. Also known as vitamin B2, sources are milk, liver, yeast, cheese, fish, eggs and leafy greens, but alcohol reduces absorption.

## GRAPE NEWS

If you want the benefits of red wine without the alcohol, drink a glass of red grape juice, which is also high in the antioxidant resveratrol and doesn't have the obvious negative effects of alcohol.

## PEPPER YOUR DISHES

Why not use a sprinkling of cayenne pepper to help season your sauces? Derived from the plant Capsicum annum, it has been reported to improve circulation and to lower cholesterol. As it's a mild stimulant, it can also be added to hot water with lemon juice as an alternative to coffee.

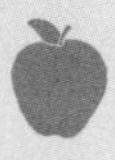



## THE RED LIGHT TO WINE

If you want to drink alcohol with your evening meal, choose red wine instead of white because it contains higher levels of the antioxidant resveratrol, which can offer protection against coronary heart disease. Try to stick to one unit a day for women and two for men.

## THE RIGHT RATIOS

Omega-6 is added to foods during processing and is the main component of most low-quality oils. As a result, the average dietary omega-6 to omega-3 ratio is about 20:1, whereas it should be about 4:1. Getting this ratio right is an important step in preventing cancer through diet.

## BOOST CONCENTRATION

If you want to give yourself a pre-exam boost or sharpen your brain before an important meeting or presentation, get yourself a steak-and-egg sandwich which contains high levels of concentration-boosting choline. It can also assist in learning and help fight infection. Other foods high in this substance are beef liver, peanut butter and wheatgerm, or take a 2000 mg supplement 20 minutes before you need to perform.

## THE SOURCE OF THE Q

If you suffer from high blood pressure, and particularly if you are taking cholesterol-lowering drugs which can deplete the body's natural stores, make sure your diet is high enough in Co-enzyme Q10 (CoQ10). Studies suggest it can help lower blood pressure as well as protect against heart disease, breast cancer and gum disease. Good sources include organic meat and eggs, rice bran, wheatgerm, peanuts, spinach, broccoli, mackerel and sardines. Try to include it in your diet every other day.

## PICK THE PITH

Don't be too careful about peeling off the pith of your citrus fruits. Although the white flesh can taste bitter, leaving a bit attached to your citrus segments is a good idea because it contains high levels of bioflavonoids like rutin, which enhance vitamin C absorption and act as antioxidants. Bioflavonoids are also found in apples, blackberries and apricots.

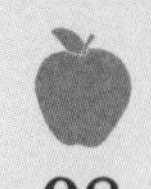



### GEN UP ON GINSENG

Many people like to take a ginseng supplement, or drink ginseng tea, which has been reported to increase mental and physical performance. Vitamin C may hinder absorption, however, so don't take the tea with lemon juice and try to leave two hours between ingesting the two substances. Ginseng should be avoided by those with heart problems as it can interfere with the effectiveness of certain prescribed drugs.

### GET YOUR QUINOA QUOTA

If you want to add a tasty source of low-fat protein to your diet, try quinoa, dubbed by some as a supergrain (although it's not a grass, and therefore not a true grain). It's high in fibre and other nutrients and has an extremely high protein content of 12–15%, making it especially useful for vegetarians. Quinoa has a mild, nutty flavour and must be soaked for a few hours before use to remove potentially toxic seed coatings. Use it in place of rice in cooked dishes or in salads or stuffing.

### THE PERFECT PARTNERSHIP

The mineral selenium and plant-based chemical sulforaphane have been found to be 13 times more effective at fighting cancer when eaten together than apart. To reap the benefits of this partnership, combine selenium-rich nuts, poultry, fish and eggs with sulphoraphane-high broccoli, sprouts, cabbage, watercress and rocket.

## minerals & vitamins

### A STRAIGHT-A STUDENT

Excess vitamin A intake increases the risk of bone fractures and can cause poisoning of some internal organs, like the liver. For optimal bone mineral density vitamin A (retinol) intake should not exceed 2000 to 2800 IU per day. A good idea is to take less vitamin A and more carotenes (found in fruit and veg), which are precursors to vitamin A but have no negative effects if you take more than you need.

## CUT BACK ON THE FIZZ

The body doesn't just need calcium to build strong teeth, skin, hair and bones – it also requires phosphorous. Keep the two minerals in balance for effectiveness (best sources are meat, dairy, fish, nuts and eggs). The recommended phosphorous dose is 1000 mg a day but too much is thought to prevent calcium being used properly. Fizzy drinks are high in phosphorous and don't contain calcium, so it's best avoid them if you want healthy bones.

## BECOME AN OYSTER EATER

Chromium is a trace element that the body requires for sugar metabolism and to control blood-sugar levels. It also lowers LDL cholesterol, triglycerides and body fats. It is found in high levels in oysters, potatoes, brewer's yeast and liver, and the RDA is at least 200 mcg a day.

## MEAT MATTERS

The best way to increase your intake of iron – particularly important in young women and those who have heavy periods – is to eat red meat. This is because the type of iron bound to muscle fibres in red meat is the most easily absorbed form.

## BALANCE YOUR CALCIUM

Magnesium is used by the body in partnership with calcium to help lower cholesterol and build strong bones. In most calcium-containing foods, magnesium is present in the correct ratio (1:3), but if you're taking a calcium supplement take magnesium as well – roughly 500 mcg a day to balance 1500 mcg calcium.

## GO SILLY FOR SILICON

The silicon content of the aorta, thymus and skin tends to decline with age so it's important to make sure you get enough of this mineral as you grow older. It will help prevent skin sagging and keep your hair, nails and bones healthy. Find it in grains such as oats, barley and rice.

## PICK PICOLINATE

Zinc is essential for all-over health, including giving important protection against cancer, Alzheimer's disease and diabetes, but it is estimated that 90% of people's diets may not contain enough. Zinc picolinate is the most easily absorbed form, found in meat and shellfish. But caffeine, bran and dairy products can reduce absorption, so try to avoid eating them with your zinc sources.

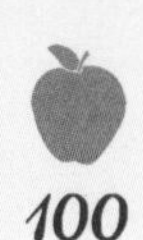



## BOOST VITAMINS WITH TEA

People who drink lots of coffee have lower levels of vitamin C and B vitamins and higher levels of homocysteine, a blood chemical linked to heart disease, than those who drink tea, which is thought to have some beneficial effects on the heart.

## C THINGS CLEARLY

Humans are one of the few animals on earth unable to make their own vitamin C. Make sure your supply is topped up with a daily supplement for optimal nutrition, or opt for a diet rich in fruit and vegetables to boost your levels.

## BUILDING BONES

Calcium, which is essential for building healthy bones, teeth and muscles, is best sourced from dairy products. Research suggests that dietary fat can reduce the amount of calcium absorbed by the body, so choosing low-fat or skimmed milk will help boost calcium as well as reduce cholesterol levels.

## SEE YOURSELF RIGHT

Foods containing vitamin A, like melons, mangoes and watermelon, can help give your eyesight a boost as the vitamin is important for optimum vision. Try to include these in your diet every day.

## MISS OUT THE MARGE

Some studies have shown that people who eat margarine have a slightly increased risk of cancer compared to those who don't – perhaps because of the saturated fats it contains. A high intake of selenium and vitamins E and C, however, found in natural polyunsaturated oils such as canola, soy, safflower and flaxseed, is thought to offset this risk.

## GET A BIT OF BETA

Betacarotene, which is found in dark green, yellow and orange vegetables such as squash, sweet potato, broccoli and greens, is converted in the body to vitamin A, which is vital for growth – so it's especially important for young people under 18.

## SUMMER DANDY

Don't forget the humble dandelion when you're making up a healthy summer salad. High in many vitamins and minerals including the B-vitamin complex, it's a healthy and tasty way to make summer dishes a bit different.

## BRAIN BOOSTER

Omega-3 fatty acids – found in fish, nuts, and flax and hempseed oils – are essential for maintaining good function in a range of body systems, including the brain. Nutritionists often recommend a supplement to keep levels up. A higher dose may be recommended for a few months to build up levels. No RDA has been established so check the manufacturer's recommendations.

## BE GOOD TO YOURSELF

If your skin's feeling a little dry and jaded, give it an injection of vitamin E, which is an antioxidant vitamin essential for healthy skin, hair, nails and the immune system. Alcohol and lack of sleep deplete body levels, so if you've been out partying, try taking a supplement before bed.

## DRINK IT FRESH

The vitamin-C content of fruit juices halves after a few days in the fridge, so if you're drinking juices at home, it's best to drink them as freshly squeezed as possible to make the most of the nutrients.

## START WITH AN A

Adults should avoid taking more than 3000 mcg (μg) per day of vitamin A. Found in livers and food derived from them, such as pâté and fish liver oils, too much can cause health problems and you should be able to get all you need from your diet. Pregnant women should be extra careful.

## BE A HEALTH NUT

Selenium is essential for preventing free radical damage in the body, and is available in a range of foods from grains to meat. It's just been discovered that the body uses selenium best when it's in a selenoprotein form, which is found in nuts (especially Brazil nuts).

## THE WHOLE STORY

When you drink orange juice, you get the vitamin C but not the beneficial fibre and phytonutrients that come from the pulp. Even if you buy orange juice with pulp, you're still not getting any of the fibrous white membrane, which is where many of the phytonutrients hide, so eat the pith too!

## QUIT THE WEED

If you smoke, you probably won't be getting enough essential nutrients from your diet because tobacco decreases the absorption of many vitamins and minerals, including vitamin C, folate, magnesium and calcium. The best health advice is to give up, but if you can't it's worth taking a dietary supplement.

## CUT BACK ON THE BOOZE

Drinking excessive amounts of alcohol can impair the body's ability to absorb vitamin B1, iron, zinc, magnesium and folate. Many people are surprised that excessive drinking is defined as more than two drinks a day for men under 65 and more than one drink a day for men over 65 and women. Aim for at least two alcohol-free days a week.

## SPICE IT UP

It might sound old fashioned, but a pestle and mortar is actually thought to be a healthier way to prepare spices than a food processor. This is because crushing retains more nutrients than whizzing.

## BERRY GOOD FOR YOU

Although tomatoes are the best dietary source of lycopene, there is an alternative if you don't like them – strawberries. These summer berries are the only other fruit or vegetable to protect against prostate cancer, and unlike tomatoes they are as potent raw as they are cooked.

## COOK CONVENTIONAL

Think twice before you microwave your beef, pork, eggs, milk and cheese as you may well be reducing their health benefits. Microwave cooking (as well as alcohol, oral contraceptives and sleeping pills) is thought to destroy vitamin B12, which is essential for carbohydrate and fat metabolism.

## SWIM OUT TO C

We all know the health benefits of vitamin C, labelled by some as the wonder vitamin for its far-reaching, positive effects on the body. People who smoke, drink alcohol or are taking aspirin, oestrogen or oral contraceptives should take more, as these can all limit uptake.

## GO GREEN

Green tea is reported to contain a variety of antioxidants and to offer protection against cancer, heart disease and stroke. Black tea, which is oxidized green tea, is not as effective. If you don't like green, try oolong tea, which is only partially oxidized. But remember, all tea contains caffeine, so unlimited amounts aren't recommended.

## SEEK OUT THE SYNERGY

Certain chemicals in the body work more powerfully when combined. This is thought to be the case for selenium and vitamin E, which have better antioxidant properties when present together. Selenium is destroyed by processing, so choosing unprocessed nuts and fish is essential.

## WHERE'S YOUR BOTTLE

Tap water containing chlorine can soak up vitamin E and prevent its absorption in the body, so if you're taking a supplement or eating a healthy meal and your water is chlorinated, it's best to drink bottled or filtered water instead.

## YOUR HEALTH IS OH-K

Don't forget about vitamin K, which is essential to maintain healthy bones and has been found to be lacking in people with osteoporosis. Antibiotics and the ageing process lower absorption, so in these cases it's even more important to get enough. Find it in green leafy vegetables, egg yolk and safflower oil.

## SEEK OUT THE SUNSHINE

The body manufactures its own vitamin D as a result of being exposed to sunlight. People who work long hours and can't get fresh air every day might find a supplement beneficial, especially as lack of vitamin D is linked to immune deficiency and osteoporosis.

## GET A HEALTHY U

As well as the well-known health-giving vitamins like vitamin C, there are a range of lesser-known substances which also have health benefits. Vitamin U is found in raw cabbage (used in coleslaw and salads) or cabbage juice, and is great for healing skin and membrane problems and ulcers.

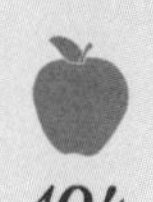



### HAVE A TEA PARTY

The caffeine in coffee is thought to deplete calcium levels, contributing to osteoporosis but the same isn't true for tea, which actually has the opposite effect. Drinking tea can reduce fracture risk by 10 to 20%, probably because of its oestrogen-building isoflavonoid chemicals.

### BE A TART!

Choose tart fruits like plums, blueberries, cranberries and sour cherries, which contain the highest levels of the bio-flavonoid proanthocyanidin (also known as pycnogenol and adoxynol), which is thought to reduce cholesterol, prevent cancer and fight the signs of ageing on skin and internal organs.

## supplements

### A GRASS INJECTION

Superoxide dismutase is a potent anti-inflammatory and one of the most powerful antioxidants found in your body. Although it is present in certain foods, including cabbage, broccoli, wheat and barley grasses, it is difficult to boost levels through diet alone as it is broken down during the digestive process. However, a new type of supplement made from wheat grass has been shown to improve levels.

### SWALLOW IT EARLY

If you take a daily vitamin supplement, take it with breakfast rather than later in the day, as studies have shown it to be better absorbed earlier in the day. And you should always take supplements with water, which helps absorption.

### BONE UP ON BORON

Studies have shown immunity benefits and the prevention of autoimmune reactions (like eczema) in people who take 3 to 6 mg of boron per day. Boron also assists in calcium absorption, which maintains healthy bones, helps prevent osteoporosis and increases the synthesis of vitamin D.

## READ THE LABELS

Vitamin C (ascorbic acid) is often made from corn, and vitamin E is usually made from soy. Both of these are heavily genetically modified crops, particularly in the USA, and vitamins A, B2, B6, and B12 may be derived from GM crops as well. Check your supplement and vitamin labels.

## REMEMBER THE CARRIERS

Even if vitamins and mineral supplements aren't derived from GM sources, some of them – such as vitamins D and K – may have "carriers" derived from GM corn, such as starch, glucose, and maltodextrin. In addition to finding these vitamins in supplements, they are sometimes used to fortify foods.

## SWIM LIKE A SHARK

There aren't many stranger supplements than shark cartilage, but some people swear by it as an anti-cancer pill, inhibiting new blood vessel growth and stopping tumour spread. It has also been reported to reduce some arthritis pain, but it can be high in mercury so make sure your supplement is purified.

## KEEP AN EYE ON THE IODINE

If you eat a healthy diet and are moderately active but don't seem to be able to shift excess weight, it's worth getting your thyroid checked – people who lack iodine or other nutrients could have an underactive gland, which leads to a slower metabolism. Taking 150 mcg of iodine a day could help.

## PROTECT THE PROSTATE

Saw palmetto is a great supplement for men as it can help reduce some prostate problems, and for women because it has been linked with improvements in urinary tract infections. It is available as single supplements which can be taken as needed.

## SUPPLEMENT YOUR TEENS

One of the most important times to give your child a vitamin supplement is during the teenage years when diets often become unhealthier. Choose one with vitamin A, riboflavin (vitamin B2), zinc, potassium, magnesium, calcium and iron, all of which have been shown to be lacking in teenagers' diets.

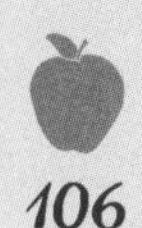


## FOLIC ACID BLOOM

If you're pregnant or thinking about getting pregnant, make sure you take a daily supplement of folic acid (vitamin B9), which has been shown to help prevent neural tube defects in babies' brains. At least 400 mcg a day is recommended.

## COLOURFUL CONNECTIONS

Eating lots of red and yellow onions, broccoli and squash is a good idea as it's important to get around 500 mg a day of quercetin, a bioflavonoid that can inhibit bowel cancer and protect against heart disease, cataracts and allergies. It may also have anti-inflammatory qualities.

## GET PRO-HEALTH

Honey isn't the only bee product that's useful for keeping you healthy – propolis, a kind of resin produced by bees to protect honey stores, has anti-cancer, anti-oxidant effects as well as boosting immunity. Aim for at least 500 mg a day.

## SUP SOME SEA HEALTH

If you just can't face the prospect of eating seaweed or plants harvested from the world's oceans, you can cheat the system by taking a supplement of phycotene. A natural extraction from spirulina algae, studies have shown it to support healthy eyes, to have anti-cancer properties and to protect the skin from sun damage.

## BLOOD-THINNER WARNING

Not everyone benefits from taking omega-3 fish oil supplements – if you're taking blood thinners you should consult your doctor before taking these oils as they can also have a blood-thinning effect. In such cases it's probably best to get your dose from the whole fish instead.

# herbs & infusions

## TUMMY TEA

If you are suffering digestive problems or diarrhoea, try blackberry tea. As well as a fruit tea, you can buy black tea infused with blackberries. The tea is rich in iron as well as easing stomach aches and diarrhoea and helping to control fevers.

## DETOX WITH LEMON

Lemon juice is a great flavour enhancer and mixed with hot water is a really healthy (and detoxifying) alternative to heavily caffeinated hot drinks. Get twice as much juice out of your lemons by heating in the oven or hot water, or by rolling until slightly soft, before squeezing.

## BREW YOUR OWN

Make yourself a herbal infusion from anise seed (Pimpinella anisum), a member of the parsley family that has a pleasant, liquorice-like flavour and is thought to improve digestion, freshen breath, calm flatulence and nausea, and help to settle coughs.

## TRY ALFALFA TEA FOR C

If you don't like citrus fruit but want to boost your vitamin-C intake, try alfalfa leaf (Medicago sativa), which is an excellent source of vitamin C a well as chlorophyll and other minerals when made into a refreshing tea or infusion.

## PUT YOUR PEDAL TO THE NETTLE

Nettles often get a bad press because of their itchy stings, but cooking denatures the sting. Brewed up to make a tea or added to soups and stews, they are extremely rich in nutrients, including iron and beta-carotene, and are thought to improve kidney and adrenal function and help cure allergies.

## RASPBERRY REPRODUCTION

Many pregnant women and those who are menstruating drink raspberry leaf tea, which is rich in nutrients, especially calcium, magnesium and iron, and is thought to help the regeneration of the reproductive system. But men can also benefit from its nutritious qualities, and often enjoy the tea-like flavour.

## MAKE A MINT

A great post-dinner choice instead of caffeine-rich coffee is a peppermint herbal infusion. Peppermint reduces the more extreme movements of the digestive system, helping to relieve feelings of fullness, nausea and flatulence. It also has antiseptic properties.

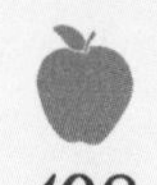



## DRINK YOURSELF COOL

If you want the cooling, calming properties of a peppermint tea but don't like the slightly medicinal flavour, try spearmint instead. The flavour is milder but it still aids digestion, and also headaches, and has mild antiseptic properties. It also tastes great as an iced summer refresher.

## TAME YOUR TANNINS

For the taste of a good strong cuppa but without the caffeine of normal black tea, try drinking Rooibos, or red bush, a traditional South African plant infusion that tastes much like black tea but contains no caffeine and is low in tannins and high in vitamin C, minerals and antioxidants.

## MAKE A NEW MATE

A great alternative to caffeinated hot drinks is tea made from yerba mate, a member of the holly family, which is rich in vitamins C and B, calcium and iron, It also contains mateine, which is similar to caffeine but less likely to interfere with sleep, cause anxiety or be addictive.

## WATER YOUR OATS

A great alternative to dairy products for calcium intake is water infused with oat straw (*Avena sativa*), the young stem of the oat plant. The infusion has a pleasant, sweet flavour, is high in calcium and is thought to relieve depression, insomnia, and stress. Try making up a batch and drinking it straight or using in cooking.

## GET A FEEL FOR FENNEL

Try adding fennel to roasted vegetable dishes or salads – a member of the parsley family, fennel helps stabilize blood-sugar levels, thus curbing appetite. It also works to relax the muscles of the digestive system, reducing indigestion and wind pains.

## INFUSE WITH FLOWERS

Instead of fizzy drinks and sugar-filled fruit squashes, try an infusion of elderflowers. These tiny flowers have a delicate taste, can be drunk hot or cold and have the added benefit of helping control body temperature – making them great as winter warmers or summer coolers.

## COLD CURE

Many people recommend not drinking milk or eating dairy products if you have a cough or cold as it is thought to increase mucus production. A great alternative is tea made with lemon balm (*Melissa officinalis*), which has a calming, anti-anxiety effect as well as anti-viral properties – making it suitable for treating colds and flu in children as well as adults.

## ZING WITH GINGER

A great herbal infusion to choose for an after-lunch energy boost, without caffeine, is ginger root (*Zingiber officinale*), a pungent herb that's not only good for digestion but also relieves nausea, improves circulation, warms the body, and has antiseptic and anti-inflammatory properties.

## SIP A SUMMER COOLER

For a fantastically effective summer cooling drink, try an iced infusion of hibiscus flowers, which have a tart, slightly sour flavour and are rich in vitamin C as well as working to help the body cool itself when served cold.

## CAMOMILE FOR CALM

Next time you're struggling to sleep, try brewing yourself a calming camomile infusion, which has been shown to have a mild sedative effect. Or if you want something with more flavour, catnip has also been shown to aid sleep.

## PICK YOUR OWN

Collecting plant foods, flowers and mushrooms from the wild yourself is a pleasurable way to ensure your food is as fresh as possible. However, many edible foods look similar to those that contain toxins so make sure you take the time to train yourself to identify them correctly, and don't eat anything unless you're absolutely sure it's safe.

## COFFEE CHIC

If you can't live without the taste of coffee but want to cut down your caffeine intake, try an infusion of roasted chicory root instead. It has a delicious, coffee-like flavour without the addition of caffeine and helps to cleanse the liver and colon.

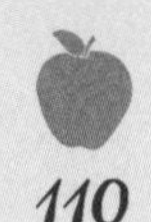



## A WINTER LIFT

A great herbal tea to brew up if you're feeling a little depressed, especially in the darker winter months, is an infusion of St John's Wort. This plant is thought to help depression by stimulating the production of the "happy" brain chemical serotonin. The standard way to make the infusion is to pour a cup of boiling water over the leaves and flowers, leave it to stand for 5 minutes, then strain and drink. See your doctor if you suffer from severe or long-term depression.

## FIGHT OFF INFECTION

Help your body fight infection naturally by drinking tea made with the herb echinacea, eating the edible flowers or taking a supplement. The herb is thought to fight colds and to boost immunity by stimulating the production of lymphocytes, but it has not been proven.

## GOOD PICKINGS

Don't eat flowers from florists, nurseries or garden centres or those picked from the side of roads. If they're not being sold for consumption, the flowers may be high in toxic pesticides and not labelled as is required for food crops. Stick to those properly identified and sold as foods – such as nasturtiums, dandelion and angelica. Always remember to use flowers sparingly in your recipes, as digestive complications can occur for those with sensitivities.

# superfoods

## GARLIC CRUSH

Garlic is great because it reduces the risk of stomach and colon cancer, helps lower blood cholesterol and reduces blood pressure. The ideal amount is 2–3 cloves a day. Crushed garlic has the strongest flavour, then chopped – roast is mildest.

## A SAUCY TOMATO

Tomatoes contain high levels of lycopene and betacarotene and have been shown to reduce the incidence of prostate cancer in men if eaten ten times a week. The best way to get your dose is to eat a mix of cooked and raw to maximize nutrient absorption.

## SPRINKLE SOME SEEDS

Seeds are packed with nutrients and beneficial oils and won't add too many calories to your diet. Sprinkle seeds on cereal salad, or, if you don't like their hard texture, grind a mixture of pumpkin, sunflower, sesame and linseed in a coffee grinder, and use whenever you can.

## DON'T LOSE YOUR TEMPEH

For an alternative to tofu, try tempeh, which is made from fermented soya beans and has a meaty texture with a nutty taste. Tempeh contains all the essential amino acids and phytochemicals such as isoflavones and saponins, which are thought to help fight disease, as well as natural antimicrobial agents.

## SEEDS OF HEALTH

If you can, choose ground flaxseeds over flax seed oil as although the oil contains just as many health-giving omega-3s, the ground seeds contain much more fibre, which is also good for health – giving you a double benefit for the price of one!

## STICK WITH SALMON

Salmon is a great protein source because it contains fewer calories than many other protein sources, and it's rich in omega oils that help the development of the brain, heart, skin and joints. For the greatest health benefits, though, it's best to go for wild or organic versions.

## EAT UP SOME SEA VEG

Sea vegetables such as arame and kelp are virtually fat-free, low calorie and one of the richest sources of minerals in the vegetable kingdom – they contain high amounts of calcium and phosphorous and are extremely high in magnesium, iron, iodine and sodium.

## SIP AN ICED GREEN TEA

Home-made iced tea is a great summertime drink because it has flavour but no sugar and it contains antioxidants. Keep a jug in the fridge so you've got it on hand, or experiment with other herbal or black teas.

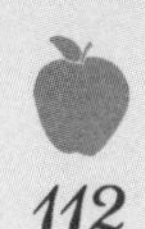



## TOMATOES SAUCED

Tomatoes are high in vitamin C and also betacarotene, which is converted into essential vitamin A in the body. They also have high levels of the antioxidant lycopene, which the body absorbs better when tomatoes are cooked.

## CAST A SPELT

If you find wheat hard to digest and are worried about food intolerance, try replacing it with its ancient cousin, spelt. This tasty grain cooks in the same way as wheat but contains slightly more protein and is usually well tolerated by people with wheat allergies.

## GET A GOLDEN PLATE

Try replacing your usual grain with amaranth, a tiny golden seed first cultivated by the Aztecs which is high in protein and calcium and an excellent source of iron. Amaranth is great as a hot cereal because it retains its crunchiness, or smuggled into baked goods or casseroles to add texture.

## SPREADING GERMS

Sprinkling a couple of tablespoons of wheatgerm on top of cereals, casseroles or yogurts is a good health-giving habit to get into because it boosts the fibre content by nearly two grams but adds a paltry 54 calories. For a nuttier flavour, use toasted wheatgerm instead of plain.

## CLEANSE WITH SEAWEED

One of seaweed's most prominent health benefits is its ability to remove radioactive strontium and other heavy metals from our bodies. Whole brown seaweeds such as kelp contain alginic acid, which binds with toxins in the intestines (rendering them indigestible) and carries them out of the system. They are also sources of fibre.

## CHOOSE NORI FOR TIREDNESS

Nori is a cultivated seaweed used to wrap sushi. It is exceptionally high in vitamin A and protein and a great source of selenium and iodine. It has anti-cancer effects and provides soluble fibre and omega-3 fats, as well as regulating the thyroid gland by balancing iodine levels.

## GET A RYE DEAL

Did you know that barley and rye contain five times more fibre than other wholegrains? This is what makes wholegrain speciality breads such a great choice for your complex carbohydrate quota. Look for bread with these ingredients where you can.

## SHARE A SHIITAKE

Shiitake mushrooms are thought to lower cholesterol, to stimulate the immune system and to help fight cancer. They are high in B vitamins and are low in calories so you can eat as many as you like.

## GET YOUR OATS

Oats are a genuine superfood because they have a low glycaemic index, which means they release sugar in the body slowly and help you to feel full for longer. They are low in cholesterol and high in fibre and protein. The easiest way to include oats in your diet is in breakfast porridge. For extra nutrients, top with dried fruit.

## BE BERRY HEALTHY

Blueberries are a great source of the antioxidant anthocyanin, which improves blood circulation, skin and the immune system and has also been reported to improve balance, coordination and short-term memory.

## BEANS MEANS HEALTH

For a great fill-up food that's good for your heart, releases energy slowly into your system to keep you fuller for longer, and is high in fibre but low in calories, choose beans. A recent study also suggests that eating beans and soy can cut the risk of lung cancer by as much as 46%. Experiment with the many varieties to find the ones you like.

## GOBBLE A HEALTHY FEAST

Turkey is a great source of protein because it's very low in fat. It's also high in B vitamins, which help boost your body's health, and in the amino acid tryptophan, which aids restful sleep – making it a great late-night snack.

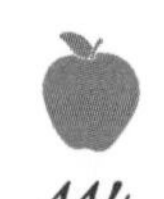



## BUY BROCCOLI

Broccoli is one of the richest sources of antioxidants and vitamin C known, and the fresher the better. If you can't get it really fresh, choose frozen as it keeps its goodness for longer.

## BE A WATER BABY

Watercress is being hailed as the new superfood because the chemical compounds it contains have been shown to help stop cancers developing by slowing down the degradation of cells. Use it in salads, sandwiches, soups and pasta.

## TEA-OFF WITH CONFIDENCE

Next time you settle down with a nice cup of tea, relax in the knowledge that you're not only having a break but giving your body an antioxidant boost as well. Drinking it without milk is best, or with a slice of lemon to add extra flavour.

## GO NUTS FOR GOOD FATS

Walnuts have lots of fibre and also contain high levels of polyunsaturated fats so although they are high in calories, the calories come from good fats which help balance cholesterol.

## DO LIKE POPEYE

Eat spinach – it's rich in vitamin C, calcium and beta carotene, boosts folic acid and helps keep blood and bones healthy. Steam lightly and add to sauces or wash and use instead of lettuce in salads.

## SWALLOW SOME SOY

If you're worried about cholesterol, add some soy to your diet. It's been shown in some tests to boost omega-3 fatty acids and strengthen the immune system as well as

## A YOGURT BOOST

Live yogurts contain high levels of bone-boosting calcium and also probiotics, which improve balance in the digestive system. Low fat, natural yogurt is best.

## PLUMP FOR PUMPKIN

Pumpkin has really high levels of potassium that can help control blood pressure problems. It's also high in vitamin C and beta carotene, which both help keep the immune system strong.

# health boosters

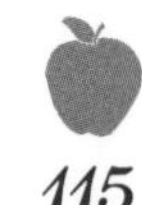



### WARM IT UP

Your digestive system works best when food is at room temperature, so get in the habit of removing chilled food from the fridge a little while before you eat in order to let it warm up slightly. Food also tastes better if it's less chilled, so there's no excuse!

### EAT LESS MORE OFTEN

Eating consistently throughout the day provides your brain and body with a constant source of fuel. This 3–4 hour eating strategy can dramatically prevent dips in your blood-sugar levels, something which is especially important in preventing premenstrual stress.

### WATER IT DOWN

Drink water with your meals as well as throughout the day. As well as helping your body to absorb the nutrients from food, it also causes the fibre within food to swell, activating stretch receptors in the stomach lining to signal when you've eaten enough.

### CHEW GUM

Chewing stimulates signals in the learning centre of the brain, which could help to preserve memory. Chewing gum also may, in a small way, help to keep you slim as it boosts the metabolic rate by about 20%. Choose sugar-free versions to prevent tooth decay and damage.

### FEAST ON FLOWERS

Flowers are a great way to add colour to food as well as boosting health. For example, add the delicate blue flowers of borage to summer drinks to help boost brain function and immunity.

### DON'T BE ACIDIC

Some scientist believe that for optimal health the body should be slightly more alkaline than acidic. For this, 70 to 80% of the food you eat should be alkaline-forming foods such as leafy greens, most fruits, soy products and seeds, and only 20 to 30% should be derived from acid-forming foods like grains, red meat and dairy products.

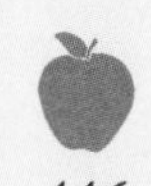



## GO LIVE

For the best bacterial health kick, make sure the yogurt you buy contains live, active cultures and lists the Latin names of these beneficial bacteria. Many of the health-promoting properties of yogurt come from these bacteria.

## MAKE A NATURAL CHOICE

Nutrition science research is finding increasingly that it is not one particular substance or another that gives foods their disease-fighting power, but the interaction of all the food's vitamins, antioxidants and other chemicals. To get the most benefit, try to eat food items in their natural form whenever possible.

## FISH FOR VARIETY

When we're told to eat oily fish, salmon and mackerel immediately spring to mind, but don't forget there are plenty of other fish containing health-giving omega-3 oils in varying amounts. If you're bored with the usual suspects, try trout, sardine, tuna, pilchard, eels and herring.

## REDUCE THE PROCESS

In general, the healthier choice is to eat foods as near to their natural state as possible. Choose organic and eat food raw, or lightly cooked. The fewer processes your food has been through, the better and generally tastier it is.

## ALL RIGHT PETAL

A great way to add colour to salads is to sprinkle over some fresh nasturtium petals, which are high in vitamin C, or the seeds, which are high in iron and phosphorous. Both leaves and seeds – which are used in place of capers – are thought to help chest complaints and aid digestion.

## CHOOSE CARBS FOR ENDURANCE

The body extracts energy more easily from carbohydrates, which it converts in to sugar, than from protein or fat, so if you have a really physical job or have an active day planned, it's best to eat a diet high in carbohydrates. Get them from vegetables, grains and legumes (peas and beans).

# healthy habits

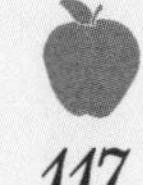



## QUIT PROCESSED FOODS

A diet heavy in processed foods can lead to numerous problems. As well as the better-known obesity, cancer and heart disease, it causes rotten teeth, bad skin, bad breath, constipation, digestive problems, headaches, poor concentration, depression, tiredness and anaemia. Need any more impetus to give them up?

## GO BACK TO THE ORIGINAL SOURCE

For each pre-packaged item of food you buy and serve, try to make it a rule to add at least one food from its original source. For instance, if you buy coleslaw from the supermarket, add your own fresh carrot, tomato or spring onions for a healthy boost. Or if you buy a ready-prepared pasta, serve it with a fresh spinach salad.

## GET DRESSED

To avoid harmful processed fats, get in the habit of mixing your own healthy salad dressings. Try a mix of extra virgin olive or flaxseed oil, white wine or balsamic vinegar, and a little black pepper or mustard. Yogurt is a tasty alternative for creamy dressings.

## VISIT THE GREAT PLAINS

If you have a daily chocolate addiction, choose dark chocolate as it contains less fat than milk chocolate and is higher in cocoa solids, which makes it richer and means you're likely to eat less. However, it does have double the caffeine of milk chocolate, at up to 50 mg a bar.

## DIGESTION BEGINS IN THE MOUTH

Chew your food thoroughly – chewing, which breaks down the food into small chunks and mixes it with saliva, actually kick-starts the digestive process. In this way essential nutrients are extracted from the food and digestion is more effective.

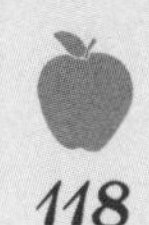


### CAN THE TUNA

In order to limit your mercury intake, which has been linked to brain damage in unborn babies and is thought to be toxic to adults, don't eat more than two tuna steaks or four medium-sized cans of tuna a week. Tuna, marlin and swordfish have been found to be high in mercury deposits and should be avoided by those who are intending to become pregnant.

### BE A GRAZER

If you're looking for long-term energy, for shift work or prolonged exercise, for example, the best way to eat is to graze on small meals or snacks. This will keep blood-sugar levels up without having to divert too much energy to the gut for digestion.

## reducing fat

### SWAP HALF YOUR BUTTER

Instead of cooking with butter, choose oils that are low in saturated fat like sunflower and olive oils, which will help keep your cholesterol levels down at healthy levels and are lower in calories, too. If you want the taste of butter, try swapping half and see if you notice the difference.

### IT'LL BE ALL WHITE

White fish is an excellent healthy food and although it isn't high in omega-3 oils, it is still a fantastic way to fill up on protein and essential minerals and amino acids without adding fat. Try halibut, skate, sea bass and plaice as well as the usual cod and haddock.

### BET ON THE BUTTER

Don't automatically choose margarine instead of butter if you want to reduce calories – margarine doesn't actually have fewer calories than butter, unless it is specifically labelled as such. It simply has less saturated fat.

### REPLACE WITH RICE

Reduce fat, increase fibre and save money by replacing half of the meat or poultry in a casserole recipe with brown rice, bulgur or cooked and pureéd dried beans or lentils.

## DON'T BE LILY LIVERED

Check the source of your omega-3 oils carefully. If possible, try to avoid those made from fish livers in favour of those extracted from the flesh of deep water fish. Pharmaceutical grade is the purest as it undergoes a variety of purification processes, so choose that for children or if you're pregnant.

## HALF YOUR FAT INTAKE

All the different fats in foods can be confusing, but make your diet is simple and give yourself a head start in the health stakes by aiming to make half of your fat intake polyunsaturated, and at least half of this oil containing omega-3s.

## LIMIT THE CHEESEBOARD

High meat and dairy product diets generate excess methionine in the body, which is converted into the blood factor homocysteine that has been shown to damage arteries and cause heart disease. Reduce your intake of these foods or increase your intake of vitamins B6, B12 and folic acid, which help restore the balance.

## OIL YOUR VEGETABLES

Instead of adding cholesterol-building butter to your steamed vegetables, make them even healthier by using a low-fat dressing or a dash of olive or flaxseed oil.

## AVOID HYDROGENATES

Most UK supermarkets are starting to remove hydrogenated oils from some own-label ranges, but there's still a long way to go. These killer oils are even more harmful to health than saturated fats. Avoid them whenever you can.

## CREAM OFF THE CREAM

Instead of using full (heavy) cream, which is high on calories and saturated fat, use evaporated skimmed milk instead, or low-fat yogurt. Or try mixing the two together for a slightly creamier texture.

## GET YOUR EGGS WHITE

It is the yellow yolk of the egg which contains the most calories, which explains the Hollywood trend for egg-white omelettes. In recipes containing lots of egg, try substituting two egg whites for one whole egg, or three whites for two whole eggs to cut calories.

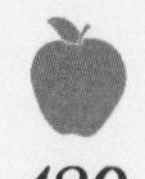



### CHOOSE OILS CAREFULLY

While most vegetable oils contain unsaturated fats and are therefore healthy, some – such as the coconut, palm and palm kernel oils found in many processed foods – contain high levels of saturated fats. Limit them in your diet, again, by avoiding processed foods.

### TRANS-FORM YOUR EATING

Saturated fats are bad in excess but our bodies do need some for optimal health. Trans fatty acids (commonly called trans fats), however, are the real villains of the food world. Formed when vegetable oils harden and seen on labels as hydrogenated oils, they raise cholesterol and have been linked to heart disease.

### ADD AN APPLE

Reduce the fat content of recipes by substituting half of the vegetable oil with apple sauce. You're unlikely to taste the difference and you'll not only be cutting the fat by half, but adding a dose of vitamins and antioxidants as well.

### SWAP MEAT FOR FISH

If you pop to the sandwich bar at lunch-time, choose something healthy like smoked salmon instead of more fattening sausage, salami, ham or beef and you'll get a helping of omega-3 oils into the bargain.

## reducing sugar

### TASTE THE HONEY

Honey and syrup don't raise your blood-sugar level faster than fruits, vegetables or foods containing complex carbohydrates as long as they are eaten with a meal, where they are absorbed as part of the whole mix.

### TOP UP WITH FLOUR

Try decreasing the sugar in your recipes by a quarter, and substituting with flour to make up the volume. Most recipes won't taste any different and they'll be lower in calories. But don't reduce sugar in recipes containing yeast as it plays a part in helping the dough to rise.

## SWEET ENOUGH

Look for unsweetened pure juices. Avoid products that are labelled as "juice drink", which may contain as little as 5% juice and be sweetened with even more sugar than is found in a can of cola. Even pure unsweetened fruit juices contain natural fruit sugars, which can cause tooth decay, but they are much healthier.

## CUT OUT THE FIZZ

Unbelievably, despite all the media publicity about fizzy drinks being linked to skin problems, bad teeth, obesity and poor concentration due to their high sugar and additives content, they still account for 20% of the drinks bought for home consumption. Do your family a favour and make the switch to healthy alternatives now.

## WHITE LIES

For a low-sugar option that's lower in calories replace white wine in recipes with apple or carrot juice, vegetable or chicken stock, with a little white wine vinegar or a dash of white grape juice.

## BE A SPORT

Don't be fooled by sport drinks, which are often marketed to appear as if they are a healthy choice but in actual fact usually contain as much sugar as other fizzy drinks. Isotonic drinks can be useful for refuelling after exercise, but water is a better choice throughout the day.

## COUNT YOUR CARBS

If you're diabetic or are being careful to regulate your blood-sugar levels, remember it's total carbohydrate intake that counts rather than sugar. If you want a dessert, for instance, drop some of the carbohydrates from your main course to keep the balance.

## SWEET-TOOTH ALTERNATIVE

If you simply can't cope with cutting out the sugar, artificial sweeteners like acesulfame potassium, aspartame, saccharin and sucralose offer the sweetness of sugar without the calories. They are especially handy as a sugar replacement in coffee and tea, on cereal or in baked goods – but it's healthier to go without.

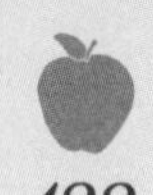



## CLOCK THE CALORIES

Artificial sweeteners don't necessarily offer a free pass for eating sweets, biscuits and cakes. Products made with artificial sweeteners still contain calories and carbohydrates that can affect your blood-sugar level and some may even contain sugar as well. Check the label.

## TAKE CARE WITH SWEETENERS

Although sugar alcohols like isomalt, maltitol, mannitol, sorbitol and xylitol – which are often used to flavour chewing gum and puddings – are lower in calories than sugar, foods containing sugar alcohols still have calories. And take care because for some people, as little as 50 g of these substances can cause diarrhoea, gas and bloating.

## DITCH THE WHITE BREAD

Swap white bread or pasta for wholegrain versions. Not only are they higher in fibre, they have a more beneficial effect on your blood-sugar level, releasing their energy slowly to help you feel fuller for longer.

## DON'T BE FOOLED WITH BROWN

Most people believe brown sugar is a healthier option than white sugar but, in reality, the majority of brown sugar is simply refined white sugar with molasses added to change its colour. For healthier options, demerara and muscovado are good choices. Both are unrefined and suitable to add to hot drinks or for cooking, and have reasonably good shelf lives.

## DILUTE YOUR JUICE

Instead of fruit squashes or cordials, which can often be loaded with sugar, dilute a little pure fruit juice with water instead. Fruit juice does contain sugar, but because it is natural fructose, the body doesn't suffer the same blood glucose peaks.

## LOWER YOUR SUGAR

To regulate blood-sugar levels the best vegetables to choose are fibrous varieties like broccoli, cauliflower, celery, cucumbers, tomatoes, spinach, peppers and courgettes (zucchini) and fruits such as raspberries, melon, papaya and cherries.

### SPREAD AWAY SUGAR

Instead of jam, which can be packed with sugar, try no-sugar jam or make your own very healthy apple spread. Cook sliced sweet eating apples and a dash of cinnamon in a little water (it will keep for two months in an airtight container).

### A SOUR TASTE

Along with refined sugar and white potatoes, overprocessed white bread is one of the worst foods for blood-sugar control. If you want white bread without the sugar rush, choose sourdough bread. It contains lactic acid, which slows down digestion and gives sourdough its tangy flavour.

## reducing salt

### GO LOW-SO FOR HEALTH

If you like the taste of salt but don't want to damage your health by taking in too much sodium, try the low-sodium varieties – it's the sodium in salt that's thought to contribute to hypertension.

### MAKE YOUR TABLE HEALTHY

High salt levels can affect blood pressure and heart health. Instead of using regular table salt in cooking, why not choose a low-sodium table salt, and leave the real salt for garnishing only? That way, you'll reduce the sodium in your diet to an absolute minimum.

### CHANGE SALT HABIT

More than one teaspoon of salt a day has been shown to raise blood pressure, but for many people adding salt is a habit rather than a preference. Don't put salt on your food as a matter of course, and make sure you taste it before you sprinkle to see if the food really needs it.

### BE A ROCK

Rather than buying standard table salt to add taste to dishes and on the table, choose rock salt instead. It has a distinctive salty flavour, which means you will use less of it, and gives all the taste with less of the damaging sodium. Plus, it contains 83 minerals and nutrients.

### SWITCH TO PEPPER

Pepper is a healthier alternative to salt as a flavouring – it is said to aid digestion by stimulating the tastebuds and to reduce the formation of intestinal gas. It has antioxidant and antibacterial properties, too. Pepper loses its flavour quickly, which is why freshly ground is recommended.

### SALT AS YOU SERVE

Instead of adding salt when cooking, allow people to season their own plates when you serve the food. This will help cut down on the amount of salt in home-cooked food.

### USE HERBS WISELY

Instead of seasoning with flavoured salt such as garlic, celery or onion salt, try using herb-only seasonings to reduce your sodium intake. Try garlic powder, finely chopped garlic or onion or celery seeds.

### DON'T SALT YOUR SOUPS

Sodium from salt can be a contributor to high blood pressure, so make sure you choose low-sodium varieties when you can, particularly in "hidden" salt products like soups, stock cubes and sauces.

### SWEET AND HOT

If you eat a lot of stir-fried food, try substituting soy sauce, which is very high in salt, with sweet and sour sauce or hot mustard. Do this every other meal to help keep your sodium intake down.

### CHOOSE UNSALTED NUTS

Nuts are a healthy, nutritious food but remember to choose unsalted varieties as salted versions can contain high levels of salt. Beware too of those coated with soy sauce or other salty products.

## alcohol advice

### RED REPLACEMENT

If you want the taste of red wine in your cooking but don't want to use alcohol, opt for grape juice, beef stock or water mixed with balsamic vinegar instead.

### BEER WITH YOUR MEAL

Instead of wine with your meal, how about a glass of beer? Some studies have shown that drinking a small amount of beer with dinner helps reduce homocysteine, a blood factor that is thought to cause heart disease, by boosting the body's levels of vitamin B6 by 30%.

### TAKE CARE OF YOUR HEART

Many studies suggest light to moderate drinking discourages heart disease, but this may not be true for men who already have it. Light drinking (less than half of the recommended maximum on an ongoing basis) was shown to cut the odds of death in men who did not have heart disease, but didn't show benefits in those who did.

### DON'T LOSE THE BUBBLES

Instead of champagne in dessert recipes, try sparkling grape juice instead, which has no alcohol and fewer calories than its more expensive relative. Or, for a stronger taste, ginger ale works well.

### REDUCE THE SPIRIT

Next time a recipe calls for brandy, think about ways to reduce the alcohol in your food by using apple, white grape, peach or pear juice instead, or mixing half and half. You'll get the full, fruity taste without as many calories.

### SAY BYE-BYE TO BEER

Instead of using beer to make a gravy for casseroles and stews, use beef or chicken stock. Stock will add flavour without boosting the calories as much as beer. For a kick, add a dash of Worcestershire sauce.

## boosting fertility

### PEAS IN THE BOD

For a nutrition boost which will aid fertility, add fresh or frozen cooked peas to your tuna salad and use spinach or watercress instead of lettuce as a base. As well as being low fat and high in protein, they contain the B vitamin folate, which is essential for reproductive health.

## SPERM HEALTH

Men hoping to boost their fertility should eat more fruit and vegetables as a diet low in these fresh products has been linked to sluggish sperm. Any fruit or vegetable will help sperm health, and it's important to have five portions a day.

## MORE THAN AN APHRODISIAC

There's some scientific proof that eating oysters can boost fertility because they are packed full of zinc, which plays a role in sperm production in men and ovulation and fertility in women. Aim for no more than the RDA of 9 mg a day as excessive amounts may actually reduce your fertility.

## STEER CLEAR OF SOYA

A few studies suggest that women who are trying to conceive should avoid soya products because they contain a component that is similar to the female hormone oestrogen, which can affect the length of the menstrual cycle. Soya also lowers the levels of two hormones necessary for ovulation.

## FIGHT THE PHYTATE

To maximize their fertility, men are advised to avoid soy because it contains phytate, which affects the absorption of the mineral zinc, essential for healthy sperm production. Another reason to limit the amount of soy consumed is that it is also thought to reduce the male sex drive – Buddhist monks have traditionally used it to lower libido!

## EAT LEAN FOR SPERM

Lean meat in the diet releases ammonia as it is broken down by the digestive system, which can make the body slightly more alkaline. Sperm are well known to favour alkaline conditions, which means that eating meat a few times a week is a good choice to boost male fertility.

## CITRUS STIMULATES

Oranges and lemons are a good food choice for women who are trying to conceive because they contain folic acid, which stimulates the development of female sex hormones, while reducing the risk of spina bifida in infants. Drink freshly squeezed juice.

## KEEP MEAT TO A MINIMUM

If you're a woman trying to conceive, meat can be helpful but it's best not to eat it more than two or three times a week. Too much can reduce blood flow to the uterus and prevent the egg from implanting successfully.

## CHOOSE THE WHOLEGRAIN

Eating wholegrains is especially important if you have polycystic ovary syndrome (PCOS), a hormonal imbalance that increases insulin levels and can affect fertility. This is because wholegrains have been shown to reduce the symptoms of PCOS. Choose unrefined wholewheat breads with seeds for breakfast and sandwiches.

## STAY OFF THE FIZZ

If you're trying to get pregnant, you should avoid diet fizzy drinks containing aspartame, which can affect fertility. Caffeine should also be limited as it constricts blood vessels, reducing blood flow to the uterus and preventing eggs from implanting.

## DRINK ENOUGH

A high fluid intake is also important when trying to conceive. In order to stay hydrated, a woman trying to get pregnant should make absolutely sure she drinks at least 6 to 8 glasses of water and natural fruit juices (that do not contain added sugar) per 24 hours.

## FISH FOR FERTILITY

Pregnant women should make sure they eat two portions of oily fish every week, or take a supplement containing omega-3 fish oils. Studies have shown that children whose mothers consumed these oils when they were pregnant perform better physically and mentally.

## BOOST YOUR E DOSE

A powerful antioxidant, vitamin E is essential for fertility because it protects the egg from damage, which can lead to problems conceiving. It is also important in male fertility. Safflower, avocado, sunflower and wheatgerm contain high levels, or take a supplement to be sure.

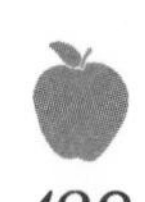



### C THE DIFFERENCE
Increasing vitamin C to 500-1000 mg a day may help boost fertility in men by increasing the number and quality of sperm produced and reducing abnormalities. Get it naturally in fresh fruit or take a supplement daily.

### CRESS THE RIGHT BUTTONS
Deficiencies of both vitamin B2 and folic acid have been linked with infertility, so women planning a pregnancy should ensure they eat plenty of foods rich in folic acid for at least three months before conception to build up levels. Cress and watercress are particularly good sources.

### GIVE YOURSELF AN A GRADE
Vitamin A is essential for reproductive health as it maintains the health of the epithelial tissues that line all the external and internal surfaces of the body, including the linings of the vagina and uterus in women. Liver, egg, yolk, cheese, butter and carrots are good sources but stick to the RDA as too much vitamin A can cause health problems.

## beating depression

### EAT YOURSELF HAPPY
There are a number of foods that can help with depression. Eating a high carbohydrate (wholewheat) diet boosts the production of serotonin in the brain, making you feel more positive. Eating plenty of protein to increase amino acid intake has the same effect.

### B-EAT DEPRESSION
B vitamins, especially B12, B6 and folic acid, can help combat psychological disturbances, so if you're suffering from depression a complete vitamin and mineral supplement containing these substances might help.

### CANOLA CAN HELP
Some studies have shown that people who suffer from depression also have lower levels of the antioxidant vitamin E. Canola oil is rich in vitamin E so try substituting it for vegetable oil in cooking.

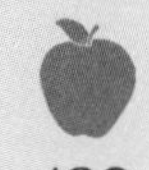



## OIL AWAY WORRIES

Omega-3 has been shown to help depression by altering the way the brain functions and reducing negative thoughts. It is not known exactly how this works, but some scientists believe it makes the uptake of brain chemicals such as serotonin more efficient.

## GO LOW-GI

Too many fluctuations in your insulin levels can lead to mood swings and fatigue, and these will be much worse if you already suffer from depression. To combat these ups and downs eat carbohydrates with a low glycaemic index such as basmati rice, couscous, oats or bran.

## CONCENTRATE ON CARBS

People who suffer depression should steer clear of low-carb diets, even if they want to lose weight. Instead, eat wholegrain carbohydrates and swap unhealthy foods for salmon and mackerel, spinach, fresh peas, chickpeas, chicken and turkey.

## SCOOP A GOOD MOOD

It's official – children have known it for years, but scientists now admit that eating ice cream can actually make you feel better. Eating a spoonful of ice cream lights up the same pleasure centre in the brain as winning money. Unfortunately, eating more doesn't give more pleasure and, as it's high in fat, one spoonful is enough!

## BOOST MOOD WITH FOLATE

Folate (also known as folic acid or vitamin B9) – found in many vegetables but most readily in the dark green, leafy varieties – is essential for the production of serotonin in the brain, which helps to regulate mood. Get happy with broccoli, spinach, kale and watercress. Some breakfast cereals are also fortified with folate/folic acid – check the label.

## GET REGULAR

Vitamin B6 plays an essential role in regulating brain chemicals, particularly when it comes to ensuring serotonin levels are high enough. Chicken and turkey are great sources of B6, which means they're good food choices to help regulate moods.

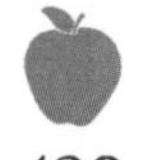



# pregnancy & menopause

## SMALL FRY

If you're worried about mercury levels in fish and want to eat oily fish, choose those lowest down the food chain, where the toxic metal hasn't had a chance to accumulate. Sardines, mackerel, anchovies and pilchards are good choices.

## TAINTED WITH TOXINS

Mercury is toxic to an unborn foetus and can stay in the bloodstream for over a year. Fish high in mercury include shark, swordfish and marlin. Fish that contain low levels include salmon, flounder, trout, haddock, tilapia and yellow fin tuna so choose these to be safe if you're pregnant or trying to conceive.

## SUP A SUPPLEMENT

After menopause, women experience a sudden drop in oestrogen levels which increases bone loss. To keep bones strong you need calcium and also vitamin D, which helps the body use calcium. If your diet isn't rich in these substances, a vitamin supplement is a good idea.

## BREAST-FEEDING EXTRA

Remember that if you're breastfeeding you'll need to consume an extra 300 calories a day to ensure your child gets the most benefit from your breast milk. This is the equivalent to a piece of wholemeal toast with butter, a full fat yogurt and a banana.

## ALL FOR ALFALFA

Alfalfa sprouts are rich in phytoestrogens, especially isoflavones, which help relieve menopausal symptoms, as well as osteoporosis, cancer and heart disease, while cress is high in folic acid. Add sprouts to your salads and sandwich fillings for all-round women's health.

## FLAX FACTS

Many pregnant women and vegetarians feel wary about eating fish but may be concerned they're not getting enough omega-3 fats. For these women, flax seeds are another good source, and extra omega-3 is now being added to many foods, including yogurts and breads.

## DROP NUTS FOR YOUR BABY

If you're pregnant, it's worth avoiding nuts, particularly peanuts, if the baby is at risk of developing allergies. Avoid them if you or the baby's father, brothers or sisters have certain allergic conditions such as hayfever, asthma and/or eczema.

## IRON OUT PROBLEMS

Low iron levels at the onset of pregnancy increase the risk of developing anaemia after the baby is born. This affects almost a third of women, reducing energy. It can also contribute to postnatal depression. To maintain good iron levels eat lean red meat, fortified breakfast cereals, eggs, pulses, green leafy vegetables, dried apricots and prunes and wholegrain bread.

## GRATE SOME GINGER

A great way to stave off nausea caused by pregnancy or other illness is to make yourself an infusion of ginger and lemon juice – not only will it calm your stomach, it will give you a vitamin boost too. Fresh ginger is the most beneficial.

## HAPPY GRAZING

If you're pregnant or thinking of trying to conceive, it's important to snack regularly if you're hungry – pregnancy isn't the time to watch your weight. Women with regulated blood sugar levels (ie, who didn't let themselves get hungry) are thought to have children who perform better in brain function and memory.

## KEEP UP THE CALCIUM

Pregnant women should aim for at least 1000 mg of calcium a day, which is more than women who aren't pregnant. Dairy products are a great source, avoiding those that are made with mould, and there is also calcium in meat and fish and green vegetables. Low-fat yogurts, cottage cheese and dried apricots make good snacks.

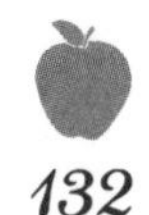



### CAFFEINE CONSCIOUS

Pregnant women should limit their intake of caffeine as more than 300 mg per day (three cups of coffee, 6 cups of tea or 8 cans of cola) has been linked to miscarriage and low birth weight.

# ailments & conditions

### REDUCE INFLAMMATION

Not only is oily fish great for brain function and skin and organ health, it's also likely to be beneficial if you have an inflammatory type of arthritis (such as rheumatoid, reactive or psoriatic arthritis, or ankylosing spondylitis), as it contains anti-inflammatory essential fatty acids.

### EAT TO SLEEP

If you have sleep problems, choosing the right foods and drinks in the evening might help. Steer clear of high-GI foods that boost energy and caffeine drinks, opting instead for foods containing the amino acid tryptophan such as lettuce, brown bread and turkey.

### PROTECT YOUR GUMS

Not only is gum disease unattractive and painful, it has also been linked with other more serious problems like strokes and heart disease. Eating a diet as low in refined sugars as possible helps.

### CUT THE ACIDS

There is no scientific evidence to prove "arthritis diets" work, but many sufferers swear by cutting out acidic fruit and solanaceous plants like potatoes, tomatoes, peppers and aubergines, or by adding honey and cider vinegar to their diet.

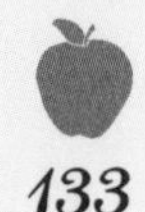



## SO SOYA FOR THE LACTOSE INTOLERANT

Soy milk is an ideal alternative to cow's milk for those who suffer from an intolerance to lactose. Soy protein has also been found to actively lower cholesterol and help to maintain a healthy heart. Substitute soya milk for cow's milk in your daily latte and reap the benefits.

## SLEEP LIKE A BABY

For a healthy, sleep-inducing midnight snack choose foods high in melatonin, which is said to protect against cancer and the damage caused by ageing and the sun, and has been shown to be good at treating insomnia. Try sweetcorn, rice, ginger, tomatoes, bananas and barley.

## EAT FOR YOUR EYES

It isn't only good for your heart and brain – eating fish can also protect your eyes from age-related macular degeneration, a potential cause of blindness. People who eat fish more than once a week are only half as likely to develop the disease as those who don't.

## FIGHT FUNGUS WITH LINSEED

Health problems that are due to yeast or fungus overloads in the body – like thrush or athlete's foot – can be reduced by taking a few teaspoons of linseed oil once or twice a day.

## GO FOR GARLIC

Adding garlic to sauces is a great health booster because it contains high levels of germanium and allium, thought to have anti-inflammatory, anti-viral and tumour fighting properties, as well as fighting arthritis. Some people choose deodorized garlic, but the smelly kind has more health benefits.

## TURN OFF THE TAP

People who drink too much tap water (more than the daily recommended dose) have been shown in some countries to have an increased chance of developing bladder cancer than those who drank other forms. Tap water contains chlorine, which has been linked to cancers, and the toxin arsenic, which has been linked to bladder cancer.

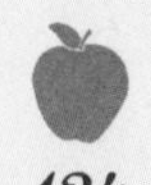



## OIL YOUR JOINTS

We all know that fish oils help fight arthritis, but olive oil can also help protect against this inflammatory disease. It is said that those who eat it every day reduce their risk by 2.5 times, possibly because of its high levels of antioxidants.

## PROTECT YOUR BREASTS

Milk doesn't only contribute to health by adding calcium and – if low-fat versions are drunk – reducing the body's absorption of fat, it has also been shown to reduce breast cancer risk by almost half in women who drink the equivalent of three glasses a day.

## KEEP SUGAR LOW

The body needs some sugar in the diet, so it's best not to cut it out completely, but high levels of sugar, especially snacks between meals, which lead to dramatic insulin peaks, have been linked with breast cancer and colon cancer as well as cholesterol levels. Cutting down is best.

## GRAPEFRUIT WARNING

The juice of grapefruits has chemicals in it which have been shown to cause harmful side effects if taken with certain medicines. If you are taking medications on a regular basis, and if you want to drink grapefruit juice or eat grapefruit regularly, check with your doctor or pharmacist to see if you are at risk.

## CURRYING FLAVOUR

Sprinkling meals with turmeric is a good idea because the herb has been reported to prevent blood clots, reduce the pain and inflammation associated with arthritis and lower cholesterol. It's good on spicy foods and with vegetables.

## CRAM IN THE CRANBERRY

A couple of glasses of cranberry juice a day can help prevent urinary tract infections, especially in older women, by preventing bacteria from sticking to the walls of the bladder. It can also help prevent cystitis in younger women. Buy the highest concentrate you can find.

## HAVE A GOOD EVENING

Evening primrose oil contains around 9% omega-6 fatty acids, which are needed by the body for hormone production and to reduce inflammation. This wonder oil is also credited with reducing blood pressure, helping fight depression and reducing the symptoms of PMS.

## SMOOTH OUT JOINT PROBLEMS

One of the best food supplements for healthy joints, especially in older people, is glucosamine sulphate, which has been shown to help the body replenish the cartilage in joints, reducing joint pain dramatically if 1000 mg is taken daily.

## FIGHT FATIGUE

If you spend a lot of time feeling tired, or you have whole days where you just can't seem to wake up, think about reducing your caffeine and sugar intake. They both drain your adrenals, whose job it is to regulate energy. It is easier to cut down a little at a time rather than going cold turkey, which can lead to headaches.

## REDUCE STRESS WITH FISH

Eating oily fish has been shown to reduce stress hormones by almost a quarter as well as boosting anti-stress hormones in the body – making it the perfect choice for a working lunch to set you up for a productive afternoon.

## CUT THE COFFEE

People who drink three cups of coffee or less each day are half as likely to develop rheumatoid arthritis as those who drink four or more, and oils in unfiltered coffee can raise cholesterol levels. Cut down coffee intake or switch to decaf to be sure.

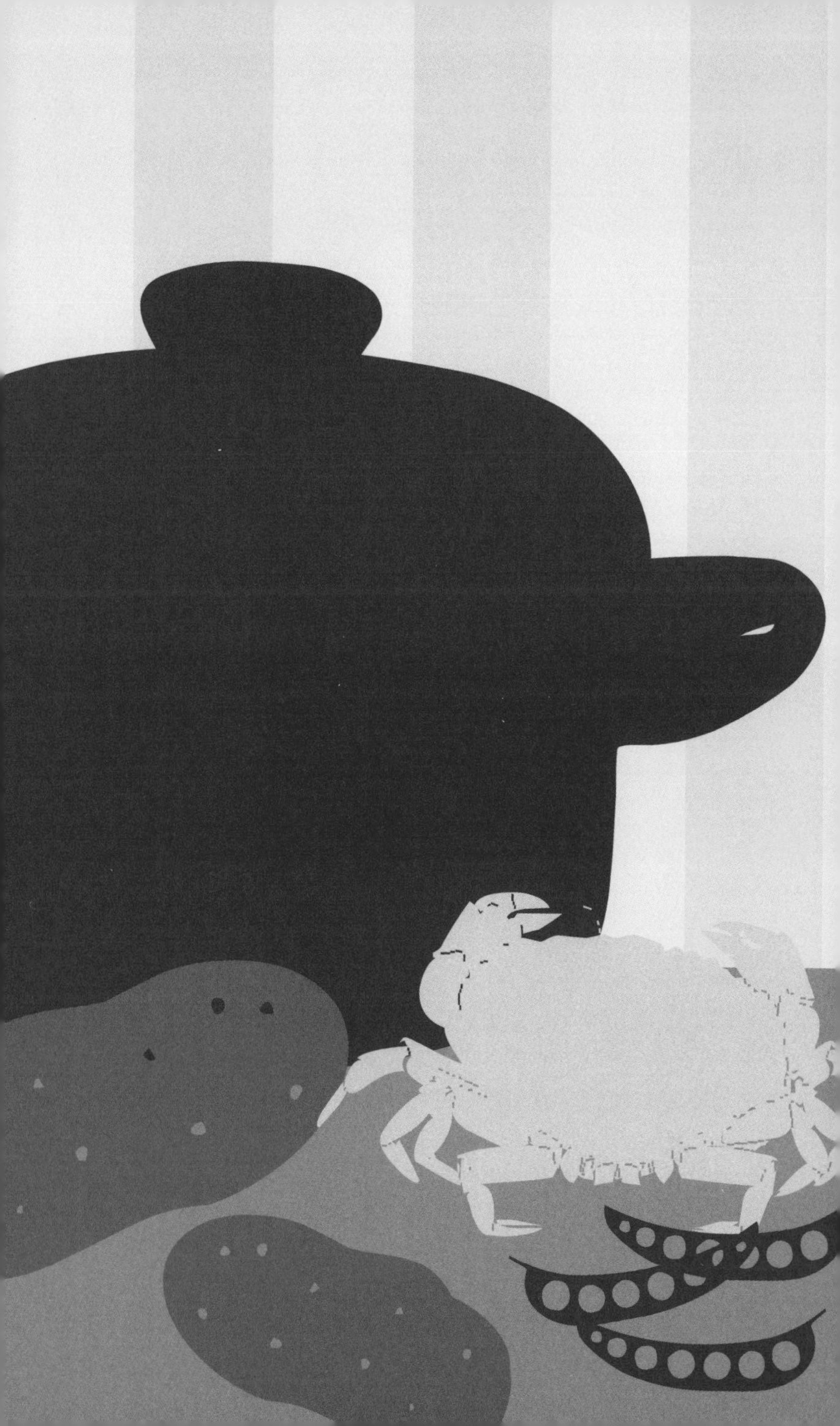

# Buying & Cooking Food

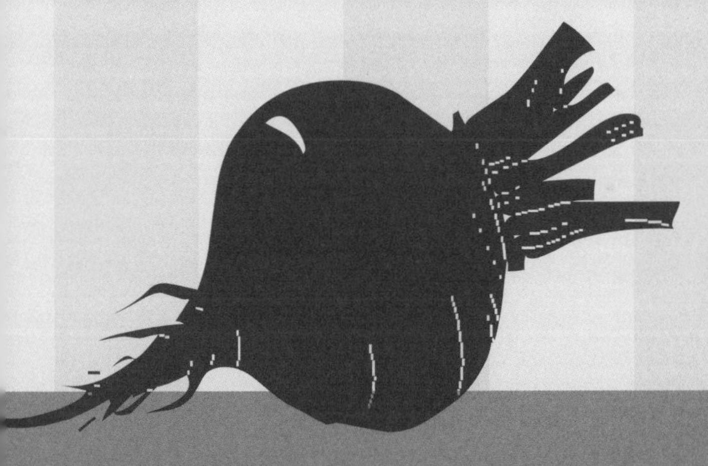

Choosing, storing and preparing fresh, wholesome food is the cornerstone to good health and here you will find not only buying and shopping advice but information on storing, shelf life, freezing, reheating, kitchen hygiene and organic food. Whether you buy your produce from a local merchant or a supermarket, this chapter includes detailed tips on how to select the freshest fruits, vegetables, meat, fish and flavourings.

# choosing fruit

## RIPE STRAWBERRIES ONLY

With strawberries, pick only the cartons with the reddest, plumpest berries. Strawberries that are showing patches of green or white are not yet ripe and once strawberries are picked, they will not continue to ripen – if they're unripe, they'll stay that way!

## A TRUE BLUE

Select cartons of blueberries that are wholly blue. Blueberries with a reddish tone will taste overly tart, and those that are too purple are probably overripe and will be too soft and low on taste. They're called blueberries for a reason!

## POP YOUR CHERRY

Cherries should be firm to the touch, not squashy, and should be a uniform red or scarlet in colour with no brown patches. Those which have been in storage too long develop bruising, which means they're not as good for you.

## AN APPLE A DAY

When you're choosing apples, go for the crispest, hardest, most blemish-free fruit you can find. Any wrinkling of the skin means the apple is too old. The skin should hold firm against your finger with no bruising. This is particularly important for Braeburn, Granny Smith and Pink Lady varieties.

## SMELL YOUR BERRIES

The best way to check if berries are fresh is to smell them. They should smell fresh and fruity. If you're buying in cartons, make sure the carton is still dry and that no juices are in the bottom. Store them on kitchen paper towels in the fridge.

## PLUMP IS BEAUTIFUL

With peaches, nectarines and plums, plumpness is key. The more plump and full the fruit feels, the juicier it will be. If you apply pressure on the skin of the fruit, the fruit should give way a little. If you have bought them unripe, leave them in a loosely closed brown paper bag for a day or so at room temperature to ripen.

## GET A POP-EYED PINEAPPLE

When you're choosing pineapples, look for a bright colour, a small, compact crown with bright green leaves and protruding eyes. Also, the pineapple should smell sweet and fragrant – like most fruit, if it doesn't smell it isn't usually ripe.

## PUMPKIN HEAVY

Pumpkins are a great source of vitamins and betacarotene, especially in the autumn (fall). Make sure you choose those that are plump and heavy for their size with a clean, firm rind with no cracks or bruises. Those that are too light may have been in storage for too long.

## GO MAN-GO

Mango is packed with vitamin C. When buying, don't worry if the mango is almost all green or red, as colour doesn't make any difference to how ripe it is – it's simply down to a difference in varieties. Put a little pressure on the fruit and if the flesh gives way a little bit, the mango is ripe.

## SMELL MELONS

Cantaloupes are the easiest of the melons to judge for ripeness as they give off an aroma that's hard to miss when they're ready for eating. Always look for the most symmetrical melon and if you buy a not-quite-ripe cantaloupe, let it sit out and ripen at room temperature for a few days.

## PICK A PAPAYA

It's hard to go wrong with papayas, but be sure to pick one that has changed from its original, unripe green to a richer yellowish or orangey colour, particularly around the larger end of the fruit.

## BERRY GOOD

Choose raspberries that have a rich berry scent. Raspberries that still have green stems on them are not ripe. They can be expensive, so it's even more important to be discriminating.

## CANNED TYPES

If you're buying fruit in cans, it's healthier to choose fruit preserved in its own juice, or in other fruit juices, than syrups. Syrups are high in sugar and contain more calories.

## SQUEEZE YOUR AVOCADOS

For immediate use, select slightly soft avocados that yield to gentle pressure on the skin. For use in 4–5 days, buy firm fruits that do not yield to the squeeze test and leave them at room temperature to ripen.

## RIPE WITH WRINKLES

Unlike most fruits, passion fruit is best when the skin sags and is wrinkly. Those with smoother skins will be too sour to use for anything but cooking. They should still feel dense, though, as those that are too light could be overripe.

## BE FIRM

Tomatoes are an excellent source of vitamins and cancer-fighting antioxidants. Look for smooth-skinned, firm fruits with uniform colour. They should be firm rather than soft, and shouldn't have scarring on the skin surface – this can indicate sun damage that can reduce nutrient quality.

## SHAKE YOUR GRAPES

The best way to pick the freshest grapes in your supermarket is to hold a bunch by the stem and shake them gently. If the grapes drop off the stem they have been in storage for too long. The ideal bunch is one where most of the grapes are plump, clear and firmly attached.

## A TASTE OF HONEY

Look for honeydew melon with a yellowish-white to creamy rind colour, with a little bit of spotting on the rind and no cracks or bruises. Honeydew that feels sticky to the touch is ripe and ready, and if the skin is giving off a faint, pleasantly sweet scent, it's ready for eating.

## GET HEAVY

Select watermelon that has few bruises or cuts to the flesh. A good watermelon is dense with water, so a smaller watermelon that is heavier than a larger-sized one will be a better choice. Make sure the watermelon has a slightly yellow belly, meaning it was sun-ripened, and a hollow sound if you knock on the rind.

## RATTLE AND HOLD

It might make you look odd in the supermarket aisles, but there are two ways to check if a melon is fresh – for the perfect ripeness, all (except watermelon) should smell sweet at the stem end and you shouldn't hear the seeds rattling inside when you shake them.

## AVOCADOS TO AVOID

Don't worry about the irregular light-brown markings that are sometimes found on the skin of avocados – these generally have no effect on the flesh inside. But avoid those with dark sunken spots or cracked or broken surfaces as these are signs of decay. Slow down ripening by refrigerating.

## FLICK THE STALK

To test whether an avocado is ripe, flick off the small stalk at the end – if it comes off easily, the fruit is ripe. If there's no stalk, use a light squeeze instead to test for ripeness.

## GREEN SKIN

Nectarines shouldn't have any green tinges to their skin, because green patches are unlikely to come up to ripeness before the rest goes bad. If you have green nectarines, why not turn them into a delicious dessert – split in half and roast in a low oven, then drizzle with maple syrup or natural yogurt.

## A HARD STEM

In general, ripe melons smell pleasant and fruity when they are ready to eat. The stem end should be indented and a little soft. If the stem looks hard or withered, the melon has been in storage for too long and won't taste fresh.

## GET HEAVY HANDED

If you're looking for the freshest citrus produce, go for those that feel heaviest. Fruits that feel light are likely to have been hanging around too long and may have started to lose their juice.

## BERRY FRESH

Berries are a great way to give yourself a vitamin and antioxidant boost, but it's important to get them as fresh as possible. Visit farm shops or pick-your-own farms for the freshest, straight off the plant.

## A GOOD APRICOT

Apricots should be uniform in colour, which shows they have been harvested at the right time and are fully ripe. Store at room temperature to further ripen, or in the fridge if they are already soft enough.

## DON'T BE A SOFTIE

Don't choose melons that are too soft because they will continue to ripen and the very soft patches will go bad before long. Choose them when they are a little bit harder if you want to wait before eating.

## CHERRY RIPE

There are many different varieties of cherries. Sweeter varieties (for eating) should have a stem and be firm to the touch. When choosing sour cherries for cooking, the stem should pop off easily when pulled.

## FIRM PLUMS

Plums taste best when they're not too soft – there should be some firmness to the skin when pressed with the flat of your thumb or finger, so the flesh springs back from the touch. Avoid relatively hard or shrivelled fruit.

## RIPE FOR THE PICKING

Make sure you choose the ripest fruit, if possible those which have matured on trees as plant-ripened fruit have the most nutrients. Find this information on the label – it usually applies only to organic fruit.

## SAY NO TO MOULD

Don't buy strawberries with any trace of mould on them, because it spreads fast between berries even if stored correctly. The freshest, healthiest strawberries don't lose their hairs when touched or washed and are red in colour and firm. Avoid those with large uncoloured or seeded areas.

## DON'T BIN THE BANANAS

Don't throw away overripe bananas. Use them in cooking (for banana cake or loaf) or for smoothies with other fruits or yogurt. You can also freeze them and use as an alternative to fruit sorbet or ice cream (over-ripe bananas freeze better than ripe ones).

# choosing vegetables

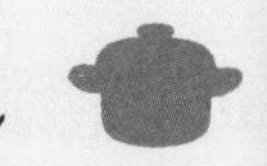



## LET US BE CRISP

Lettuce should be crisp to the touch when you buy it, and there should be no see-through patches on the leaves, or moisture. It's best to buy it in open packets or brown paper and keep well refrigerated.

## CORN COLOUR

Contrary to popular belief, it doesn't matter if sweetcorn is yellow or white. Sweetness isn't determined by colour, which is naturally varied – it's determined by freshness, so make sure you choose a freshly picked ear.

## DARK SECRETS

Green, leafy vegetables are a great addition to any diet, but if you want to make sure you get the most goodness out of them, avoid those with wilted leaves or those that are too pale or yellowed in colour.

## CHECK YOUR TASSELS

There is only one surefire way to tell if an ear of corn is fresh (and they don't stay fresh for long) and that is by the tassel at the end of it. If the tassel is soft and silky then the corn is fresh. If, on the other hand, it's starting to get hard and brittle or if it has been removed, don't buy it.

## THE CRUNCH

For the best flavour, look for deep-orange coloured carrots with smooth-skinned roots. Fresh-looking tops mean they have been recently harvested. Avoid those with purple or green shoulders or those that are pale in colour, and steer clear of those with forked or oversized roots.

## SNAP A SUGAR SNAP

Avoid sugar snap peas with dry-looking, rusty, wilted or damaged pods, as they might have been hanging around for a while. Pods should be plump, uniform in colour and crisp – reject them if you can see large seeds through the skin, which means they will have lost their freshness.

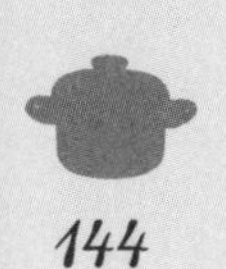





## ARTFUL CHOKER CHOICE

The head of artichokes should be tightly closed and feel firm and heavy with no discolouration. Keep fresh in a brown paper bag or wrap in plastic in the fridge.

## WASH YOUR LEEKS

For leeks to taste their best and give you the best dose of healthiness, they should have long white shanks and dark green leaf tissue. Avoid dry or yellowish leaves or discoloured shanks. And remember to wash inside the outer layers, where dirt and grit can accumulate, under cold running water.

## FIRMNESS IS KEY

If you're choosing aubergine (or eggplant), go for firm, shiny dark purple fruit with small blossom scars. Avoid soft, bronze or green-coloured fruits or those with a dried stem, or calyx – it should be bright and green. Older aubergines tend to have a bitter or acidic taste.

## GREEN SHOULDERS

Parsnips and turnips should have clean, smooth, firm and well-shaped roots with light, even-coloured skin. Those that are sunburned (which have green shoulders) are likely to be low on flavour and if they're soft they'll be woody.

## CHOOSE TIGHT BUNCHES

If you want to make sure you're choosing the best broccoli, Brussels sprouts or cauliflower, choose tightly compacted flower clusters on broccoli and cauliflower, and compact, uniform sprouts. Avoid wilted, yellow, or dirty heads, and avoid loose, open sprouts or those that are yellow or pale green.

## AVOID ARTICHOKE FLOWERS

If you're hunting for the perfect artichoke look for tight, solid buds on fruits that are heavy for their size. Avoid ones with loose buds or purple flowers forming, which are overmature. If they're fresh, they'll be squeaky when rubbed against each other.

## DON'T SUPERSIZE YOUR RADISHES

Choose radishes with medium-sized firm crisp roots. Avoid wilted or soft roots, which is a sign of them being too old, or oversized roots, which will taste pithy. And choose smoother skins, because those with growth cracks retain fewer nutrients.

## GO GREEN WITH ASPARAGUS

Asparagus should be mostly green in colour (those with white colouring are invariably less tender, even when fresh) and choose firm stalks with close, compact tips. The sooner it's used the more tender it will be, but don't forget to cut off the woody white end before cooking.

## GET WITH THE BEET

For beetroot, the key to flavour is in appearance – look for smooth round uniform bunches with small to medium roots. Avoid beetroots that are blocky or angular in shape, rough-skinned or oversized. Freshness of tops or leaves is not necessarily an indication of quality.

## PEPPER SPOT

For the healthiest addition to your lunchtime salad, choose peppers that have a uniform colour. Those that have contrasting colour spots may have had sun damage, which can reduce the nutrients and vitamins they contain.

## PACK A PUNCH

Cauliflower is freshest and healthiest when the tops are light in colour without any discoloured patches, and when the florets are tightly packed. If the stalks bend when you touch it, it's been in storage too long.

## A GOOD BEET

Beetroot should be used quickly, before its sugar turns to starch, which can make it taste fluffy. It should be hard to the touch, and if you're buying it with the greenery attached make sure there's no wilting.

## SWEET BROCCOLI

If your broccoli smells like cabbage, it's probably been hanging around too long. Broccoli should be completely green and not yellowing, and should smell sweet and fresh.

## GARLIC HEAD

Garlic tastes best when the heads are firm and plump with no green shoots. Green shoots coming out of the bulbs means the garlic has been in storage too long and will taste less fresh and may be slightly bitter. The bulbs can still be used for cooking, although they won't taste as good, but discard the green bits.

## HIDE THE SPINACH

Spinach contains many great nutrients and antioxidants and is a really versatile vegetable, so it's great for adding a "hidden" vegetable kick to dishes. Spinach should have bright green leaves when it's fresh, not yellowed or dry looking, and is best kept airtight or with stalks wrapped in damp paper towels.

## COOL YOUR SPUDS

Try to buy potatoes as close to cooking them as you can, but if you have to store them for a while, keep them in a cool dark place away from sunlight and preferably in paper. Potatoes which have sprouted tubers have less flavour, and green tinges prevent them cooking well.

## SPROUT A FRESH CHOICE

The best way to buy Brussels sprouts is to buy them still attached to the stalk – that way they'll keep more of their moisture. Cut or break them off the stalk just before use for maximum health benefits.

## DON'T SPLIT YOUR PEAS

If you're buying garden peas in the pod, the pods should be whole but not split at the sides, which means they're overripe. One of the healthiest ways to buy them is frozen because peas hold a lot of their nutrients that way.

## PICKING PARSNIPS

With parsnips, the general rule is that the fresher they are, the whiter the flesh. Try to avoid those that are yellowing or brown around the central core as these are likely to have been in storage for too long.

## GET RID OF THE GREENS

Rhubarb, carrots and other vegetables you buy with greens attached will store better if you remove the green tops to prevent them absorbing the vegetable's water and reducing nutrient content.

## CHOOSE CRISP CELERY

Choose large, firm celery stalks with a uniform shape and a clear white bottom. Avoid spindly, wilted stalks, or those that are too green, as these can have too strong a taste.

# buying meat & fish

## BUY FREE-RANGE BIRDS

Always buy free-range chickens, which will have been reared with enough space to move around freely and develop muscle tone. The meat will be leaner and better for you than the meat from less-mobile birds.

## BEEF IT UP

When shopping for beef, choose sirloin or topside as they are the leanest cuts. Sirloin has only 3.8 g fat per 100 g serving and topside 5.2 g, compared to 24.1 g fat for minced (ground) beef. Spend the same amount of money – just buy less of the leaner, more expensive cuts.

## LEAN CUISINE

If you're looking for meat or poultry that will last longer, go lean. Lean cuts last longer than fatty meats because it's the fat on meat that first starts to decay.

## YOU CAN'T BEAT A BUTCHER

Most people think butchers are more expensive than supermarkets for buying meat, but the opposite is often true. A good butcher will be able to help you get the best meat for your money, so ask for advice.

## FISHY ISN'T DISHY

If you want to check your fish is fresh, look for light scales and a slightly slimy sheen to the skin. Fish that looks dry or where the scales are dark or peeling is too old. Above all, it shouldn't smell too "fishy"– really fresh fish has very little odour.

## THE RIGHT LIGHTING

If you buy your meat in a supermarket, try to examine your choice away from the brightly lit meat counters, which are often too bright for you to see the real colour of the meat. Take it to a different aisle and make your choice there.

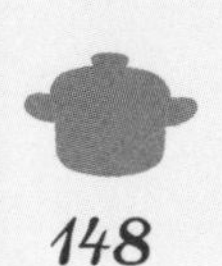



## PIG ON PORK

Pork is often thought to be a fatty meat but it's healthy because not as much of it is saturated as with other meats – the level of fat depends entirely on which cut you choose, so go for leaner cuts like tenderloin (3.6 g fat per 100 g/3.5 oz), which has half the fat of other cuts.

## IT'S IN THE EYES

If you're buying fresh fish whole, look at the eyes, which should be clear, and the gills, which should be transparent and bright red in colour. Don't be afraid to ask the fishmonger to show you the fish close up – they might give you a fresher fish if they think you know what you're looking for!

## DON'T BE GREY

Lamb should never be grey or sweaty, which means it's either been hanging around too long or has been in and out of hot and cold environments too much and won't have retained its characteristic aromatic taste. The flesh should be pink and the fat white.

## BEEF UP THE DARK

The best-tasting beef should be a dark red colour with slightly yellowish fat. If the fat is too white or the meat is bright red, the beef hasn't been hung for long enough and will be lower on taste and tougher. It's better if there's some fat marbled throughout, as this makes it more tender.

## DON'T DITCH THE FAT

It might sound counter-intuitive, but buying fattier meat can actually help you take smaller portions, because (as long as you cut off the fat on your plate) you are likely to eat less. Also, fattier meat generally has a better taste, so it will be more satisfying.

## PINKY AND PORKY

Pork is one of those meats which can harbour salmonella bacteria, so it's important that you buy fresh meat which has been properly stored. Look for meat that is pink and firm to the touch with very white fat. If the fat is too yellow or the meat is grey, you should reject it.

### GET FRESH FISH

It's difficult to know how fresh fish is when it's on the rack – even if you visit a specialist fishmonger, it could be three days old if you're in the city. The best way to ensure fish is fresh is to buy really fresh in bulk from a market and freeze. Buying frozen fish can also be a good option, as it is often frozen quickly and therefore has less time to deteriorate.

### DON'T BE A FARM FAN

Salmon and trout are great choices if you're eating fish because they're high in omega-3 oils and low in the damaging mercury deposits that can build up in other cold-water fish. Farmed fish, however, are lower in omega-3s and the flesh is less lean. Choose wild or organic whenever you can.

## buying flavourings & condiments

### BUY SMALL

If you don't use spices and dried herbs very often in your cooking, buy the smallest quantities you can. Ground, blended and chopped spices last around six months in your cupboard before they start to lose their potency, while whole spices can keep their taste for up to a year.

### BE AN EXTRA VIRGIN

Labelling of olive oils can be confusing, with early and late varieties, single estates and different extraction methods. The most important label to look for is "extra virgin", which means it's taken from the first pressing of the olives and is therefore finer in flavour and best for dressings.

### SEND FOR THE SALSA

Instead of buying commercially prepared tomato ketchup, choose fresh salsa – or buy tomatoes, red peppers and chilli and make your own. Chop them up and mix together to make a great alternative to ketchup for meat, eggs and burgers.

# buying organic

## TWO SHOPS ARE BETTER THAN ONE

Organic fruit and vegetables often don't keep as long as non-organic so you'll have to think about how you shop as well as how you eat. It might mean two trips instead of one and making better use of your freezer.

## TOTALLY FREE TIPPLE

If you want to be sure your wine and beer is free of pesticides it's best to choose organic. However, some health experts say it doesn't make any difference as the time the alcohol is stored for fermentation means the chemicals break down anyway.

## BECOME A CONVERT

Organic meat is often more expensive, especially if you buy it from supermarkets. Look for "in conversion" labels (also labelled "free range additive free"), which is food from farms undergoing the two-year conversion to organic status.

## COCOA LOCO

Don't deprive yourself completely of chocolate but do choose dark organic varieties, which are high in cocoa solids. They're expensive, but so rich that a few squares is usually enough to satisfy, and they contain antioxidants so will give you a health kick, too.

## PRIORITIZE FOR PRICE

The decision to buy organic food can be restrictive as it's often more expensive than non-organic. Solve it by converting bit by bit rather than in one go – each time you shop, bring home one more organic item so you build it up slowly. Choose meat, dairy, fruit and vegetable organics above other kinds of food to start with.

# shopping tips

## ON SPECIAL OFFER

Take time to compare fresh, frozen, and canned foods to see which is cheapest. Buying what's on special offer can be a great way to get cheap, healthy food and is often linked to what's in season. Many of these foods can be bought fresh and then frozen for longer-term value.

## ORDER YOUR LIST

Before you go shopping, make a list of all the foods you need, then you won't forget anything. If you know your supermarket well, arrange your list according to where foods are placed, so you can go through the list in order as you work your way through the shop.

## AIR-CON THE CAR

If you have air conditioning in your car, put your summer shopping on the back seat rather than in the boot, because it's likely to be cooler there, which will help food stay at the right temperature.

## STORE YOUR VOUCHERS

In order not to forget those all-important money-off and discount coupons when you're doing your supermarket shop, write out your shopping list on an old envelope and put your vouchers inside.

## STICK TO YOUR LIST

Make yourself a list before you go shopping and stick to it – that way, you won't be tempted to indulge in all those high-sugar treats the supermarkets leave by the till.

## GO STRAIGHT HOME

Cars heat up in the summer months, which means that your shopping heats up too if it's stored in the car for any significant length of time – not a good idea for fresh and frozen food. Solve the problem by doing your food shop last so it's not left hanging around, then head straight home. Alternatively, use your own insulated cool bags, which are useful for smaller shops.

## SHOP ONLINE

If you're short on shopping time, why not try ordering your basics on the internet? Many supermarkets and local shops now have internet ordering and delivery sites and you can make sure you're always stocked up with the basics.

## DON'T BE FOOLED

Ready-prepared convenience foods often appear to be good value, and may even claim to be healthy choices, but they are rarely as healthy as fresh foods because they contain more fat, sugar and salt. If you must buy pre-packed and processed foods, make sure you read the nutrition labels carefully and choose those lower in fat, sodium and calories and higher in vitamins, fibre and other nutrients.

## TWO-FOR-ONES

Don't be tempted by two-for-one or three-for-two offers on unhealthy foods as studies have shown people with more in their cupboards generally tend to eat more. Buy only as much as you need.

## BUILD UP THE BASICS

Often, people resort to ready meals and take-aways because they just can't get to the shops. Make sure your cupboards are always stocked with the basics for producing a quick meal – such as canned or frozen vegetables, meat and fish, and dried pasta and rice.

## CHECK OUT YOUR LOCAL

Many people don't use their local shops – which can offer really good quality and value – because they haven't got time to visit during working hours. But it's worth paying them a visit to check if they do a home-delivery scheme so you can get the best of both worlds.

## BACK BOX SCHEMES

Instead of buying your fruit and vegetables off the supermarket shelves, where they might have been imported from all over the world, why not subscribe to a local organic fruit and vegetable box scheme? Most areas have them, where fresh foods are delivered weekly often from local farms.

### THE WHOLE SHOP

Remember that shopping in local healthfood and wholefood shops is a different experience to the local supermarket, and often, things aren't labelled as clearly. But don't let that put you off – the assistants expect, and are usually more than willing, to give advice.

### MAKE A COMPARISON

If you're worried about comparing how healthy foods are, it's easier to compare the fat, salt and sugar content of 100 g of the product with the same amount of another product rather than to rely on serving size, which may alter between products.

### HONESTY IS THE BEST POLICY

If you're looking at the labels of a food to see how healthy it is, be realistic and honest about your serving size. If you always find yourself eating three biscuits, don't just look at the fat and sugar content of one. Remember to multiply!

## storing your food

### KEEP IT COOL

Keep your fridge below 40°C (104°F) if you want to make sure your food is kept as safe as possible, because eating food that has been stored in refrigerators warmer than this temperature can increase the risk of food-borne illness.

### DON'T BE A BRUISER

Take care to avoid bruising or mashing fruits and vegetables when transporting or storing them. It doesn't just make them look bad, it also oxidizes antioxidants and destroys nutrients. And one bruised fruit or veg will cause others to become rotten or ripen much faster, so remove any that are and use them straight away.

### GET THE LOW DOWN

It's best to store raw meat and fish covered on a tray on the bottom shelf of your fridge or in the boxes at the bottom. This will make sure none of the juices escape and drip on to other foods. It is also usually marginally colder at the bottom because cold air is more dense.

## MAKE SOME SPACE

Avoid overfilling your refrigerator – cool air must be allowed to circulate to keep food at the proper temperature wherever it's placed. Try to space food evenly throughout and avoid stacking too many items on top of each other. Most people tend to over-buy anyway, so buy less more frequently.

## EGGS-TRA SAFE

Eggs don't have to be stored in the fridge. A cool place will do, especially as most recipes assume that the required eggs will be at room temperature. They should be stored, thin-end down, away from strong smells because the shells are porous and can absorb strong flavours.

## SPUDS YOU LIGHT

Store your potatoes in a cool dark place. If you leave them exposed to too much light, they will turn a greenish colour. The substance that causes this to happen can be mildly toxic and therefore should not be eaten, especially by children.

## CHECK FOR DAMAGE

Never eat any foods from jars or tins which appear damaged or look as if they might have been opened. If stored food has come into contact with air, it is likely to have been spoiled and is best returned or disposed of.

## SUN SENSITIVE

Light is the enemy of oil! Buy olive oil in dark glass bottles and keep it in a cool dark place to preserve quality. Sunlight can oxidize the oil, turning it rancid.

## KEEP DRY DRY

Store all your dry foods like flour and pasta on one dry shelf, and make it a higher shelf than for wetter ingredients such as oils and vinegars. This way, the humidity levels will be just right for keeping foods at their best for longer.

## HUMIDITY CHECK

The cupboard under your sink can be more humid than other cupboards because of the water going through the pipes. Remember this when you're considering storage, as fruit and vegetables rot quicker in humid environments.

## DON'T CLING TO PLASTICS

Clingfilm (plastic wrap) contains plasticizers which are said to leach into food. Use paper, foil or reusable sealed containers, especially for high-fat foods like cheese which are highly absorbent. Or choose food wrap which is made without toxins.

## BE A HONEY

If you're looking for the ultimate food to keep in your cupboards for years, choose good old-fashioned honey, which is the only food that doesn't spoil. In fact, archaeologists have even found edible honey in the tombs of Pharaohs!

## TOO COLD FOR COMFORT

Potatoes will actually keep for longer outside the refrigerator as being too cold causes the starch in them to turn to sugar. A cool, dry, dark place is best.

## KEEP CHEMICALS CLEAR

Don't store foods near household cleaning products and chemicals. It's unlikely, but possible that chemicals could leach into foods, especially if the foods are to be eaten raw or if they're absorbent, like dairy products and vegetables.

## SEPARATE DRAWERS

Store fruits and vegetables in separate drawers in your fridge. Even when chilled, fruits give off ethylene gas that shortens the shelf life of other fruit and vegetables by causing them to ripen more quickly.

## CUT OUT THE LIGHT

Spices and dried herbs keep their flavour better if stored in a cupboard away from heat, light and moisture, all of which impair flavour, change colour and shorten life. Try attaching a spice rack to the inside of your cupboard door. As a general rule, herbs and ground spices will retain their best flavour for a year. Whole spices can last for up to one year.

## LOOK FOR STORAGE ADVICE

Always check the labels on cans or jars to determine how the contents should be stored. If you've neglected to refrigerate items that should be kept cold, it's usually best to throw them out.

# extending shelf life

## CLEAR CUCUMBERS

If you're storing cucumber in your fridge and want it to stay fresh, keep it away from apples and tomatoes, which will shorten its life. Cucumber stays fresh for up to a week, then the water content starts to drop.

## KEEP YOUR ONIONS

Yellow and brown onions keep for longer than red onions because they have a lower sugar content. Store in an open space that's cool and dry, away from bright light, which can make them bitter. Don't store under the sink or anywhere that may be damp.

## A GOOD EGG

Eggs should keep for around four to five weeks if they are kept refrigerated. However, bear in mind they might have been two weeks old when you first bought them, so keep an eye on the "best before" date. Always store with the pointed side down – this keeps the yolk in the centre and helps to keep them fresh.

## APPLE YOUR SUGAR

If brown sugar becomes solid, add a slice of apple to the container for a couple of days to restore the moisture and the balance. And keep it soft by storing a few marshmallows in the bag.

## BURIED GINGER

If you want to keep ginger fresh for adding a healthy zing to smoothies, soups and casseroles, as well as aiding digestion, follow the ancient Chinese method of storing it – fill a small clay pot with white sand or sandy potting soil and bury the ginger root inside – it will keep for months and will eventually also start to grow.

## PAIR UP POTATOES

If you want to store potatoes without them budding, put an apple into the bag with them. It will help them stay smooth and eye-free for longer in your cupboard.

## BAKING SODA FRESHNESS

Many people have a cupboard full of baking ingredients they don't have time to use regularly – baking soda, for example. Check if your baking soda is still fresh by pouring half a teaspoon of lemon juice or vinegar over a small pile of it. If it bubbles, it's still fresh enough to use.

## FRESH SARNIES

To keep sandwiches fresh right through the day (or night, if you prepare them the evening before) wrap them in a piece of kitchen towel before packing them in a sealed box or bag. The paper will soak up excess moisture, leaving the sandwich soft and fresh.

## MUD IS GOOD

If you buy organic vegetables that are still muddy, don't wash them before putting them in the fridge or larder. The mud acts as a natural preservative, preventing light from reaching the surface of the veg and helping to keep it cool. They might not look pretty, but they taste just as good.

## DE-HUMIDIFY YOUR VEG

Line vegetable drawers in the fridge with a section of newspaper wrapped in kitchen towel. This will act as a de-humidifier, soaking up the excess moisture that can cause vegetables to rot or go mouldy.

## RICE ON TOAST

Rice will keep in the fridge for longer if you store a slice of toast on top of it. The toast will absorb excess moisture and keep the rice fluffy and fresh.

## DON'T SHAKE OR STIR

If you like your yogurt thick and creamy, don't stir it. Stirring changes the consistency and makes it more runny – perfect if you're using it instead of single cream, but not if you want a healthy dollop.

## BETTER APART

If you want your potatoes to last longer, don't store them near onions, even if you're refrigerating them. Being in close proximity to onions can cause potatoes to rot more quickly.

## DON'T TOUCH THE WALLS

Take care that delicate salad items such as cucumber and lettuce don't touch the walls of your fridge, where the high moisture content and low temperatures can cause them to go off more quickly. Keep them in the centre of shelves.

## SUGAR YOUR CHEESE

Cheese can go off pretty quickly, developing mould within a week even if stored in the fridge – and tempting you to eat it up quickly! Prolong its life and help keep it mould-free by adding a couple of sugar cubes to your cheese containers.

## KEEP TABS ON THE FRIDGE

To keep the contents of your fridge healthy, don't crowd the refrigerator or freezer so that you can't see what's on the shelves and air can't circulate. Check the leftovers in covered dishes and storage bags daily for spoilage. Anything that looks or smells suspicious should be thrown out.

## BLANCH BEFORE STORAGE

To keep all the goodness and vitamin content of your vegetables, blanch them before storing – blanching kills the enzymes that cause rotting. Plunge into boiling water then straight into cold water to refresh. Cook up quickly when you need them.

## FRUIT AT THE FRONT

Be honest, how many times have you bought healthy fruit and stored it in the fridge, only to forget all about it and find it a few weeks later, rotting at the back? Store fruit on its own shelf or at the front of the fridge to remind you it's there.

## KEEP A TIGHT LID ON IT

The best way to store biscuits or other foods that you want to keep really dry is in jars with screw top lids, or press-top storage jars that keep the air out more effectively than other lids. Tins don't generally tend to be airtight once they've been used for a few months.

## STEER CLEAR OF THE DOOR

Don't put eggs or milk in the refrigerator door because the temperature fluctuates more there, and you need to keep dairy products really cold to ensure they stay fresh for longer. Place them on a shelf in their original carton, which helps them retain moisture.

## KEEP YEAST COOL

If you use a bread maker or make your own breads, store yeast in the fridge where it keeps for much longer and in much better condition than in your cupboard. Old yeast can reduce the bread's rising significantly.

## COOKIE REVIVAL

If you don't want to throw out biscuits just because they've become hard, place them in a sandwich bag with a piece of bread overnight and the next day you'll have soft cookies again – but it only works once.

## IT'S A WRAP

Store flour in a cool, dry, well-ventilated place. Keep it in the bag and wrap it in another plastic bag to prevent it from being attacked by weevils and stay fresh.

## GINGER PRESERVE

Keep ginger root for a long time in your fridge by immersing it in alcohol, which will preserve it. Sherry and vodka work well, and when it's finished you've got ginger-flavoured liquids to add to cooking as well.

## ZAP YOUR BERRIES

If you find yourself with a leftover bowl of strawberries you don't want to waste, liquidize them with a little sugar and freeze. Use as a healthy sorbet or compôte instead of ice cream.

# keeping things fresh

## PILLOW TALK

Don't throw away an old pillowcase – it makes an excellent lettuce bag to keep leafy greens fresh and crisp in the fridge. Wash and dry them thoroughly, then hang the pillowcase in your fridge.

## LEFTOVER FLESH

As a guideline, cover and refrigerate leftover fish and meat within two hours of serving. Fish should be eaten within two days, and meat within three, after being taken off the bone.

## A BUNCH OF BROCCOLI

Broccoli will keep for a couple of weeks if you store it like a bouquet of flowers in the fridge – cut about an inch off the stem and submerge the stem in a bowl or tub of water. Change the water every couple of days and if the base of the stem seems a little slimy, snip the ends off. Broccoli can also be kept in a plastic bag.

## TOFU TIPS

Once you have opened a package of tofu, you should store the unused portion in a container of water, with a tight-fitting lid. Tofu should be used within three days from when you first open the package and the water should be changed daily.

## THE YOLK'S ON ME

If you have a recipe that uses egg whites, you can refrigerate the yolks for later use by storing them, unbroken, in a small bowl, covered with cold water for up to two days.

## THE OTHER HALF

If you've used half an aubergine (eggplant) and want to keep the other half fresh, put it in a sealed plastic bag in the fridge and rub the cut side with lemon juice to stop it going brown. Make sure it's kept airtight and it should stay fresh for a couple of days.

## KEEP MILK COOL

Full milk will stay fresh for 24 days if kept cold but it is very sensitive to temperature and goes off quickly. You will reduce its shelf life drastically by leaving it out for just two hours, so get into the habit of putting your milk back in the fridge as soon as you've finished with it.

## ENHANCE TOMATO FLAVOUR

To bring out the most flavour in tomatoes, store them in a basket on your work surface as chilling them below 55°C (130°F) can harm the flavour. They don't keep as long out of the fridge, so if you're going to do this it's best to buy them no more than one or two days before use.

## MELLOW YELLOW

For unripe fruit you want to soften up in a hurry, leave at room temperature in a bowl with a couple of ripe bananas, which give off enzymes that help other fruit to ripen quicker. Conversely, if you want fruit to ripen slowly keep your bananas in a separate bowl.

## PAY ATTENTION, HONEY

If honey becomes crystallized in the jar, it doesn't mean it's gone off – it just needs a little attention. Just warm the jar up gently in a microwave (be careful of metallic labels and lids) or put in a pan of hot water for a few minutes. A quick stir and it will be as good as new.

## KEEP FLAVOUR IN PAPER

To get the most out of your mushrooms and aubergines, store them in paper bags in the fridge and only wash or wipe them just before use, which will keep them drier for longer and help them retain more flavour.

## FOIL YOUR CELERY

To keep your celery fresh and crisp in the fridge for weeks, wrap it completely in aluminium foil to keep the moisture in.

## COOKING WITH YOGURT

Preserve the benefits of the active cultures in your yogurt by not heating it above 50°C (120°F). High temperatures can kill the beneficial bacteria in yogurts so if you want to use it in cooking, try adding it at the end.

## UNDER WRAPS

Always cover your butter, as it is a very absorbent substance that will absorb fridge odours, making it taste or smell funny. The last thing you want is breakfast toast tinged with last night's curry or garlicky sauce!

## BAG A RIPE ONE

To speed up the process of ripening tomatoes, keep them in a brown paper bag or closed container to trap the ethylene gas that helps them ripen. Adding an ethylene-emitting apple or pear can also help.

## UPSIDE DOWN IT

Sour cream will keep longer in your fridge if you store the container upside down, which reduces the amount of oxidizing air that can find its way into the package. Be careful when you open it, though!

## NOT TOO RIPE

Apples are one of the few fruits which are best eaten slightly underripe, when they are still crunchy. If you keep your apples in the fridge, the cold air will slow down the ripening process but not stop it completely. It's best to buy just a few at a time to maximize your eating pleasure!

## PICK PAPER

Try to avoid food packaged in plastic as much as possible if the food is absorbent, such as meats and cheeses, which could take up toxins from the plastic. Choose paper packages instead, or buy fresh and remove packaging when you get home.

## FREEZE YOUR LOAF

Bread goes stale faster in the fridge than on the counter. Freezing, however, is an excellent way to keep it fresh if you cannot finish it in one day. Cut bread, bagels and buns before freezing, then toast to defrost. Make sure the bread is protected from freezer burn by closing the bag tightly.

## GRAPE FULL

Store your grapes in the coldest part of the fridge in a plastic bag. Make sure you wash them well before you serve them to avoid pesticide residues and other toxins, but don't wash them before you refrigerate as this can cause them to rot.

## REMOVE MOULD

While not a major health threat, mould can make food unappetizing. Don't eat the mould or food that has come into contact with it. Hard cheeses, salami and firm fruits and vegetables can be saved from mould if you cut out the mould and also a large area around it, where there might be growth beneath the surface of the food.

## WASH AND SERVE

Don't prepare your strawberries and raspberries too early if you want them to stay fresh – you can hull or slice them earlier, but only wash them just before you serve, then pat dry with kitchen towel to help them keep their fresh texture.

## PAPER MUSHROOMS

When you bring fresh mushrooms home from shopping, remove them from any plastic wrapping and put them into a paper bag. Fold the top closed and the mushrooms will last a week.

## AVOID THE PLASTIC FANTASTIC

Don't keep meat in plastic in your fridge unless you're going to eat it the same day. Instead, put it on a plate covered with kitchen roll or a tea towel so the meat can breathe but is protected.

## BLEACH WITH LEMONS

Lemon juice is a great way to stop pre-sliced fruit turning brown and unappetizing, and it will give it a fruitier, more intense taste too. Use it on apples, pears and bananas.

## DON'T COVER STRAWBERRIES

The moisture content of fresh strawberries is high, so store uncovered or loosely covered – covering the berries up can cause them to rot, even when refrigerated.

## LEAVE SEEDS ATTACHED

When using only part of a red, green or yellow (bell) pepper, cut it from the bottom or the sides, leaving the seeds attached, and it will remain moist for longer. You can put the rest in a resealable plastic bag and use it 3–4 days later.

### FISH FOR SAFETY

Seafood is responsible for a lot of food poisoning, but it's perfectly safe and very healthy if treated correctly. If you can't use it immediately, remove it from its original wrapping and rinse in cold water. Wrap loosely in plastic wrap, store in the coldest part of the refrigerator, and use within 2 days. Store ready-to-eat fish such as smoked mackerel separately from raw fish.

### FOOD POISONING

Although you might be tempted to keep foods in your fridge and cupboards for a long time, there are certain foods which you should never keep more than a few days – most importantly fresh or thawed meat and fish, and cooked rice.

### A QUICK REFRESH

If your lettuce is looking a little droopy, try a restaurant trick by refreshing it before you serve it. Fill a bowl with ice cubes and water and plunge the lettuce into it to give it back a bit of its lost crispness.

### KEEP LETTUCE DRY

To keep lettuce fresher longer wrap a dry paper towel around the root end of the lettuce head and store in a freezer bag or in a sealed plastic container in your fridge. The paper towel will absorb the excess water.

## freezing & reheating

### MEAT-FREEZE ZONE

If you want to freeze raw meat at home, make sure you do it before the "use by" date, and preferably as soon as you get it home. Defrost properly, try to use within one day of defrosting and make sure it's cooked right through before serving.

## USE THE RIGHT SETTING

If you're defrosting meat or fish in the microwave, choose the defrost setting or use low power to stop the outer edges of the food cooking before the middle defrosts. Arrange loose pieces of fish or meat in a single layer with thickest parts or largest pieces towards the outside.

## CAN'T FREEZE EVERYTHING

You can freeze any food except canned or preserved food or whole eggs. Some foods, however, do not freeze well. High-fat dairy products like cream and mayonnaise tend to separate when defrosted, and high water content vegetables, such as lettuce and cucumber, will go soggy.

## THE BIG FREEZE

The freezer should be below -18°C (0°F). If items are not frozen solid, then the temperature is too low. Check from time to time and throw food away the minute you notice any slight defrosting, because harmful bacteria could be thriving in the too-warm conditions.

## DON'T DOUBLE YOUR JEOPARDY

You can refreeze frozen food that has partially thawed as long as it still contains frozen areas. If it has thawed through, however, or has been at room temperature rather than refrigerated, you shouldn't refreeze it and it should either be cooked or discarded.

## ICE IN SOME FLAVOUR

Don't worry that freezing your meals will harm them or lessen the flavour – in fact, for dishes such as lasagne and stews freezing can be beneficial as it increases the diffusion of antioxidant-rich herbs and spices.

## WARM UP SLOWLY

It is not ideal to defrost food at room temperature. The best way to defrost is by planning ahead and allowing the food to defrost slowly in the fridge. If you're not organized enough to do this, use the microwave. But as it can partially cook food, it's best to cook the food directly after defrosting as it is not safe to keep partially cooked food in the fridge.

## COOK IT THROUGH

Contrary to popular belief, freezing doesn't actually kill bacteria or other food microbes, but what it does do is put them in a dormant state so they won't be active or reproducing until the food is thawed again. This is why it's important to cook food thoroughly after defrosting.

## TAKE A BATH

If you don't want to use the microwave – or you're defrosting something too big to fit in – you can submerge the food in cold water, remembering to change the water every 30 minutes to speed up the thawing process. Certain types of food can become watery with this method, but it's great for joints of meat and poultry.

## FREEZE YOUR EGGS

The best way to make sure you don't waste eggs, especially if you cook or bake a lot, is to separate the eggs and freeze whites and yolks separately in a lightly oiled ice-cube tray. When frozen, pop them out and store in separate Ziploc bags in the freezer.

## GET A THERMOMETER

Don't just rely on your inbuilt thermometer to ensure that your fridge is at the right temperature. Invest in an appliance thermometer and check regularly that your refrigerator is at 4°C (40°F) or colder and your freezer is at -18°C (0°F).

## STORE UP A TV DINNER

Instead of ordering a takeaway when you can't be bothered to cook, make your own "emergency" TV dinners using leftovers by investing in a three-section reusable plastic container. Fill up each section with protein, vegetable and starch respectively. If all three sections aren't full after one meal, fill up with leftovers from your next meal.

## TURN UP THE HEAT

If you're using leftovers, make sure they are piping hot throughout when reheating, to ensure that any bacteria or microbes are killed off – bacteria are destroyed very quickly with heat. Gravies and soups should be heated to a rolling boil, and other food to 74°C (165°F). Refrigerated leftovers should be used within 3 days.

## THAW IT COLD

Thaw meat in the refrigerator rather than on your kitchen surface, where food is more susceptible to bacteria and might thaw too quickly. Store meat and fish on a dish on the bottom shelf as they defrost, so that the juices don't drip on to other foods and contaminate them.

## CRUMBS!

If you have unused digestive biscuits (graham crackers) in your cupboard, crush them up and add melted butter to make a cheesecake base, then freeze. Simply mix together cream cheese, condensed milk and lemon juice to make a quick topping.

## HERB CUBES

One of the reasons so many people like shop-bought sauces is that they never have the right ingredients to hand. Stock up with herbs that won't last in the refrigerator, like basil or parsley, by finely chopping and freezing with a small amount of water in ice-cube trays. When you need herbs for a recipe, just toss in a cube.

## SHUT THAT DOOR

In case of a power cut, keep the fridge and freezer doors closed as much as possible. Food should last in the fridge for 4 to 6 hours and in the freezer for 1 to 2 days, depending how full the freezer is – the fuller it is, the longer the food will last.

## HAVE YOUR CAKE AND FREEZE IT

If you want to freeze a cake or dessert but aren't sure you're going to want the whole lot in one go, why not cut it before freezing. Then you can take out one or two slices at a time, as and when you need them. If buying frozen, though, it's not safe to defrost to cut, then refreeze.

## REHEAT YOUR RICE

Freeze leftover cooked long grain or brown rice (other varieties tend to get sticky) for quick use later. Cool the cooked rice before packaging in plastic freezer storage bags and freeze flat. Remember, rice can only be reheated once, so only defrost as much as you need. Also, cooked rice should never be stored at room temperature.

## BAG THE CUBES

If you're freezing food leftovers or baby meals in ice-cube trays, put the trays in a large plastic bag before you freeze them. This will cut out the air and stop the tops of them from drying out as they freeze, which means they'll keep longer.

## BATCH YOUR BROWNING

Browning beef mince (ground beef) can be time consuming, and also messy. Try browning a large batch all in one go when you've got a spare hour or so, then freeze it in your usual-sized portions. Remove it from the freezer and defrost as you need to. Remember not to refreeze it.

## NO NEED TO CRY

Many people object to chopping onions because it makes them cry. Put a stop to regular tears by preparing 20 or so onions at a time – peel and chop them all, then freeze in a plastic bag. Be aware, though, that they may soften and lose a little of their flavour in freezing.

## ACCUMULATE A STEW

When you have a spoonful or so of vegetables such as beans, peas or corn left over after a meal, put in a freezer container or bag in the freezer instead of throwing them away. Then, once you've accumulated enough, use your veggie leftovers to make a stew or soup.

## FLATTEN BAGS

Freeze ground meat in 500 g (1 lb) portions and place in freezer storage bags. Flatten out to the edges of the bag and remove all the air before sealing then freezing. These flat bags of ground meat stack neatly in the freezer, thaw quickly, and it's easy just to break off a bit and reseal.

## DON'T WASTE WINE

Next time you have a glass or so of wine left in the bottle that you just can't finish, don't throw it away. Freeze it in an ice-cube tray then pop the cubes into a sealed bag and use in recipes that require a little wine – and avoid having to open a new bottle before you need to.

### GO GINGERLY

Fresh ginger is a great addition to many recipes, but you only need a little and it can be messy to grate. Try freezing it when you buy it then grating as much as you need straight from frozen.

### KEEP IT TIGHT

The tighter you wrap foods before freezing, the better they will last because fewer ice crystals, which dry the food out, will form. Make sure air is removed from bags and larger items are well wrapped.

### BULK UP YOUR BACON

Bacon is a great protein-filled snack, but the mess it creates in the kitchen can put people off cooking it. Try buying in bulk, cooking, cooling and then freezing. When you want a snack, you can simply microwave a few rashers.

### BABY PUREES

Instead of buying baby food in jars, which may contain preservatives, make up a big batch of puréed vegetables and freeze it in ice cube trays. Defrost one or two ice cubes for each meal.

### A STRONG BASE

Frozen sauce bases are great for when you don't have time to cook. Try freezing small portions of white sauce that you can defrost, and add cocoa for a chocolate sauce or cheese to make a cheese sauce. You can also freeze a tomato-based sauce.

### SQUEEZE OUT THE AIR

When you're freezing foods, reducing the amount of air in packages not only helps your freezer to work more efficiently by making packages less bulky, but also prevents ice crystals forming on foods.

## meal planning

### COOK UP A STORM

If you live alone, it can be difficult to muster up the energy to cook a healthy meal for yourself. Try cooking up meals in batches and freezing them, or cook extra and use the leftovers for the next night or two.

## MAKE GRAFFITI

Don't be afraid to annotate your recipe books when you make changes – instead of using them as food bibles, think of them as starting points and use your own creativity to make healthy changes, making notes as you go. It's usually a good idea to make the original recipe first so that you can compare with any alterations.

## ONLINE ADVICE

If you're having problems making a meal or menu plan for you or your family, visit one of the increasingly popular menu-planning websites online. Some of these even suggest weekly menus and shopping lists, which means all you have to do is the cooking!

## ONE-POT COOKING

If you're cooking for one or two, preparing one-dish meals such as beef, barley and vegetable stew, chicken or turkey casserole, vegetarian chilli con carne, or fish and vegetables roasted in a foil package will give you the benefits of home cooking without the hassle.

## TICK THE RIGHT BOXES

To make sure you and your family are getting the right levels of nutrients in your diet, make yourself a weekly or fortnightly meal planner. Include tick boxes for essential nutrients – that way, you can check at a glance whether your diet is balanced and healthy.

## PLAN YOUR SHOP

Planning your meals for a week or two at a time and then putting together a grocery list with everything you need to cook those meals will cut your trips to the supermarket down to one a week – giving you more time to cook up all those fresh ingredients. You'll be less tempted by fast foods, too.

## BE AN EARLY BIRD

It might be tempting to lie in for a few extra minutes each morning and skip breakfast, but studies have shown that breakfast eaters are slimmer and perform better at work. Set your alarm five minutes earlier than normal and sit down to eat before you leave the house.

## MEALY MOUTHED

Redefine a "meal" – if you're short on time or energy, make a nutritious snack rather than a full meal, but make sure you serve it on a plate rather than eating it on the go. Try healthy snacks such as rice cakes with cheese, olives and tomatoes, or oatcakes with apple and cheese slices.

## SAVE YOUR PLANS

Keep hold of each week's menu plans, especially when you feel they have worked well, and you will soon be able to start using previous plans for reference, or even repeat successful weeks in their entirety.

## BE RIGID

A really rigid meal plan and schedule makes the early days of a diet much easier to stick to because it eliminates choice, helping you to deal more easily with temptation. Try to stick to it for at least five days, preferably two weeks, before you get in the swing.

## NO GOING OFF

Plan your meals around the things that go off most quickly. To avoid soggy veg, for instance, if you buy a big bag of carrots, try to include them in several dinner recipes. Eat them as snacks, too, and use them up by making a carrot cake towards the end of the week.

## FREE UP FIVE MINUTES

Many people have a problem with meal planning, because they can never find the time. Make a five-minute slot in your day or week to sit down with a cup of tea or cold drink and plan at least your day's, if not your week's, meals. The more you do it, the easier it gets.

## MEAL FILE

Make yourself a family meal planning file. Keep your previous week's plans in it as well as blank paper for shopping lists, recipes you want to try and any coupons you might have cut out and saved.

## TEAR OUT A PAGE

Many magazines and newspapers now contain recipes which you may want to try, and these are often aimed at healthy eating. Create a "healthy eating" recipe folder or scrapbook to keep them all in once place, and use different headings to make the recipes easy to access.

## CHECK YOUR STORES

Don't forget what's already in your cupboards. Every week or month, look through your kitchen store cupboards to see if there are any foods you can use to plan your meals around. That way, you'll reduce food wastage and give yourself some ideas as well.

## THINK OF THE FREEZER

Think ahead when planning meals and use your freezer. If you're making something that freezes well like a lasagne or a spaghetti sauce, a stew or casserole, make double and freeze the second portion for those days where you just don't have any time to cook.

## ADD FRUITY FLAVOUR

Get a vitamin boost by adding fruit to flavour main meals as well as puddings – cook rice in a mixture of water and apple juice, sprinkle broccoli or spinach with raisins, sunflower seeds or chopped almonds, or simmer carrots and parsnips in orange juice.

## SLIP IN A QUICKIE

Although going to the supermarket once a week is a good way to save time and avoid overspending, it may not always be possible for all items. If you buy a lot of fresh fruit and vegetables you may want to include only half a week's worth of items on your list, and to make a second quick trip during the week for the rest.

## BE REALISTIC

When you're planning meals, remember to make allowances for days when you don't have a lot of time. If you know Tuesdays are always stressful, plan something simple for that day like leftover meat and steamed vegetables or salad.

### BALANCE YOUR INTAKE
Planning meals is a great idea because you can make sure you balance your meals both nutritionally and in terms of cost. If you plan an expensive meal one night, balance it with a pasta dish or a cheaper vegetarian meal the next.

### IN FULL VIEW
Stick your weekly or bi-weekly menu on your fridge or other prominent place and plan ahead every day. Make a note on your plan if you need to take something out of the freezer, for instance, or if you can prepare part of the meal in advance.

## tastes & flavours

### FRUIT UP YOUR FISH
Don't just stick to serving vegetables with your evening meals – fruit tastes good with fish and meat and is a great way to increase your vitamin and antioxidant intake. Try mango and papaya with tuna, apple with chicken, or pineapple with pork.

### ADD FLAVOUR LATER
For dishes that take a long time to cook, beware of overflavouring with herbs and spices, which often develop stronger flavour the longer they cook. Add very few herbs and spices at the beginning and an hour before serving add more if you think the dish needs it.

### DRIED MEANS LESS
Fresh herbs are a great way to get flavour and an added fresh vitamin boost into your dishes, but they're not always available. Remember if you're using dried herbs they're much more pungent than fresh – you need on average one third of the fresh amount.

### TOAST YOUR SPICES
Whenever possible, grind whole spices in a grinder or mortar and pestle just prior to using. Toasting whole spices in a dry skillet over medium heat before grinding will bring out even more flavour, but be careful not to burn them.

## SHAKE A FLAVOUR FEAST

Add flavour to your food on the plate without using oils and other calorie-filled flavour enhancers by creating your own flavour shakers. Choose your favourite dried herbs and spices and combine in a sugar or salt pot to give flavour without fat – try chilli and chives or basil and oregano.

## STICK WITH STEVIA

Instead of using refined white sugar as a sweetener, go for a natural-sweetening option with the no-calorie herb stevia, a herb from Paraguay with a slightly liquorice aftertaste that is approximately 100 to 400 times sweeter than sugar. It can be purchased in most health food shops and can be used for cooking or baking.

## MORE CINNAMON LESS SUGAR

In baked spiced recipes like muffins and biscuits, try reducing the amount of sugar in your recipes by half and doubling the cinnamon. Not only will the cinnamon taste help retain sweetness with the least calories possible, it has also been shown to help control blood sugar levels.

## HEALTHIER SWEETNESS

Try natural alternatives to sugar in baking and for sweetening drinks and desserts. Barley malt, rice syrup and granulate cane juice all contain as many calories as sugar, but they also have added minerals and vitamins so are slightly healthier.

## MUNCH A MACADAMIA

If you love shortbread or buttery biscuits, try closing your eyes and snacking on a handful of macadamia nuts instead. With a rich, buttery taste because of their healthy unsaturated fats, they are filling as well as being low in carbohydrates and high in magnesium, iron and calcium.

## OREGANO AND GO

The herb oregano is high in antioxidants, and tastes great finely chopped and scattered over salads, grilled meats and fish. Fresh oregano is also very good added to Italian dishes like pizza, pasta and Bolognese sauces.

## TREAD GINGERLY

Dried ginger is quite different from fresh. It has a slightly sweet flavour and a hint of citrus as well as the characteristic ginger kick. It can be used to replace sugar in recipes containing fruits like apple and pear, and instead of salt to enhance the flavour of chicken, turkey and rice.

## MAKE IT WITH MACE

Experiment with spices to replace salt and complement your food. If you find nutmeg too overpowering, try mace. Mace is ground from the covering of the nutmeg seed and is warmer and more delicate in flavour. Use in sauces and meat stews and sprinkled on to vegetables.

## STAR SUGAR SUBSTITUTE

Instead of piling sugar into your puddings, think of alternatives like star anise and liquorice, which can add a delicious tang without piling on the calories, especially if you combine it with using low-fat yogurt or crème fraîche.

## GO NATURAL

Replace high-fat sour cream in recipes and as a garnish with low-fat natural yogurt instead. Not only does it contain fewer calories, but if you buy a live version it also contains bacteria which are beneficial to your digestive system. Or substitute half and half if you want to keep the taste but reduce the calories.

## SPRINKLE SOME SPICE

To easily reduce sugar in sweet recipes without losing out on taste, try substituting spices like cardamom, cinnamon, nutmeg or vanilla, which will enhance the impression of sweetness without adding calories. You can replace the sugar in recipes between a half and a third without altering the result.

## DON'T CAST AWAY THE CARAWAY

Caraway seeds add a nutty, almost liquorice flavour to foods and are often used in rye breads and other speciality baking. Use them instead of salt to flavour cooked vegetables such as parsnips, carrots and beetroot. They're delicious in parsnip soup and pork and tomato casserole.

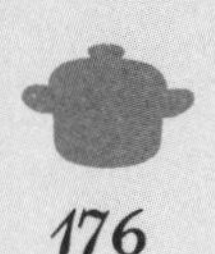



### CLOVES FOR MEMORY

Cloves are not only great for adding their characteristic flavour, they also contain chemicals which aid digestion. Cloves are also believed to improve mental clarity and memory, so adding them to slow-cooked, spiced dishes like stews and curries is a very good idea all round.

### GARLIC ON A STICK

For the flavour and health benefits of garlic in cooking without actually having to bite through the flesh, stick a whole clove of garlic on a toothpick and add to soups and stews – that way, you'll be able to find and remove it easily before serving.

### MAKE YOUR OWN MILK

You can make your own healthy low-fat buttermilk for recipes by mixing one cup (235 ml or ½ pint) of plain yogurt with either one teaspoon cream of tartar or one cup of milk and a tablespoon of vinegar.

### ADD MUSHROOMS TO TASTE

Instead of mayonnaise and creamy dressings, think about ways you can add interest to your salads without adding fat. Raw, chopped or whole mushrooms are a great way to add taste.

## quick fixers

### GET IT RIGHT WITH RICE

If you want a boost of energy in a hurry, which will keep you going for hours until you next eat, try whipping yourself up a simple and healthy carbohydrate treat – mix cooked brown rice with herbs and lemon juice and sprinkle with toasted sunflower or pumpkin seeds.

### COOK UP AN OMELETTE

If you've only got a few minutes for supper, an omelette with vegetables like spinach, onion and broccoli makes a quick healthy meal. Use lots of vegetables and just enough egg to hold it together, then add salad for an extra health boost.

## A QUICK FIX

For a quick, nutritious TV dinner, bake or microwave a sweet potato and instead of butter, drizzle with a little honey or maple syrup and sprinkle with cinnamon and/or nutmeg. Then serve with salad and a protein source such as fish or meat. Kids love it, too.

## TASTE THE TABOULLEH

For a fresh and healthy alternative to pasta or rice, make up a bowl of Lebanese taboulleh, which is made from cracked wheat and traditionally contains large amounts of healthy parsley as well as tomato, onion and extra virgin olive oil.

## GLAZED FRUIT DESSERT

Cook yourself a decadent dessert that's a lot healthier than it might seem by glazing pineapple with rum or brandy and frying or grilling until warm. Serve with a sauce made from reduced orange juice, cinnamon and nutmeg and a spoonful of natural yogurt.

## GET SAUCY

Make your own light pasta sauce using fat-free or low-fat cottage cheese puréed or whisked together with a touch of evaporated skimmed milk, lemon juice and a little rosemary. Shred some spinach into the dish just before serving for colour and an added health boost.

## BIND WITH BEANS

Instead of creamy dips, use the binding power of beans to knock up healthy eastern-style hors-d'oeuvres. Purée kidney beans with garlic, red chilli, powdered cumin seed, lime juice, olive oil and tomatoes, then stir in chopped onion and coriander leaves.

## A HEALTHY BLEND

To make a healthy breakfast smoothie, blend strawberries and papaya (low-GI foods with a high antioxidant content) and half a banana (for blood sugar regulation) with skimmed milk (for calcium) ice cubes and a squeeze of maple syrup (for taste!).

## BAKE A WHOLESOME TREAT

Bake up a batch of healthy muffins for family breakfasts and snacks. If you make your own you can include only the best ingredients – and you'll know they won't contain preservatives and artificial flavourings or colourings. Choose ingredients like oats, banana, honey, raisins, bran and blueberries.

## START THE DAY WELL

For a great carb-free breakfast, have a bowl of yogurt – which has digestive benefits as well as calcium – and fresh berries for a morning vitamin boost. Add some flaxseed oil or ground flaxseeds for a dose of omega-3 oils for a perfect start.

## BOOST BREAKFAST ENERGY

Don't only use fruit for your morning smoothie. Kick start the day with an energy-giving blend of green tea (for a healthy caffeine boost), carrot juice (for carbohydrates) and your chosen fruit (try mango and banana or apricots and plums). Add low-fat natural yogurt as a filler.

## HOME IS BEST

Make sure you eat breakfast at home rather than on the go, as take-away breakfasts are often laden with calories and sugar. A regular latte with a flapjack adds up to an astounding 750 calories, compared with around 250 for a bowl of cereal and a cup of tea or coffee with skimmed milk.

## GRILLED FRUIT

For a quick, healthy pudding, try making fruit kebabs. Peel and chop fruit into similar sizes, then alternate on a skewer and grill for a few minutes on each side. Serve alone or with natural yogurt and a dash of honey or maple syrup.

## TAKE A CHEESY DIP

Instead of dipping crudités and raw vegetables into dips like taramasalata and sour cream, which can be fattening, try making your own healthy version using cottage cheese, spring onions and garlic.

## BREAKFAST ON MUESLI

Set yourself up for the day with a bowl of muesli with low-fat milk, fruit and low-fat yogurt. The oats and wholegrains will help you to feel full until lunchtime.

## BUTTER AN APPLE

Cut one apple into thin slices and top with 1–2 tbsp of peanut butter. Include a glass of milk or a small carton of low-fat yogurt for an unusual, all-round healthy breakfast.

## NOT MUSH-ROOM FOR MEAT

Mushrooms have a great meaty texture and are an easy and cheap way to cut down your meat intake. Choose grilled portabello mushrooms in place of a burger (or in place of the bun if you're cutting out bread).

## COOK WHEN YOU RISE

Don't be afraid to use your oven in the morning. Eggs with wholemeal bread are a great way to start the day, giving you a good measure of protein and carbohydrate. Add a piece of fresh fruit for total balance.

## PICK THE RIGHT PASTA

Substitute wholewheat pasta for plain pasta in recipes, particularly in the evening when you don't want a quick release of sugar into your system.

## GET THE GREEN BENEFITS

Instead of iceberg lettuce in your salad, which has fairly low levels of nutrients (but is still better than no salad) choose leafier, darker greens like chicory, kale, rocket or watercress, which contain higher levels of nutrients.

## BULK UP WITH VEG

If you're making a meat stew or casserole, halve the amount of meat required and substitute it with vegetables. That way, you'll cut the calories and give yourself a bit of added vegetable goodness, not to mention reducing the costs.

## DITCH THE GRANOLA

Granola might seem like a healthy breakfast choice because it's packed with fruit and carbohydrates, but unfortunately it's also full of fat and sugar, and is one of the most calorific cereals on the market. Stick to low-fat muesli instead, or dilute it with some healthy oats or bran. It's also delicious used as a topping for low-fat yogurt.

## SKIM OFF SOME WEIGHT

Skimmed milk contains about half the calories of whole milk (80 compared to about 150 for one cup), and semi-skimmed milk sits somewhere in between. Lower-fat versions also provide the body with more calcium, so they're the healthier choice, unless you're underweight or a child.

## BAKE YOUR OWN BREAD

Bread is often full of additives such as palm oil and even hormones, so one of the best ideas for family cooking is to invest in a breadmaking machine. They're relatively cheap and very easy to use – and you'll know exactly what your kids are eating.

## LOVE YOUR LENTILS

Serve brown or wild rice or lentils instead of white rice as a filler with your meals. The rice doesn't taste very different and because you're choosing wholegrains they're better for your digestive system and have a lower GI.

# healthy preparation

## SPLIT YOUR EGGS

To help your low-fat diet, separate out the yolks and whites of your eggs so that you only use the more calorific yolks if you really need them. Do this by breaking the egg in half then transferring the yolk from one side of the shell to the other, while collecting the white that falls out in a bowl below.

## CHOOSE QUALITY INGREDIENTS

Choosing quality, rather than quantity, when it comes to cooking can help you stay healthy because you'll get a great deal of flavour without having to pile up your plate. Try a dash of balsamic vinegar for dressings or truffle oil instead of butter in mashed potato.

## TAKE A WORLD VIEW

Think global and try incorporating the healthiest part of other cultures' eating habits into your diet – the olive oil and fresh vegetables of the Mediterranean, Japan's variety of small, tasty portions, the fish of Scandinavia, and Latin America's fibre-filled wholegrains.

## UP-TEMPO EGGS

When you're going to beat egg whites for a recipe, let the eggs sit at room temperature for 30 minutes before using them. The egg whites will then beat to a greater volume.

## BE A FRESH PHYT-ER

Adding a variety of fresh herbs to cooking is a great idea because each herb contains different types and levels of health-giving phytochemicals, which are used in the body to help mop up free radicals and fight damage. Add them freshly picked just before serving for the best effect.

## RUN THE COARSE

It's healthier to use coarse ground salt than powdered varieties in measured recipes. This is because the lower surface area to volume ratio means the food absorbs less of the potentially damaging sodium.

## SKIM OFF THE CALORIES

Preparing your desserts with skimmed milk instead of whole milk will save around 63 calories and 8 g of fat per serving, so use skimmed milk whenever you can, and use single (light) cream instead of double (heavy) where possible, too.

## BASE IT ON STOCK

If you want to marinade but don't want your fish or meat swimming in oil, use fruit juice or stock to form the base instead. You'll still help the meat retain flavour and tenderness without using extra oil.

## USE DRY MARINADES

Instead of marinating meats in oil and your favourite spices, rub the dried spices into the meat instead. That way, you won't be adding any extra fat to the meat and you'll get the same yummy taste.

## LET IT EXPAND

To ensure the optimum taste of meat, allow it to come to room temperature for half an hour to an hour before cooking. This will allow the meat to expand, helping the taste to spread evenly during cooking.

## MEASURE THE OIL

Don't splash oil into the pan before frying or stir-frying without measuring it – you might use more than you need. Most frying only needs a teaspoon or less of oil per serving.

## FLOUR YOUR RECIPES

Instead of using egg as a thickener in recipes, use a tablespoon of wholewheat flour, which will play the same thickening role but with far fewer calories. If the egg is being used as a binding agent, use flour and oil instead.

## BAG THE DRESSING

To limit the amount of oily dressing you use on salads, don't pour it directly on to the salad in a bowl. Instead, start by putting all your salad ingredients into a Ziploc bag. Add a small amount of salad dressing and shake the bag before dividing into individual bowls.

## OAT ROLLING

Rolled oats are quicker to cook but not quite as good for you as unrolled oats, which have a very low GI rating (meaning they release energy very slowly). If you want the best of both worlds, blitz your unrolled oats in the blender to turn them into instant oatmeal!

## MIX IN SOME OIL

If your recipe requires eggs but you don't want the calories of egg yolk, use the egg white mixed with a teaspoon of olive oil instead. This gives a better consistency than using the whites on their own, which can make the mixture too light, plus extra health benefits.

## THE WHOLE STORY

Whenever possible, avoid buying salad leaves in ready-prepared bags available in supermarkets, as they have often been washed with chlorine products to kill bugs. Buy lettuces whole instead, and wash them yourself.

## AN OATY COAT

Use rolled oats or crushed bran cereal instead of breadcrumbs on your fish fillets or chicken drumsticks – you'll use less because it's more powdery and it will give you a wholegrain boost into the bargain!

## HOW TO CHOP ONIONS

To chop onions the easy way, start by cutting off the stem end, then peel the skin back to the root, but keep it attached. Holding the skin to steady the onion, cut towards the root end but not through the root, then slice finely across the onion from the stem end.

## DITCH THE SALT

Unsalted butter can be substituted for normal salted butter in most recipes. You won't usually notice any difference in taste, but you will be cutting down on salt.

## MAKE DO WITHOUT MAYO

Instead of mayonnaise, combine low-fat yogurt with low-fat cottage cheese and mix well together. If you like, you can add extra flavour with a little mustard, garlic or some fresh or dried herbs.

## STUFF A MUSHROOM

Instead of filling your poultry with a stuffing that's heavy on breadcrumbs, substitute half the breadcrumbs for chopped mushrooms. They'll keep their form, taste really good and cut down your carbohydrate intake.

## BAN THE BOOZE

Alcohol is an optional ingredient in many recipes like stews and pasta sauces and gives a distinctive flavour. If you'd prefer a lower-calorie option, you can substitute with stock in most savoury dishes, and fruit juice in most sweet recipes.

## KEEP IT LEMON FRESH

When preparing ripe avocados, to avoid the flesh turning brown and looking unattractive when exposed to air, immediately place the cut fruit (flesh side down) in lemon juice until ready for use. Covering the cut surface tightly with clingfilm (plastic wrap) and putting it in the fridge will also stop it changing colour. Use within a couple of days.

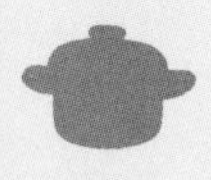



# equipment & utensils

## RACK UP YOUR HEALTH

Invest in a roasting rack for your Sunday dinners. The principle is that the rack elevates the meat or poultry, allowing fat to drip into the pan below and reducing the amount of fat on the roast. A rack is also a good idea for cooking sausages and chicken pieces in the oven.

## PUT A LID ON IT

If you're stir-frying, invest in a lid for your frying pan or wok. Covering will increase the humidity of your cooking, meaning you can use less oil to achieve non-stick results.

## BUY QUALITY

Invest in a set of quality non-stick pots and pans so you can bake and sauté without adding extra oil. If you can only afford one or two, go for a frying pan first, then a large pan for pasta, and so on.

## ACHIEVE GRATE THINGS

Instead of relying on slices of cheese, use a cheese grater, which will help you use smaller portions because it adds air to the cheese. Your grater should also have a thin slicer with which you can cut thinner slices than you would by hand.

## MAKE THE CUT

Invest in one good quality kitchen knife rather than an array of cheaper ones, and keep it sharp. It will help with healthy eating by allowing you to cut nearer to the skin of fruit and vegetables, where more nutrients are stored, and to cut the fat off meat without wasting the flesh.

## GET A GRILL

To cook your food more healthily, especially if you rely on fried foods, consider investing in one of the many varieties of fat-free electric grills on the market, or a simple griddle (grill) pan. There's no need to add any oil to these – just get the pan nice and hot and cook as you would do when pan frying.

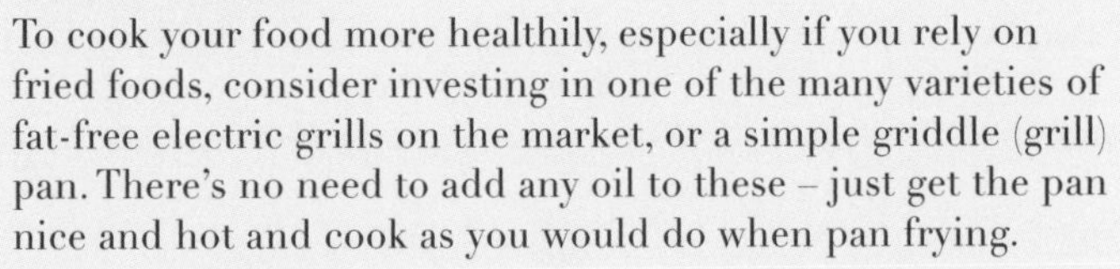


## STICK TO THE SKINS

Next time you plan on serving mashed potatoes, just stop for a minute and consider that the act of mashing will raise their glycaemic index as well as causing loss of healthy vitamins. Serving them baked in their skins with a low-fat filling such as cottage cheese is much healthier.

## ROAST POTATOES

Instead of using your deep-fat fryer to make chips (French fries), create a healthy version by roasting thick slices of sweet potato in olive oil – leave the skins on for added goodness.

## ADVICE OF A MEDIUM

One of the main benefits of eating fish and meat is the essential amino acids they provide, which help the body with energy and the growth and repair of cells. Moderate cooking enhances this benefit, but overcooking can kill them off, so choose medium-cooked meat and fish.

## ADJUST TIMINGS

It's important to cook grains for long enough for the body to absorb their nutrients, but be aware that cooking times aren't set in stone. Grains that have been in storage for a long time will take longer to cook through than recently harvested ones, and toasted grains often cook faster because the breakdown process has already begun.

## A CAKEY COOKIE

If you're making biscuits or cookies, choose to make the soft drop, more cakey version rather than the rolled variety – they generally contain more air per serving and therefore fewer calories.

## BUY PRE-SOAKED

It can be difficult to add wholegrains to recipes because of the soaking or cooking time required. Many supermarkets now sell pre-soaked varieties which cook in 30–45 minutes, or try cooking up a batch at once and keeping it (for 2–3 days in the fridge or several months in the freezer).

## WOBBLE YOUR FRUIT

Instead of fattening puddings, why not serve fruit set in jelly? It's a favourite with adults and children alike and looks smart and sleek served in individual portions, with the added bonus of being very low in calories. Use apple juice instead of sugar to sweeten.

## COOK UP A JUS

Instead of serving your roast meals with traditional thick gravy, which can add calories to a meal because of the flour and fat it contains, try a small amount of meat juices. Add a dash of lemon juice or white wine for poultry and a little red wine or balsamic vinegar for red meats.

## OIL QUALITY TEST

Test the quality of your olive oil by frying a few drops in a pan – really good quality oil which has the most health benefits will stay green and light. If it turns dark and loses its shine, it's not a good quality oil.

## BRAISE THE FLAVOUR

One of the healthiest ways of cooking meat, particularly tougher cuts which need longer, is braising. This method involves browning in a pan, then slowly cooking with a small quantity of liquid such as water or stock, to retain tenderness without adding fat.

## DOUBLE YOUR DISH

If you're preparing a family meal such as shepherd's pie, beef stew or lasagne, make double and freeze half of it so you've got a healthy emergency family meal to hand if you ever need it.

## COOK THINGS SLOWLY

If you're busy all day and don't have the time or energy to cook a healthy meal when you get home every night, think about investing in a slow cooker or slow steamer. You'll have a healthy meal to come home to – and you're less likely to think about snacking when you get back.

## FLAKE YOUR FISH

For added crunch with fewer calories, use cornflakes instead of breadcrumbs to coat fish fillets. Not only do cornflakes contain fewer calories than breadcrumbs, they are less absorbent and give a lighter covering, so will absorb less oil.

## SQUASH WINTER BLUES

Butternut squash is a fantastic winter food that can store its healthy nutrients and betacarotene for months, but it can be hard to cut and prepare. Prick a few holes in the skin and put it into the microwave oven on high power for 1 minute. Let it sit for a minute and it should be easier to cut – now there's no excuse!

## AFTERNOON ZEST

Citrus fruits are a great way of getting a vitamin boost and their aromas are thought to help boost energy and alertness, so they're a great afternoon pick-me-up. The zest is great sprinkled on yogurts for pudding – grate and store the rinds of your oranges, lemons or grapefruits instead of throwing away.

## TOWEL AWAY GREASE

When grease settles on broth or soup, float a piece of paper towel lightly on top of the liquid and it will absorb grease. Don't allow it to become sodden – you may have to use more than one piece – and lightly lift to remove excess oil.

## LET MEAT STAND

After cooking a joint of meat, you should always let it stand for 10–15 minutes (depending on the size of the joint) to "rest". The meat will actually continue to gently cook during this time, which allows the juices to permeate the meat and makes it taste more full and tender.

## LETTUCE ON STAND-BY

If you don't like washing your salad leaves every time you prepare a salad or garnish, keep a ready-washed store in your fridge. Wash and dry whole lettuce leaves (breaking them up causes them to go limp quickly) and dry carefully with kitchen towel (being careful not to squash them), then store in a large plastic bag in the fridge.

## RINSE YOUR MINCE

When making meals using beef mince (ground beef) at home, try this fat-reducing tip: put the browned mince into a strainer and rinse with hot water until the water runs clear, removing the fat in the process.

## REDUCE YOUR OIL

Use your microwave to cook foods without covering them in oil. Microwave cooking relies on water content, not fat, so is often lower in calories than oven-cooked food. It's especially useful for fish and vegetables.

## MASH WITH WATER

Save on fat when making mashed potatoes by setting aside some of the water the potatoes were cooked in and adding it to the potatoes when mashing them. The potatoes will be just as fluffy without butter.

## USE A VINEGAR SHIELD

If you're making a pasta salad, cut down the amount of dressing or mayonnaise your pasta soaks up by tossing it in a little vinegar first, to coat it with a fat-repelling layer.

## TOSS IN HOT WATER

Instead of tossing your cooked pasta with oil to prevent it sticking, use stock instead, or a little hot water. That way, you won't be adding any extra calories to your meal, and you can enjoy a little more sauce instead!

## ALL BY ITSELF

Balsamic vinegar makes a great fat-free salad dressing. Try it sprinkled on ripe tomatoes with some fresh basil on top. For extra taste try the really thick varieties – they're expensive but you only need a few drops.

## SKIM OFF THE FAT

For a low-fat soup, the best way to remove all the excess fat is to cool then refrigerate the soup. Then simply skim off the hardened fat when it's cold.

## USE A LEAF TO CUT FAT

If you're making a quick soup and you want to get rid of the fat from the top, but haven't got time to refrigerate it, try throwing in a large lettuce leaf. The fat will stick to it, then you can remove and discard it.

## NON-BISCUIT BASE

If your recipe calls for biscuits, such as crushed digestives (graham crackers) for the base of a cheesecake, try crushed oatcakes with no added sugar instead. They're a healthy alternative, made from wholegrains and full of fibre and vitamin B. Muesli is another good alternative.

## CUT THE ICE

Ice cubes are another great soup or casserole de-greaser. Simply drop in a few ice cubes and watch the fat and grease cling to them, then remove (before they have time to melt) and throw away. Or wrap them in muslin and drag over the surface instead.

## DITCH THE ALCOHOL

Contrary to popular belief, alcohol in recipes doesn't burn off entirely with cooking. Even after an hour, 25% of the alcohol can remain, and three hours later there is still a residue of 5%. Choose alternatives like dealcoholized wine, vinegar or fruit juices instead.

## NON-STICK SPAGHETTI

To make sure you don't pile your plate too high with spaghetti, stop it sticking together (especially if you're using fresh rather than dried pasta) by washing off the starch with boiling water once it's cooked. The sauce won't cling as well, but you'll be able to better control portion sizes.

## SOAK UP FAT

Place a few pieces of dry bread in the grill (broiler) pan when grilling meats to soak up dripping fat. This not only means your meats will be leaner, it eliminates smoking fat and therefore reduces fire risk.

## DON'T OVERCOOK FISH

Fish tastes best when it's cooked just enough, and not overcooked. As a general rule, cook for 4–5 minutes each side for every inch of thickness. When it's done, the flesh should just start to separate into flakes when tested with a fork, and should appear opaque throughout. Some fish, such as tuna and salmon, can be served medium rare.

## SAUTE IN WINE

Instead of sautéeing in butter or oil, use wine, especially if you have some handy ice cubes of leftover wine in the freezer. Otherwise, a quick splosh and you'll have a low-calorie sautéed meal.

## JUICE YOUR MASH

It might not sound a likely combination, but try squeezing some fresh lemon juice into your mashed potatoes instead of butter or oil. Season with freshly ground black pepper for a no-added-fat mash that is flavourful and goes fantastically well with roast chicken.

# outdoor entertaining

## COOL OFF

For picnics, freeze juice or cordial in small plastic water bottles and use them to keep your other food cool and fresh. When they defrost, you'll have a cold drink.

## THE TWO-HOUR RULE

If you're planning to have take-away foods such as fried chicken or barbecued beef on a picnic, eat them within two hours of pick-up or buy them ahead of time and chill completely before packing the foods into a cooler.

## SKEW GOOD

Using skewers on the barbecue serves two great roles – first, it allows you to exercise good portion control by making a "meal on a stick" using vegetables as well as meat or fish. And second, using metal skewers heats up the centre of food, helping it to cook more thoroughly.

## PACK FOOD TOP DOWN

To help your food stay fresh and cool in the great outdoors, pack foods in the cooler in the order opposite to that which you'll be using them. In other words, pack the food you'll need last at the bottom so it stays cooler longer.

## DON'T RE-USE MARINADES

To keep bacteria at bay, never reuse marinades that have come into contact with raw meat, chicken or fish. And don't put the cooked food back into an unwashed container or dish which has been in contact with the marinade.

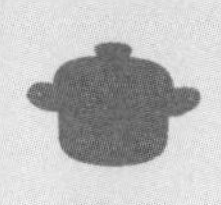



## KEEP UTENSILS APART

Make sure if you're barbecuing to keep separate utensils for raw and uncooked meat. Using the same tongs to put raw sausages onto the grill and to take cooked ones off could spread harmful bacteria. If you've only got one set of tongs, sterilize them by plunging them into the coals or flames between use.

## A CLEAN PLATE

When taking foods off the barbecue, put them on a clean plate and not on the same platter that held any raw meat.

## SEPARATE FOOD AND DRINK

If you're picnicking or eating outdoors, take separate coolers for food and drinks. The drinks cooler will be opened much more often, meaning your food can remain closed and retain its cool air as long as possible.

## LAST-MINUTE COOLNESS

When preparing chicken, egg, cold meat salads or any recipes featuring mayonnaise, refrigerate as soon as possible and keep cold right up until packing time to ensure they are extra cold.

## COOLER TO KEEP HOT

Don't forget that cool bags and boxes can be used to keep hot food hot as well as cold food cold. Line the cooler with tea towels (dish towels) for extra insulation and wrap foods well before putting them in and they could stay warm for hours, especially if tightly packed.

## COOL THINGS DOWN

If you're taking pre-cooked food to eat out at a picnic or barbecue, make sure you make it the night or morning before, so it's got plenty of time to cool right down in the fridge before transportation. Never precook meat and poultry partially before transporting. It must be cooked until done and chilled thoroughly.

## FREEZE GRAPES

If you want to keep your wine cool in the glass for drinking on hot summer days, use frozen grapes instead of ice cubes. They'll keep the drink cold and they won't dilute it or change the taste as they thaw. Make sure you wash them before freezing.

### GRILL UP SOME HEALTH

Barbecues don't have to be unhealthy. Simply choose more of the healthier foods like chicken, peppers, aubergines (eggplant), fish and bananas and less of the high-fat sausages, burgers and marshmallows.

### GIVE SNACKS THE BOOT

If you've stocked up on treats for a special occasion but are worried you won't be able to resist opening them and tucking in beforehand, use your car as a store. You'll be much less likely to snack if you have to go out to your car to get a treat!

### MAKE YOUR OWN DIP

Instead of buying fatty dips for your vegetables or crisps, make your own homemade healthy dip with low-fat natural yogurt, lemon juice, garlic and diced cucumber – delicious for summer parties.

## *hygiene & safety*

### SEPARATE FOOD TYPES

When shopping, keep raw foods away from pre-cooked items. Raw meat and fish are often wrapped but, particularly if they've been bought from a butcher or fishmonger, there's a possibility the outside of bags may also contain bacteria, so separation is safest.

### WRAP UP FISH

To keep fish fresh, securely wrap it in a plastic bag or moisture-proof paper and store in your refrigerator. You should always use fresh fish within two days, and preferably on the day of purchase. Store frozen seafood for no more than six months.

### WASH HANDS THOROUGHLY

You know you should wash your hands after handling raw fish and meat but make sure you wash them properly – studies have shown that many people neglect thumbs and the areas between the fingers, as well as the backs of hands. Check the soap has covered the whole area before rinsing with hot water (warm for children).

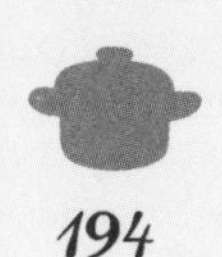



## NOW WASH EVERYTHING ELSE

Fresh raw fish can contain bacteria and microbes which can cause illness if ingested without being sterilized by cooking. Make sure you wash hands, cutting boards and utensils after coming into contact with fish.

## WASH BOTTLES

If you re-use water bottles, make sure you wash them with warm soapy water or put them through the dishwasher from time to time. Although water is clean, it does contain some microbes and you don't want bacteria to build up. You should also wash water-filter jugs between uses.

## EGG TEST

Lower uncooked eggs into a bowl of water to see if they're past their best. A very fresh egg will immediately sink to the bottom and lie flat on its side. This is because the air cell within the egg is very small. If it settles vertically, it's just about OK, but if it rises to the top, throw it away.

## THAW RUN-OFF

When meat thaws, lots of liquid can come out of it. This liquid will spread bacteria to any food, plates or surfaces it comes into contact with. Either keep thawing meat in a sealed container at the bottom of the fridge or carefully dispose of the juices and wash your hands.

## EXTRA CARE

Pregnant women, children and older people are less likely to be able to recover from food poisoning, so they should avoid products which may contain harmful bacteria. Avoid dishes made with raw or undercooked eggs, unpasteurized diary products and soft cheeses, and reheat cook-chill dishes until piping hot.

## DON'T REPEAT THE REHEAT

If you defrost raw meat and then cook it thoroughly, you can freeze it again, but remember you should never reheat foods more than once. If you want to use a bulky sauce like Bolognese for several meals, reheat individual portions as and when you need them rather than the whole pot.

## DON'T BE A TECHY

Some believe that hi-tech antimicrobial cutting boards in the kitchen could leach toxins into foods, particularly those that are absorbent like meat, fish and dairy products. Choose wood, marble or steel for safety and durability.

## A RAW DEAL FOR BOARDS

Try and keep one of the cutting boards in your kitchen for raw meat and fish only. Many people choose plastic versions but there is evidence to show that wood is actually the best choice because of its natural antimicrobial properties.

## GET OFF YOUR METAL

Don't store food in tin or aluminium cans in the fridge or cupboard as the air can cause metal ions to spread into food (unless they are designed for repeated use, such as with golden syrup). If you only want to use half a can, empty the rest into a bowl or other food container and dispose of or recycle the can straight away.

## YOUR TUM LIKES IT HOT

When you purchase a hot take-away, eat with 2 hours to prevent harmful bacteria from multiplying. If you are not eating within 2 hours, keep your food in the oven set at a high enough temperature to keep the food at or above 60°C (140°F). Check with a food thermometer.

## THE DANGER ZONE

Harmful bacteria can grow rapidly in food if it's kept in the danger zone (4–60°C/40–140°F), so remember the 2-hour rule and discard any perishable foods left in the danger zone longer than 2 hours.

## BEAT THE BULGE

If any of your cans start to bulge, throw them away immediately without opening as they could contain nasty bacteria – including the potentially deadly botulism organism which could cause serious harm.

## DON'T FOIL YOUR ACID

Aluminium kitchen foil can be useful for wrapping and covering foods, but it's best to avoid it for foods that are highly acidic, such as tomatoes, rhubarb, cabbage and soft fruits, because aluminium can affect their taste.

## CLEAN UP

Remember that housework can burn up to 300 calories an hour, so keeping your kitchen surfaces clean could not only help you prevent food poisoning, it could also help you drop those extra inches! Remember to clean door handles, where bacteria can accumulate.

## SEARCH FOR THE STEAM

Make sure you always reheat pre-cooked meats until they're steaming hot, which will kill off any bacteria that may cause health problems. You should never eat meat that's only been reheated to lukewarm.

## FIRE SAFETY

Outfit your kitchen with a fire extinguisher and teach everyone in the family how to use it, even children. Many house fires could be prevented if kitchens were prepared.

## THROW IT OUT

If you have leftovers from a picnic, only keep them if there is still ice in the cooler and they haven't been out in the sun for too long. There's one basic rule for leftovers – if in doubt, throw it out!

## DON'T FAN THE FLAMES

If one of your saucepans catches fire, use the lid of the pan to cover the flames and suffocate the fire. Then give the pan a chance to cool down before you move it as movement may cause it to re-ignite.

## PUT IT OUT WITH SODA

Humble baking soda is the best defence against small kitchen fires – simply throw baking soda at the base of the flames. But don't use this method if the fire is caused by fat or grease, as splashing could result in severe burns.

## MEASURE FOOD TEMPERATURE

To make your barbecues extra safe, invest in a food thermometer. Burgers, ribs and sausages should be at least 70°C/160°F and poultry 80°C/180°F before you can be sure all the bacteria are killed.

## GO FREE RANGE

If you're using raw eggs in a recipe, such as chocolate mousse or mayonnaise, use free-range eggs. Almost no salmonella has been found in free-range eggs.

## KEEP THEM APART

Use separate knives and other utensils for raw and cooked meat, so you don't transfer any bacteria to the cooked items. Also, if you are cooking for vegetarians remember to keep any utensils used for any meat product – cooked or raw – away from the vegetables or other ingredients that will be combined.

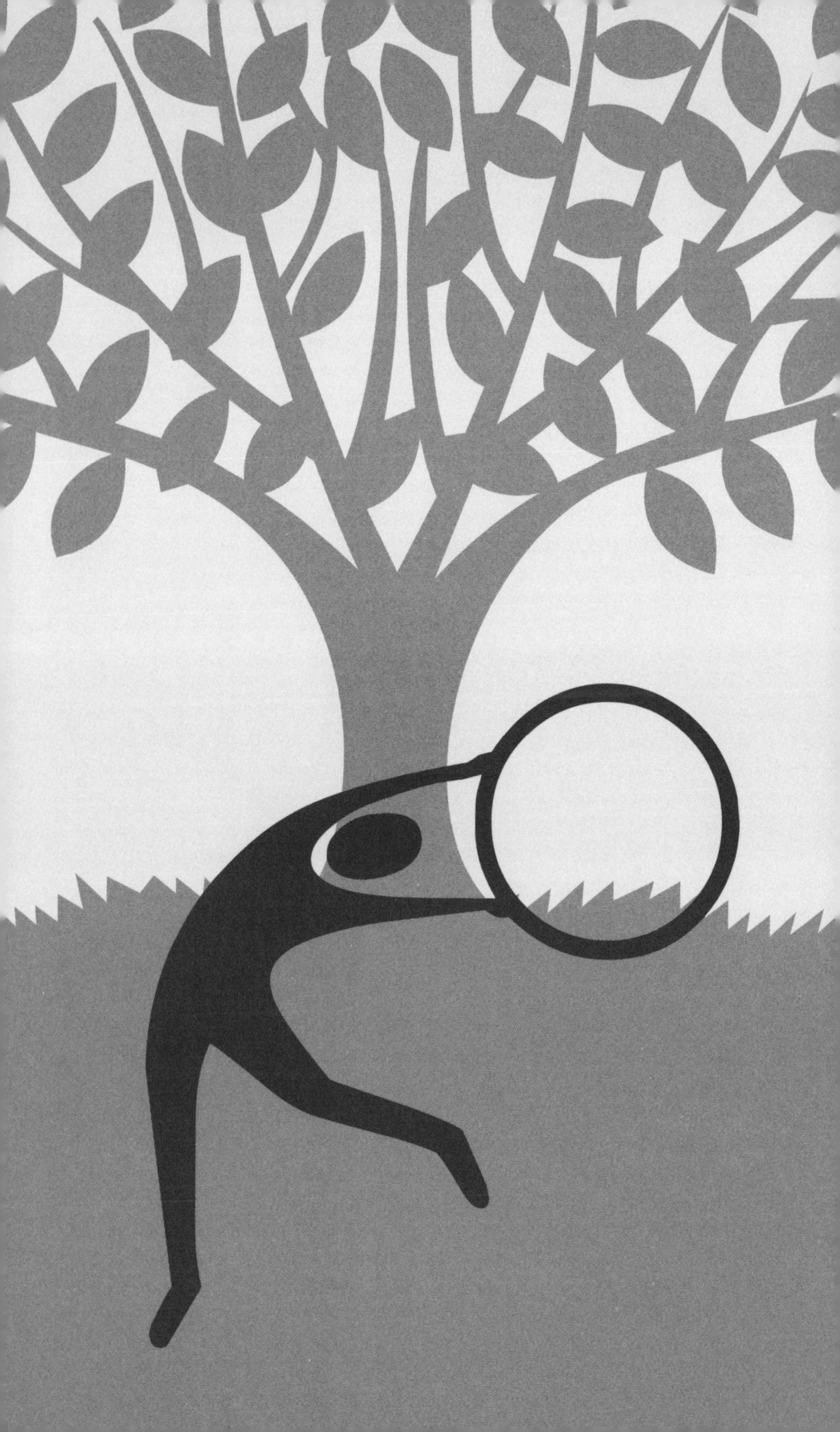

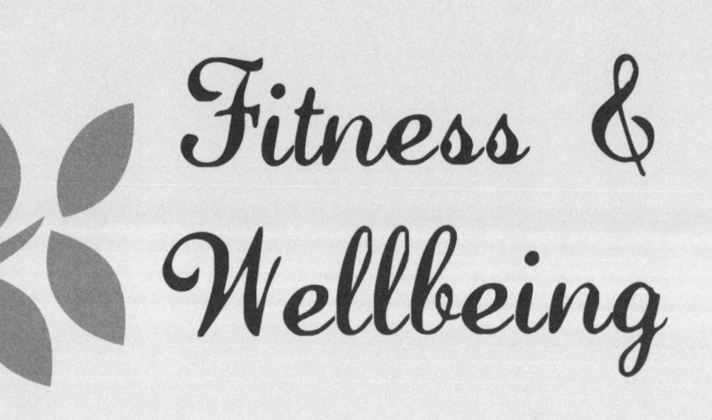

# Fitness & Wellbeing

From tips on boosting your energy and fitness levels to guidance on creating a good work-life balance, this chapter is full of expert advice on dealing with day-to-day life in a happy, positive way. Along with self-help solutions for a more rewarding personal and professional life, there are ideas for improving your physical self too – improving your balance, circulation, immunity and core strength, as well as a "workout wisdom" section.

# family favourites

## FIVE A DAY

To help your family get their five portions of fruit and vegetables a day, encourage them to snack on fruit by having a bowl full of ready-washed fruit within easy reach. Keep the blender to hand and mix up smoothies in the morning – even those family members who are tempted to skip breakfast will have time for a drink.

## SHARE THE CHORES

Make sure everyone in the house has a share in the chores. Even children as young as two or three can take some responsibility for tidying their toys, and taking a share of the housework makes everyone appreciate their home more.

## DON'T EAT ALONE

If you live alone, try to eat with friends as often as you can to boost social happiness. Eating as a family is important to cement relationships, while in shared accommodation, make an effort to eat with housemates (even if you don't eat the same thing).

## GO ON AN OUTING

Spend time with your family just doing something you all enjoy, like walking or visiting a park or museum, even going to the cinema or out for a meal to get to know what really makes them tick.

## SET A TIMER

To help your children learn to share and to prevent stressful battles in the home, invest in an alarm you can set for 5 or 10 minutes so they know when their turn has finished.

## GET OUTSIDE

Walking is not only great exercise, it's often a really good time to have conversations about feelings and other issues. Borrow a dog for weekends or family walks, or go it alone and just enjoy nature.

## GET ROUTINE

Creating a routine for your children, especially around bedtime, will not only help them to settle down more easily, it will give you more time to help tie up those loose household ends.

## BANK ONLINE

Moving your banking to online or telephone banking means you can avoid time-consuming trips to stand in the queue at the bank. Do as much of your banking as possible that way to help free up time.

## COOK IT UP

Try to cook meals that will last more than one day. For instance, stews could be served one night with potato and the next with rice, or meat could be hot one night and cold with salad the next.

## MAKE YOUR OWN

Instead of buying your coffee and snack on the way to work, take in your own and make it yourself. Not only will this save you time, you'll be amazed what a difference one coffee a day makes to your finances.

## BOARD IT UP

Instead of gathering around the TV, encourage your family to relax by playing cards or a board game, which will help you spend quality time being engaged with each other.

## SET A TIMETABLE

Have a set homework time each evening. Set aside an hour or half an hour and use it to catch up on work and administration (and set an example to your kids, if you have them). Make it public, so that you won't be disturbed.

## HAVE A HOME CINEMA NIGHT

Every few months, get your family together and have a real home cinema night. Choose a movie together, make popcorn or home-made pizza and enjoy watching and talking about a film. In the summer, why not set up an outdoor screen and move into the garden?

### MAKE JOINT DECISIONS

When it comes to big issues like where to go on holiday or what to do with the house, let your children be involved and respect their input. Working together as a team to make decisions will help them develop cooperative social skills.

## happy home

### GO GREEN FINGERED

One of the easiest ways to make your home feel like a healthier environment is to include house plants, particularly in areas you spend a lot of time in. Choose plants you like the look of and never keep dead plants.

### MAKE A STATEMENT

Don't fall into the trap of not reading your bank statements. Not only is it important to check each transaction thoroughly to ensure you are protected against fraud, it will also help you to stay on top of spending.

### STOCK UP

Make a point of keeping a stock of certain basics you need for organizing your home or home office. That way, you won't have to pop to the store every time you need them. Stamps, envelopes, notepaper and pens are all good staple choices.

### MAKE YOUR BED

Making your bed when you leave the house in the morning might sound a strange way to help yourself cope better with life, but starting the day organized is a great way to stay positive for longer. Taking a few minutes to smooth down those sheets every morning could actually help you off to a better start to the day.

### ENJOY YOUR HOME

Don't make your home a place only of chores and "to do" lists. Make an effort to enjoy spending time there doing something that makes you feel happy, relaxed and refreshed.

## FILE A BILL

Make a habit of keeping receipts and bills together so it's easy to arrange your finances and check bank statements. This will also save you hours when it's time to get your taxes filed.

## CATCH UP AT THE WEEKEND

Weekends are for enjoyment but they are also a great chance to get set for the next week. Spend a few hours making sure you have work clothes, food for lunches, etc, ready for Monday morning.

## STICK TO IT

Don't give up if your attempts at managing your time better don't work immediately. It takes a while to learn good habits, so stick to it until it works.

## GET RID OF PILES

Go through those piles of papers on your desk that have been sitting there forever, file the important documents and shred the rest. Then work out a system to stop the papers piling up again and stick to it.

## DIG YOURSELF HAPPY

Gardening has long been hailed as a way to help ease problems and reduce stress hormones. Because it combines fresh air – which boosts mood as well as improving vitamin levels – with low-level exercise, it helps the brain unwind. Aim for 30 minutes two or three times a week.

## CLEAN LITTLE BY LITTLE

There's nothing worse than having the week's cleaning or household organization hanging over you all week. Instead of leaving it all to the weekend, or your one particular time a week, clean small areas regularly. Doing a little bit each day will keep it more manageable, help you to stay relaxed and ultimately save time.

## DITCH THE OFFICE

Never allow computers or work into your bedroom. It should be a space devoted to sleep and relaxation, and a place to be together with your partner for intimacy, not a place to be reminded of work.

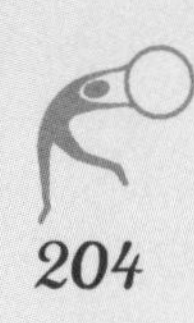



## DO A SPRING CLEAN

It might sound like a cliché, but devoting a weekend to giving your house a spring clean will help your mind feel fresh as a daisy, too. Do it in spring when the light starts to increase and you can see the dirt.

## GO SOFT

One of the best investments you can make for your bedroom is to make sure you choose sheets that are soft and made of natural fabrics that allow your skin to breathe. This will help enhance deep, healing sleep and help you feel better through the day.

## DO A DANCE

The old myth about dancing while you do the housework is really true – dancing does make you happier, so turn up the volume and get grooving (and you'll have a clean house, too!).

## LIMIT YOUR SCREEN TIME

Don't allow yourself to slump in front of the TV for hours every night, which can actually make you feel more lethargic. Instead, limit yourself to certain TV times and use the rest to achieve something.

## BUY A ROBE

A great way to enhance the feeling of relaxation in your home is to invest in a really luxurious bathrobe. Don't make it your everyday robe; save it for your special relaxation times to mark the difference.

## REFLECT IN YOUR HOME

One of the best ways to spruce up your home environment in just a few minutes is to give your windows and mirrors a clean. Not only will it improve light levels, it will make the whole place look and feel cleaner. Large clean mirrors are also good feng shui, bringing calm and refreshment while reflecting away negativity.

## GET ENVIRONMENTAL

Take a good look at the various different environments you spend time in – your home, workplace and friends' or family's houses – and ask yourself if they are positive, negative or neutral places. What can you do to make them more positive? Making a list can help.

### DON'T BE A SQUARE

Your mother used to joke that watching TV would give you square eyes, but nowadays it's more likely to be the computer screen you're staring at for hours. Don't allow yourself more than a few hours a day in front of any screen during leisure time.

### KEEP THEM HAPPY

Don't forget that everyone in your home will benefit from a bit of pampering. Next time you treat yourself, get a little something for everyone else in the house as well to enhance the feeling of wellbeing (and that includes the pets!). It doesn't have to be much, but if the thought is there it will surely be appreciated.

## decluttering

### HAVE A CHARITY MONTH

Do you feel overwhelmed by the sheer amount of stuff in your home? For one month, put away one thing every day to take to the charity shop. Not only will you be helping local charities but your house will be much less cluttered.

### ONE IN ONE OUT

To solve serious storage problems, develop a "one-in one-out" system where for every new thing you accumulate you have to get rid of something. You'll be amazed how many new things slip by unnoticed unless you pay attention. It could save you money, too.

### MAKE A DIVIDE

Divide your wardrobe into winter and summer clothes and make sure at the end of each season that clothes are cleaned, ironed and put away. This will free up storage space and help you ring the changes.

### DECLUTTER

There's nothing more irritating than a room with clutter in it. Try to develop a storage system where everything has a place to reduce those "moving from place to place" clutter problems. Stock items neatly on shelves and they will be more pleasurable to look at and use.

### DON'T BE A HOARDER

If the sight of your overcrowded wardrobe (closet) makes you run for cover, develop a clothes system – each season, put away clothes you won't wear until the next, and give or throw away anything you haven't worn for more than six months.

### DE-JUNK YOUR LIFE

It's hard to be happy unless you can think clearly, and it's hard to think clearly if you're living in a clutter bomb. Make it a rule to have a clear-out a couple of times a year and sell, give away, recycle or throw out anything you're unlikely to use.

### CLEANSE YOUR MIND

Give your mind a cleanse as well as your body and home. Invest in a book of meditations for your bathroom. Before you take a bath or shower read just one of them, and use your time in the bath or shower to think about the words and what they mean.

### PLAY IT AGAIN

One of the best ways to turn your home into a place for relaxation is through music. Play some of your favourite tunes and allow yourself to really listen to them without any distractions.

### CULL YOUR FILES

Do you really need to keep every birthday card you've been given since you were a kid, or every bank statement since you opened your account? Keep financial documents for six years and get rid of as much of the rest as you can.

## creating a sanctuary

### WATER DOWN YOUR MOODS

Adding a water feature to your room, balcony, patio or garden is a great happiness booster. It is thought that the sound of running water penetrates deep into our subconscious, helping the brain rid itself of stress.

## GET COLOURFUL

Changing the colour of your bedroom walls can give the room a completely new feel, and help you to relax inside it. Try soft blues or greens to create a relaxing space; just paint one wall if you don't like too much colour. If you don't want to paint the walls, try incorporating artwork and wall-hangings that feature those colours to help relax your mood.

## CHOOSE NATURAL MATERIALS

Invite nature into your home by choosing natural fabrics and colours. Choose wood, wicker, cotton and earthy tones as well as blues and greens to help you reconnect with the world outside. Maximize comfort levels – soft sheets, pretty cushions, pillows you can sink into, and a variety of textures and colours all aid relaxation.

## LIGHT A CANDLE

Candlelight is of a lower luminescence than electric light, so our eyes find it easier to stay relaxed by the warmer glow of candles. Use them in your bathroom or while you eat. It will help you stay relaxed and calm.

## GO HOME

At the end of a busy day, take at least 5 or 10 minutes before your evening begins just to sit or lie down in the quiet of your house or apartment. If your space is noisy, use earplugs to help you stay tranquil.

## ITCHY FEET

Instead of slumping in front of the television or going out with friends every night, make one night a week your "self improvement" night. Use it to further your skills in whatever area you'd like to develop – whether it be a new language or hobby.

## KEEP THINGS NEAT

Making your bed every morning and tidying up clothes dropped on the floor will help your bedroom feel like a retreat rather than a hovel. Try to keep surfaces as clean as possible and don't allow clutter to build up.

### BE SINGLE-MINDED

The bedroom is the most important room to keep for single use – that of sleeping. If you truly want better sleep and relaxation, don't put a computer or television in the bedroom.

### IT'S ELEMENTAL

Make your living area more relaxing by enlivening it with natural elements, such as stone and water. According to feng shui, an aquarium combines water and living energy (chi), which stimulates energy and brings good luck and wealth.

## getting organized

### DARN THE TV

Keep a sewing kit in your living room near the television so you can make essential repairs while you're watching something interesting. It will make you more likely to do the job rather than letting the mending pile mount up.

### MAKE A LIST

If your life requires multitasking, stay on top of your different responsibilities by taking a few minutes every morning to make a list of everything that needs to be done in each of your life areas. Tick them off as you go along so that you never lose track of what needs doing, and update it the next day.

### KEEP A WORKBOOK

Keep all your handy telephone numbers in one place – such as plumber, builder, car garage or repair services – and use the same place to make a note of serial numbers, guarantee numbers, etc, of your items, so you have everything you need when you need to make the call.

### GET FIRE RESISTANT

Keep your important documents, like passports, birth certificates and insurance policies, inside a flame-retardant box so you won't have to worry about losing them. Irreplaceable documents should be kept with a lawyer or at a bank, with a copy at home for reference.

## SEE DOUBLE

Why not have two laundry baskets – one for whites and one for colours? It will save you masses of time sorting out the washing loads, and you'll never have to worry about colours running again!

## GET MULTIPLE

Buy enough essential clothes items like underwear and socks for a couple of weeks so you don't have to worry about running out or rushing to do the washing.

## TIDY AT NIGHT

Before you go to sleep, make sure you spend a few minutes tidying away your shoes or putting dirty clothes into the laundry basket so that when you wake up in the morning the first thing you see is an orderly room.

## ON-THE-SPOT NOTEBOOK

Keep a notebook or a pad stuck to the fridge or on the wall in the kitchen so you can make a note of anything you've run out of. Encourage everyone in the house to use it so you don't have to remember everything.

## TAKE A COURSE

If you feel your life is constantly escaping from under your feet and you simply don't have time to do anything, think about doing a time-management course, which could help you see things differently.

## PLAN YOUR DRESS

If you find your clothes are often in chaos, why not spend a few weeks sticking to a clothing plan. Work out what you're going to wear in advance and make sure you have enough for a two-week cleaning rotation.

## KEY TO SUCCESS

Make a place for your keys so you don't keep misplacing them. Make it prominent but not too near the front or back door (which could give burglars an easy way to make their escape).

### SLEEP IT OUT

Studies have shown that couples who get enough sleep are generally happier than those who don't, so make your bedroom work for both of you.

### MAKE AN EXIT

Decide on a realistic time to leave work every day – for instance, if you know you always need to stay later on Wednesdays, be honest about it, but make sure you leave earlier on other days. Stick to your times to help you leave work behind at night.

### ORGANIZE YOUR HOME

Don't leave important home phone calls, like paying bills and organizing visits, to chance. Free up an hour a week where you can sit down with your diary and phone numbers and organize your home life so important tasks aren't left undone.

### ASK FOR HELP

Don't hide your head in the sand. There's nothing worse than feeling as if you've got too much on your plate and things are out of control. You're much more likely to be able to get yourself out of the situation by facing up to it and asking for help.

## enjoying life

### CLEAR YOUR HEAD

If you're trying to get your head around a problem, taking the time to go for a walk or a run – or simply to have a bath if you prefer – can give you valuable subconscious insight. Don't think about the problem deliberately; just give your brain space to process and you'll be amazed at the solutions that spring to mind.

### EAT EARLY

Skipping breakfast, which leads to low blood sugar in the morning, can play havoc with memory and concentration. To help you start the day thinking straight, make sure you eat something nutritious.

## GET MUSICAL

Listen to relaxing music while travelling through the city. Driving or even walking in a busy city can be stressful, and listening to light, calming music will help you to keep your inner calm among the whirlwind of people and cars.

## MAKE GOOD DECISIONS

If you've got a big decision to make, such as whether to move house or change jobs, it's imperative to write a list of goals. Make note of everything that's important to you and what your priorities are, including those of your partner, and make a decision that works towards them.

## GO BY THE LIST

Be flexible and realistic when planning your day. Work through your list in order of priority and don't allow yourself to be distracted – it will help you feel in control of your day rather than it being in control of you.

## BACK TO NATURE

Spend time at the nearest park, tree-lined path, river, lake or beach whenever possible. Being in nature, even if it is bang in the middle of a buzzing city, is calming and restorative. It will help you to relax.

## BE A BOOKWORM

Read a book while taking public transport through a city. Choose books that are funny, relaxing or calming so that you can get your mind off your commute and lose yourself in your book.

## MAKE A CHANGE

Change is refreshing, so do something different at least once a month. This could be something big like trying a new adventure sport or going away for the weekend, or something small like taking a new route for your daily walk or visiting a different pub.

## TAKE A BREAK

If you work in a city, it's even more important to take small breaks throughout the day. Step outside the office, even if only for 5 minutes, to breathe deeply, look at the sky and step out of the mayhem for a few minutes.

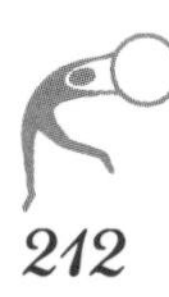



### REMEMBER TO RELAX

Don't fall into the trap of scheduling your whole life into activity slots. Make sure you incorporate leisure and relaxation time for yourself when planning your schedule and stick to it as rigidly as you would to your other time slots.

## relationships

### BE APPRECIATIVE

Learn to do the one thing that is most likely to restore good feeling in your relationship – giving your partner a genuine, loving and approving smile. A simple hug, too, can help restore contact and affection without even having to say a word.

### INVEST IN QUALITY

Without quality time, your relationship will not survive. Carve out at least half an hour a night and at least one day a month when the two of you spend time exclusively together. Talk to each other and make a pact not to bring up problems or arguments during these times.

### LEARN TO COMPROMISE

A good relationship is built on compromise on both sides. Choose three things each that you feel you really can't compromise on and agree to work with each other on those areas, then be willing to give way on the other, less significant, things.

### DON'T BE CODEPENDENT

Keep your dependence and independence in balance. Tell and show your partner how much you need them, but don't cling or try to control them as that can make your partner feel trapped.

### LEND AN EAR

Encourage your partner to listen to you by showing appreciation when they do and make an effort to let yourself hear what your partner is saying rather than assuming you know what's coming next.

## ANGER OR BOREDOM?

Remember that boredom typically covers up anger so if you're feeling bored with your partner or with your life, ask yourself what you're angry about.

## GO OUT

Make an effort to see your friends without your partner as often as you can, preferably once a month. It will remind you of the "you" that's inside, independent of partners, jobs and families.

## TEACH EACH OTHER

Don't be shy about what you want in the bedroom – save the guesswork and teach your partner (preferably early on in the relationship) exactly what you need to feel satisfied. Just don't forget to be prepared to hear the same from them.

## MAKE SOME SPACE

Don't assume your partner needs the same things as you when you're arguing or tense. You might want to talk, but many people need some "space" to get their heads straight. Being understanding about what your partner needs will lead to a more fruitful discussion in the long run.

## LIST THE GOOD THINGS

When your relationship feels really good, such as after a great meal out, or when you feel things are going well, take the time to write down what makes you love your partner so much and why you're with them. Referring back to it during the bad times or a rocky patch may help you get some perspective.

## SET THE TIMER

If you've got a issue that needs discussing, try a mediator's timing method to help clarify both sides of the argument. Set the timer for 5 minutes and take turns talking – the only rule is that during your 5 minutes your partner is not allowed to interrupt, and vice versa.

## FORGET PERFECTION

Nobody's perfect, and it's unreasonable of you to expect your partner not to have bad habits just like everyone else. Don't try to change them too much because chances are it won't work; instead, try to love them warts and all.

## COMPLIMENT YOURSELF

If your partner is bad at giving compliments, instead of letting your resentment build up, make them appreciate you. Say something good about yourself and ask for their agreement – it will encourage them to think of nice things to say.

## OUT IN THE OPEN

Hidden resentments poison a relationship so if something is bothering you, say it. But don't nag or assign blame; simply express the problem as you see it and ask your partner to help you find the answer. That way, you're working together and nobody feels blamed.

## NEVER SAY NEVER

When you have a disagreement or argument, avoid the phrases "you never ..." and "you always ..." They are rarely true and inevitably cause defensive reactions, which won't help you to move forward. Even if they are true, saying them is unlikely to lead to the person changing.

## THINK FIRST

Next time your partner tries to tell you something negative about yourself, make an effort not to respond immediately. It's tempting to jump to your own defence, but instead, try really listening to what they've got to say and let them finish before you bite back.

## BE A NEGOTIATOR

Set a rule that each of you states what you want and then both of you work together to find a way forward. If you really work together, no problem is unsolvable.

## A DUAL PARENT

If you have children, involve your partner as much as possible with the child care, even if you feel they are not as good at it or as natural as you are. It's important to present a united front to your children.

## DON'T BANK ON SUCCESS

Money is the number-one cause of couple conflict. For a relationship to work, you need to address your finances and work out a budget. Be honest about debt and spending, and come to a joint solution.

## END OF THE AFFAIR

If you do stray, don't feel it necessarily spells the end of your relationship. Most couples recover and some find that unearthing the cause of the affair helps them get closer.

## DON'T FAN THE BLAME

Learning how to argue well is an art. Try to avoid using blame words like "you make me ..." and opt for softer versions like "when you ..., it makes me feel ..." instead.

## BALANCE THE PAIN

Think about your relationship in terms of balance. If there is consistently more pain than pleasure, more hurt than enjoyment or more arguments than laughter, then something's got to change.

## BITE YOUR TONGUE

If you're arguing with your partner, keep one golden rule in mind – never say anything you wouldn't want said to you. That way, you'll learn to phrase your anxieties better and avoid causing hurt.

## GET A BUNCH OF FIVE

Research suggests that you need five positive experiences to erase the memory of one negative experience. So aim to give five kind words for each negative comment you give, even if it is done inadvertently.

## DIVIDE AND RULE

If the domestic work is not divided fairly between you, it will cause friction in your relationship. Make a list of the domestic tasks, talk it through with your partner and mobilize the whole family, your partner included, to share the workload.

## SORT THE SEX

Your sex life may ebb and flow over the years, but if the actual sex starts going downhill (rather than the frequency) don't accept it. As soon as you notice a slide, question why and work at bringing the passion back. Discuss with your partner what might be happening sooner rather than later and be honest with each other.

### SEEK PROFESSIONAL HELP

Professional help can turn a bad relationship into a great one. Don't feel that seeing a professional counsellor, marriage guidance or sex therapist means you've failed – what it actually means is that you're taking steps to work things out together and it could save your relationship.

### GET TRAINING

Instead of nagging or moaning when your partner does something you don't like, ignore it and concentrate on the things they do that you do like. Positive reinforcement works much better than punishment.

### GO WITH THE CHANGES

People change over the years so even if you think you understand your partner now, or believe you have agreements sorted, check regularly – at least once a year – to make sure neither of you has changed your mind.

### KNOW WHEN TO QUIT

If your life aims are really incompatible and you feel you can't compromise, ending the relationship may be the only option. Take professional marital advice but don't feel you must stay if you aren't happy.

### WRAP IT UP

Make your partner feel good and give yourself a boost too by writing a list of things you like about them, then giving it to them for no particular reason.

## sex

### THE SOUND OF MUSIC

Use music to get you in the mood for sex. Make a playlist of your favourite tracks – and those of your partner – and play it to help aid relaxation, promote romance and bring back good memories.

## TALK IT OUT

Talking about sex when you're stressed about it isn't easy but starting with a little tenderness will help. Ask your partner to hold you close and use that physical intimacy as a platform to talk about your sexual problems, worries or desires.

## MAKE IT WORK

Good sex starts with love and affection, and part of ensuring you both have a good time is being honest. Don't be pressured by what you see in films or read in magazines, which are often invented anyway; tell each other what works for YOU.

## CHOOSE YOUR WORDS

You want to ask your partner to do something differently in bed but you don't want it to sound like a criticism. Avoid using negative phrases like "I don't like it when you ..." and instead opt for positives such as "I love it when ..." or "we could try ...". Don't expect it to all change overnight.

## GET TOUCHY FEELY

Words make up a tiny proportion of human communication, which is mostly done through body language and tone of voice. Back up your words with behaviour by touching and holding your partner.

## BE HONEST

If your partner does something that rocks your world next time you're having sex, don't assume they will realize it. Tell them you loved what they did and not only will it boost their ego, it might make it happen again!

## TALK DIRTY

Feeling stressed and tired can make it difficult to get in the mood for sex, but talking about your fantasies can help change your mindset into one of desire. Share fantasies over dinner and then retire upstairs!

## DON'T GET STUCK IN A RUT

Sex doesn't always have to be in the bedroom – spontaneity can be really sexy, so go for it in the kitchen, lounge, garden or even on your Sunday afternoon walk. Try new sexy underwear or sex toys to spark up your love life, too.

### GET COMPLIMENTARY

Take your relationship to new heights by telling your partner what you love about them – many of us take for granted that our loved ones know what we find attractive about them, but the chances are they need to be told.

### OPEN YOUR EYES

Many people make love with their eyes shut, particularly if they feel self-conscious in bed. Try doing it with your eyes open for a change and you may feel a higher level of intimacy.

### BE GRATEFUL

Say thank you to your partner if they make you feel good in the bedroom – good sex is like giving and receiving a gift, so saying thank you is a great way to let them know it's appreciated.

### HOLD YOUR TONGUE

Never make derisory comments about your partner's sexual performance. Ridiculing him or her or making them feel bad will only lead to insecurity, which will affect future performance. Be supportive.

### BE A SOFT TOUCH

Use massage to help you relax before a sex session. Use light strokes which have been shown to stimulate the body's natural feel-good chemicals, or endorphins, and enjoy better sex as a result.

## breaking up

### ENJOY LIFE

After a relationship breakdown, help yourself see the positive side by treating yourself to all the things you like but your partner didn't. This will remind you of what you were giving up during the relationship and what you have now regained.

### TIME TO GRIEVE

For most people, it's a shock when a relationship breaks down, even if you've known for some time that things weren't right. If your relationship ends, give yourself a few months of grieving time for the life you thought you would have.

## FACE UP TO IT

Going through a divorce is a stressful time for everyone involved, all of whom can suffer damaging effects. The first step to helping you get through a breakup successfully is to acknowledge that these effects can't be fixed straight away. Healing takes time.

## DREAMS AREN'T REAL

It's not unusual for people who are divorcing, or even those who have been divorced for a long time, to have dreams about their ex-spouse. Sometimes they're even good dreams or sexual in nature. It doesn't mean you harbour secret desires for reconciliation.

## GET IN FOCUS

Don't just think about your individual problems when it comes to analyzing your relationship breakdown. Think about external factors too, and what changes you might be able to make to ensure future relationships are protected.

## GIVE YOURSELF TIME

After a relationship breakdown, many people find themselves struggling with low self-esteem and confidence, and with so many things to organize – such as children and moving house – it can be hard to find time for your own feelings. Remember you need to look after yourself and give yourself some time to heal.

## FORGIVE OR FORGET

If you know you will never forgive your partner over something important, then give them – and yourself – a break and start again, with someone else. But if you do say you forgive them, you have to mean it.

## BE HONEST WITH CHILDREN

Don't try to hide the situation from your children if your relationship is ending. As a parent, it's natural to want to protect them but not being honest can leave them feeling confused.

## ANSWER QUESTIONS

One of the best ways to talk to your children about a relationship breakup is to give them a brief explanation and then allow them to ask questions.

## GAIN UNDERSTANDING

Understanding why a relationship failed is the first step to getting over it. Don't worry about whose fault it was, which isn't constructive. Instead concentrate on what stopped you overcoming your differences.

## BE CARING

It's tough being a parent when you're splitting up, but understand that your children will need more care and reassurance than normal. Let them know they're loved and try to present a united front.

## MAKE A CHOICE

How a person handles the sad reality of separating from a relationship is a matter of personal choice. Try to have the view that it is a learning experience rather than a failure.

## SEEK ADVICE

It's normal to feel anxious and fearful when situations change, and especially if your relationship is ending, but you're not alone. Join a support group or seek advice from websites or organizations.

## GET MEDIATION

If there are children involved in your relationship split and you don't think you can work together to come to an arrangement, getting a mediator involved can help cut out emotional arguments and reach a solution.

## HAVE A CLEAROUT

If you're splitting up, clearing out your ex's belongings can help provide some closure. Holding on to items such as clothes, personal effects and memorabilia may only bring back painful memories, hindering the move to start anew.

## FOCUS ON SUCCESS

It's difficult to keep your self-esteem high if you're going through a relationship breakdown. Although boosting self-confidence doesn't happen overnight, focusing on little successes rather than big failures can help. For example, give yourself a pat on the back for that DIY job you finished or that job application you made.

## EXTEND A HAND

One of the major worries for children involved in separations is that they will lose contact with their extended family, particularly grandparents. Make an effort to include former in-laws and maintain contact with them so that your children feel supported.

## THINK OF YOURSELF

If you're going through a stressful time, like a separation, it's easy to start obsessing about what other people might think of your situation. But this is not going to help you. Instead, try to focus on healing your own feelings.

## KEEP A JOURNAL

Instead of wallowing in feelings of loneliness, use your energy to write down how you feel. Keep a notebook to hand and use it when you need to express something or when you're feeling bad. Even if you're writing about a negative feeling, the process can be positive and constructive.

## SEE A PROFESSIONAL

If things become too unbearable, don't be afraid to seek the help of a professional like a counsellor, church minister or psychiatrist. They will be able to help you see the situation from another angle without adding to your emotional burden, and they won't be giving advice based on whatever they might be going through, as friends might.

## TALK IT THROUGH

If you've been separated for a while and suddenly start having feelings about your ex, don't feel you can't approach them to talk about it. Sometimes they'll be receptive, sometimes they won't, but perhaps an effective reconciliation can be made.

## GET OVER IT

Not getting over a divorce can mean you haven't been able to take stock of yourself as an independent person but still see yourself as merged with that other person. After a period of grieving, make a decision to stop talking about your ex and the divorce and start thinking about yourself.

# communication

## PICK YOUR TIME

Don't try to initiate an important discussion when you're feeling low. Try to choose a time of day when you're likely to be feeling your best, and arrange to have the discussion then.

## TAKE CRITICISM WELL

Next time someone criticizes you, take a breath before you bite back and ask yourself, is it really a criticism and if it is, could there conceivably be a grain of truth in there?

## LISTEN AND LEARN

Empathize by restating or rephrasing what's been said: Use phrases like "it sounds as if ..." or "what I'm hearing is ...", which will open the door to further discussion.

## LISTEN TO YOURSELF FIRST

The starting point for all good communication is knowing what you want to say before you say it, and getting your point across in a way other people understand. Take a moment to listen to yourself before you speak.

## THINK AHEAD

If you're trying to tell someone something important, practise first. Think of possible barriers to getting your point across, such as interruptions or questions, and how you will deal with them if they arise. It can help to clarify things in your own mind if you write things down first. Keep rewriting until you're happy about what you want to say and how you'll deal with barriers.

## ARGUE WELL

A good rule of thumb for arguments is to make sure you stick to the point and don't drag in old grievances. If anyone starts to lose control, take time out to calm down and finish the discussion later.

### STAY CALM

You communicate most effectively when you're calm, so try to relax before the discussion and do your best not to become too emotional during the course of the conversation. If you get heated, the other person may too, then neither of you will be very effective.

### TAKE OFF THE HEAT

If things do start to get out of hand when you're trying to have a discussion, suggest that you continue the conversation later, when both of you are feeling less emotional about it. And do try to set a time and a place before you part.

### USE "I" MESSAGES

Let the other person know how you're feeling about the situation by using "I messages" – statements that start with "I feel ..." or "I felt ...". These are a stronger, positive way to start rather than "you messages", which introduce blame and can provoke a hostile reaction.

### LISTENING SKILLS

You might know exactly what you want to say if you're having a discussion with someone else, but discussion means just that – it's a two-way process. You've got to listen as well as saying your piece, and try to find a common ground. Stop yourself from jumping in with your opinion too quickly, and really listen to what's being said.

## *balance*

### KEEP SKIN SILKY-SMOOTH

Exfoliating the skin to remove dead skin cells may help you to retain a good sense of balance by heightening the sensation powers of your skin, thus allowing your body to make tiny adjustments.

### GET FIT TO STAND TALL

Fitter people have better balance, not just because of their tendency to be the correct weight but also because their nerves and muscles are used to working together to keep their body upright.

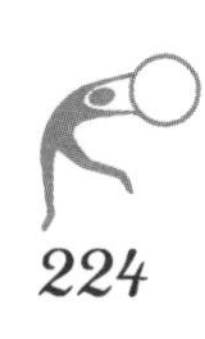



## DON'T SPILL A DROP

Don't just drink eight full glasses of water a day – use them as an opportunity to work on your balance by walking around without spilling them for a few minutes before you take a sip.

## LOOK INSIDE TO CENTRE YOURSELF

Recent studies have revealed that those people who practise techniques that involve breathing exercises and inner contemplation – such as yoga, tai chi and chi gong – have better balance than those who don't.

## AVOID CRACKS TO SPEED UP REACTIONS

Practise walking faster and stepping over or avoiding objects lying in your path, such as cracks in the pavement or tiles on the kitchen or bathroom floor. This will help improve the speed of your walking and decrease hesitancy.

## GET BALANCED AS YOU GET OLDER

Balance problems affect more than a third of people over 65 years of age, and more than half of those aged over 75. Make certain that you prepare your balance muscles with regular exercises well before you reach this stage.

## STAND UP SLOWLY TO HELP YOUR HEAD

Morning dizziness is often caused by a drop in blood pressure upon standing, particularly after a long time spent lying down. Get up slowly to give the blood time to work its way around the body.

## BE A FLAMINGO FOR BETTER BALANCE

Practise standing on one leg, with your eyes fixed on a stationary spot in front of you. Start on a hard floor and progress to carpet or foam. Once you can stand balanced for a whole minute, try changing the positions of your arms, legs and eyes without falling over.

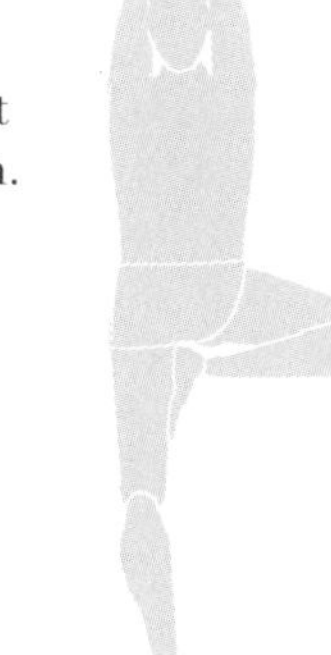

# circulation

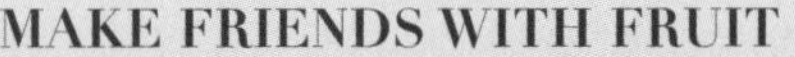

## MAKE FRIENDS WITH FRUIT

People with high levels of fruit and vegetables in their diets have lower blood pressure than those who choose less healthy foods, probably thanks to good salt and sugar regulation.

## GET UP TO SCRATCH WITH CAT'S CLAW

The herbal extract cat's claw, which comes from an Amazonian rainforest plant, has been shown to lower blood pressure in some clinical trials.

## GET A SENSE OF HUMMUS

Increasing fibre intake helps level out circulation by aiding fluid balance after eating. Pulse (legume) spreads like hummus and bean dips, in place of sour cream and cheese spreads or dips, are tasty ways to eat more fibre.

## SPRINKLE AWAY STICKINESS

Vitamin E, which is found commonly in seeds like pumpkin and linseed (flax) and in fruits such as cherries, kiwi and green peppers, has been shown to reduce the stickiness of the blood, so reducing the possibility of clotting. Sprinkle the seeds on salads for a daily dose.

## GO ORANGE FOR STRENGTH

Oranges and other types of citrus fruit contain high levels of vitamin C and bioflavonoids. These substances work in the body to strengthen the walls of capillaries to keep blood pumping fast around the body.

## TAKE IT NIACIN EASY

Niacin, which is also known as vitamin B3 and is found in liver, poultry, pulses (legumes), nuts, cereals and rosehips, boosts the circulation and blood flow to the small blood vessels, helping alleviate circulation problems.

## PRESS AWAY PROBLEMS

Massage has major benefits for circulation as it increases blood flow to the area being treated, increasing the flow of nutrient-rich, oxygenated blood to skin, muscles and underlying tissues.

## CURE COLD FEET WITH CAYENNE

Soaking feet and hands in water with a teaspoon of mustard powder or cayenne pepper for five to ten minutes can help boost circulation by dilating blood vessels.

## SOCK IT TO 'EM

Wearing elasticated flight socks, particularly on air journeys of longer than about 90 minutes, can help blood return from the lower legs and so reduce the chances of DVT (deep-vein thrombosis) and dangerous blood clots developing.

## HANG LOOSE TO STOP CLOTS

Body-hugging neoprene sports shorts, said to promote weight loss and designed for use in the gym or aerobics classes, may, however, increase the risk of blood clots developing in the legs by restricting blood flow. Choose looser clothes instead to safeguard your circulation.

## GO FRUITY

Fruit that contains high levels of lycopene helps general circulation in the body by preventing a buildup of plaque, which restricts blood flow through arteries. A tasty choice is watermelon, which contains 14mg per slice.

## GET TO THE POINT

Reflexology, a technique that concentrates on stimulating pressure points on the feet, can help boost blood flow to the feet and legs, hence improving circulation.

## POUND AWAY PRESSURE

Working out at least three times a week boosts circulation, clears out arteries and lowers blood pressure, giving the circulation system an energy boost.

## GET JIGGY WITH GINSENG

Extract of ginseng not only alleviates problems caused by bad circulation but increases blood flow to the extremities, boosting health and wellbeing.

## WEED OUT THE WEED

Smoking is the single worst thing you can do for your circulation. It narrows arteries, breaks down capillary walls and stops the heart working efficiently. There's only one answer – give up.

### STAND ON YOUR HEAD

Not for those with a health condition, head and shoulder stands boost circulation to the head and neck. For a safer alternative, try sitting with your head between your knees for several minutes.

### PUT YOUR FEET UP

Lounging about watching television for hours at a time or slumped in a chair reading can leave you in bad positions for blood drainage and impair lower-limb circulation as a result. By putting your feet up, however, you will place less stress on your system – and you might find that it's more comfortable, too!

### POUND THE PAVEMENT

Any type of physical exercise that involves impact on the feet and hands – such as skipping, running, walking, boxing and kickboxing – improves circulation to the extremities. Impact exercise can also prevent pain and the onset of problems.

### DETOX YOUR ARTERIES

Studies have shown that eating garlic can help reduce the buildup of plaque in arteries, and even clear away existing deposits. Aim to include some in your diet once a day or take a supplement.

## core strength

### COUGH UP A CORE

Your core strength relies on the muscles you use every time you cough. So, in order to find the muscles, cough gently a few times and use your fingers to feel where your abdomen contracts. These are the muscles that hold your trunk erect.

### TILT INTO SHAPE

Try this pelvic tilt, which is proven to strengthen the abdominals. Lie on your back with knees bent and feet flat on the floor. Breathe out and draw your abdominals down towards your spine, hold, and repeat several times.

## BRACE YOURSELF

Practise forming a "back brace" by pulling your bellybutton inwards without flattening your back, then tightening your pelvic floor muscles as if you were stopping the flow of urine. Keep your breathing relaxed.

## HAVE A BALL

Swiss ball exercises can help strengthen your spine and core muscles safely and easily. Try swapping the sofa for a ball as you watch television, or engaging your body fully by using one at your work desk instead of a chair.

## SWING OUT SISTER

To boost core strength, stand beside a table or wall (in case you overbalance) and stand on one leg. Swing the outer leg backwards and forwards. Make sure you don't dip, twist or rotate your pelvis.

## THINK YOURSELF STRONG

Hard to believe, but imagining yourself with strong core abdominal muscles could actually make them stronger by more than 10%. It's no substitute for exercise, but it's better than nothing!

## BE STRAIGHT WITH YOURSELF

Try this simple exercise: stand up straight with your eyes closed and concentrate on feeling the muscles in your body adapting to keep you in position. This will help core strength as well as your balance.

## WORK IT AT WORK

Don't allow yourself to fall into bad habits at work that can ruin your posture. For toning, and to remind yourself to stay strong at the core, contract your abdominals and pelvic floor muscles from time to time as you sit at your desk.

## PULL IN YOUR BELLY TO PROTECT YOUR BACK

Having poor core strength makes you many times more susceptible to injury and lower-back pain, as the spine is forced into adopting unnatural positions. To support your lower back, pull your bellybutton upwards and backwards until you feel "lifted".

# energy boosters

### BE A SUNFLOWER SEEKER

Toasted sunflower seeds are a great choice to nibble on when afternoons at work begin to drag. Not only will they stop you reaching for fatty, salty snacks, they'll also boost your energy-giving vitamin levels while you munch.

### GO HOT FOR GET-UP-AND-GO

For an instant pick-me-up at mealtimes, dust your food with chilli powder, cumin and coriander. These spices are a natural and tasty way to invigorate your body, and there is no drawback of a corresponding sugar low afterwards.

### HAVE A BRAZILIAN

No, not a bikini wax, but a healthy eating alternative instead! Brazil nuts not only boost short-term energy, but just three a day can also help cut the risk of heart disease by a third.

### CRUNCH CRACKERS FOR GOOD SNACKING

Wholewheat or rice crackers spread with peanut butter, tahini, hummus or low-fat savoury spreads like tapenade have been shown to help weight loss and boost energy levels by curbing unhealthy snacking.

### APPRECIATE THE APRICOT

Dried apricots, perfect substitutes for biscuits (crackers) with cheese, are an excellent source of fibre, potassium, iron and betacarotene. Choose air-dried, not sulphur-dried, as sulphites have been linked to different forms of cancer.

### STRETCH AND YAWN TO WORK OUT FACE MUSCLES

Stretching allows blood to flow into muscles that have become inactive, which is why it's so regenerating after sleep. Yawning gives your body a big oxygen boost, which combines with the stretching to give muscles instant energy.

### FEEL CHIPPER WITH BANANA

For a handy and tasty pick-me-up, why not try dried banana chips? They are rich in carbohydrates, iron and magnesium and, in addition, they have natural sugars to give your body an energy boost when you're on the move. Combine them with plain, natural yogurt when you're looking for a more substantial snack.

### WAKE UP TO MORNING GLORY

For a morning boost, swap your first cup of tea or coffee for an energy-giving detox drink made with hot water, lemon juice, freshly grated ginger, maple syrup and a pinch of cayenne pepper.

### LIQUIDIZE YOUR ASSETS

Make a natural power drink by liquidizing apples, banana and a tablespoon of peanut butter together. Drink a glass with your breakfast. The fruit sugars will boost your energy at different levels to keep you going all morning.

### FEEL BLOOMING GOOD

Add a ray of natural sunshine to your life by feasting on edible flowers like violets, nasturtiums, marigolds, primroses and pansies, which can benefit body and mind.

## eyesight

### LOOSEN UP FOR AN EASY VIEW

Tight collars and ties have been shown to raise blood pressure in the eyes, which is a leading risk factor in glaucoma, by constricting the jugular vein. If your neck's under pressure, loosen up!

### FISH OILS FOR NIGHT VISION

Problems with night vision can be relieved by adding extra essential fatty acids (EFAs) from fish oils to your diet. Deficiencies can also lead to retinal damage. So if you want to see in the dark, make sure you eat at least two portions of oily fish a week.

## STOP DEGENERATION WITH VITAMIN A

Very high doses of vitamin A may provide a cure for age-related macular degeneration, which is a very common cause of blindness in the over-50s. The minimum effective dosage is currently being researched, since too much vitamin A can damage the liver. Consult your doctor for advice.

## DON'T SALT UP YOUR SIGHT

Too much salt in your diet could double your risk of developing cataracts. Studies have shown that people who eat the least amount of salt are the least likely to develop the condition. Watch out for hidden salts in processed foods, soups and cereals.

## KEEP AGEING EYES IN THE CAN

Eating canned tuna more than once a week reduces the risk of developing age-related macular degeneration by more than 40%. Combine with vitamin-rich sweet potato and tomato for the best benefits.

## TREAT YOURSELF TO A BERRY GOOD VIEW

Compounds called flavonoids, found in berries, protect the sensitive cells of the eye, which are especially prone to strain from work at computers. Drink a blueberry smoothie for a bright-eyed day.

## LOOK YOURSELF IN THE EYES

If the whites of your eyes appear dull or yellowish in colour, this could be an indication of a struggling liver. Help it out with milk thistle, ginger and citrus fruits.

## COOK UP A GREAT VIEW

Carrots really can help you see in the dark. This is because the high levels of vitamins (especially vitamin A) they contain help protect eyes from daily wear and tear. The beneficial effects of carrots are easier to assimilate in the body if they're cooked (but not overcooked).

## FOCUS ON FISH

Omega-3 fish oils are thought to protect the macula lutea (the spot at the centre of the retina) from problems. Aim to eat oily fish like tuna, mackerel or salmon more than once a week and use linseed (flaxseed) and sunflower oils for cooking.

## KEEP ON THE LEVEL

Staring at a computer screen all day can be very damaging for the eyes, especially if the screen is badly positioned. Screens should be roughly 60cm (2ft) away with the top at eye level, and arms should rest lightly on the desk's surface.

## EAT SWEET POTATO FOR SWEET VISION

Although they taste rich and creamy, sweet potatoes are fat- and cholesterol-free and full of vision-boosting betacarotene and vitamin A. One medium-sized sweet potato has only around 130 calories.

## RETAIN AN EGG-CELLENT RETINA

Taurine, found in eggs, meat and fish, is an essential ingredient for keeping the retina strong and supple, enhancing vision.

## CHOCOLATE FOR FIRST-RATE VISION

A daily dose of chocolate, particularly the dark, high cocoa-solids varieties, can help vision by topping up copper levels.

## PUT YOUR EYES IN THE SHADE

The optician's no. 1 tip for healthy eyes is to make sure your sunglasses have high UVA and UVB protection, which will protect eyes against the damaging rays generated by the sun. This is guaranteed to give you a brighter future.

## CUT OUT WHEAT AND BANISH UNDEREYE CIRCLES

Dark circles under the eyes, usually considered a sign of tiredness, can also be caused by food intolerance, often to refined foods. Try cutting out processed foods for a few days and see if they lighten up.

## GIVE YOUR EYES A REST

Even if you have only a minute to spare, focus on something far away, blink several times to build up moisture, then hold the lids closed for a few seconds, pressing your palms over the sockets to rest and rejuvenate the eyes.

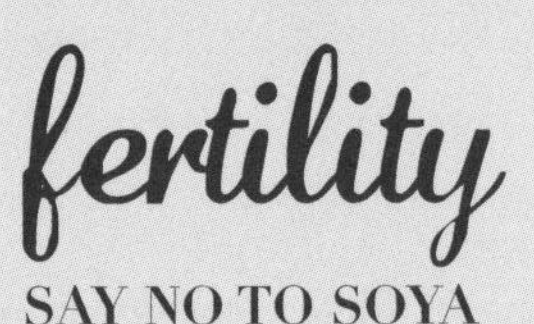



## SAY NO TO SOYA

Food products that contain soya or that are wrapped in plastics may reduce the sperm count in men, as they may have chemicals that mimic the action of female hormones.

## AXE THE ALCOHOL

Studies show that women who drink small amounts of alcohol (fewer than five units a week) double their chance of conceiving within six months compared with women who drink more.

## COUNT TEN TO CONCEPTION

Women wishing to conceive should make love every other day for a ten-day period during the middle of their cycle. Studies have shown that the five days before and the five days after the projected ovulation date are the most promising times to become pregnant.

## DON'T BE A LEMON

Calming coffee-free drinks like hot water with lemon juice may actually harm chances of conception because lemon juice has been shown to kill sperm, not only directly but also by altering the acid levels in the body.

## WAIT UNTIL THE YEAR'S OUT

It is not unusual for most women to have to wait several months before conceiving, especially if they have been on the contraceptive pill for a number of years. Experts suggest that there is no need to worry about fertility until you've been trying for a year with no results.

## RAISE A CUP TO FERTILI-TEA

Taking an infusion from 125g (4oz) or more of tea each day could double, or even in some cases triple, your chances of conception. Black teas contain slightly more caffeine than green, but either will do the trick.

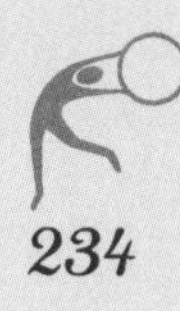



### DESTRESS TO BOOST EGG QUALITY

You can improve the quality of your eggs by cutting down on the stress in your life, which causes the body to release stress hormones such as adrenaline. These substances alter the natural hormone balance in the body and jeopardize the quality of eggs.

### CONCEIVE WITHOUT COFFEE

High-caffeine products with none of tea's antioxidant benefits, like filter coffee, cola and energy drinks, have been shown to reduce the chances of conception in both men and women.

### GIVE A FIG

Dried figs and apricots, wheatgerm, leafy green vegetables, sesame seeds and nuts are all good sources of magnesium, low levels of which have been shown to reduce the chances of conception in women.

### ACCURATE PREGNANCY TESTING

Don't test too soon. One week after your expected period is the best time to take a pregnancy test. About 25% of women who ultimately get positive results, won't tests positive on the first day they miss their period.

## immunity boosts

### GRAB A GRAPE

Grapes, especially those with seeds, could boost immunity by inducing the production of important cells known as T-cells, which play a key part in protecting against viruses and bacteria in the body.

### NATURE'S WAY

Natural immunity is something we're born with, but it can be boosted early in life by being breast-fed. Breast-feeding enables antibodies to be passed from the mother to the child.

### SHORT-TERM BOOSTS

Echinacea – available as tablets or as a liquid – stimulates phagocytosis, the consumption of invading organisms by white blood cells. The herb has maximum effect when taken in short courses to fight recurring infections, such as colds. For this reason, avoid taking it as a long-term preventive measure.

### CHINESE HERBS FOR HEALTH

The Chinese herb astragalus stimulates immune-system activity by increasing the number of stem cells in the marrow and lymph, and stimulates their development into active immune cells. Research suggests that it can also trigger immune cells from a "resting" phase into an "active" phase.

## posture

### IF AT FIRST YOU DON'T SUCCEED...

Practise really does make perfect. It might sound staggering, but you may have to repeat a postural change around 10,000 times before it becomes sufficiently engraved on your brain to become a subconscious action.

### DON'T LET SHOULDERS CREEP UP ON YOU

A common fault is to let shoulders creep up towards your ears as muscles tighten and the back bends forward. Gently hold shoulders back and try to keep space around the sides of your neck.

### SUMMON SOME LUMBAR SUPPORT

A lumbar support should fit snugly into your spine at the point where it curves inwards at the waistband. If it is too low, it can put pressure on the sacroiliac joints, pushing the pelvis forwards.

### WALK TALL TO FREE YOUR BACK

As you walk around, lift your head until you're looking straight ahead of you, with a relaxed neck and shoulders. Press your shoulders back (not up) so your chest is pushed out, and straighten your spine so you are standing straight, but not too rigidly, like a ramrod.

## KEEP CIRCULATION HEALTHY WITH THE THREE-FINGER GAP

If your feet are hanging or tucked under when you sit down, the increased pressure on the backs of the legs can impair return circulation from the feet. This can lead to or aggravate swollen ankles and varicose veins. Keep both feet on the floor and aim for no more than a three-finger gap behind your knees.

## GET FIRM AT NIGHT

Make sure your mattress is firm enough to support the contours of your body, to reduce pressure on the spine.

## PULL YOUR KEYBOARD CLOSER

By holding your elbows away from your body you set up continuous tension in the muscles of the neck and shoulders, thus creating a buildup of lactic acid and other unwelcome by-products. If you're typing, make sure the keyboard is positioned so that your elbows fall to your sides, not in front of you.

## SLEEPING SUPPORT

If you lie on your side in bed at night, consider putting a pillow between your knees to keep them at the same width as your hips, and so reduce twisting and strain on the pelvis. This will also help you avoid the discomfort of hip pain.

## GIVE IT THE ELBOW

By bending your arms at the elbow when you walk, and using them to work your stride pattern, you will burn at least 5%-10% more calories than if you let them hang by your side.

## DON'T STRETCH TO FIT

For perfect posture, your neck should not be straight or stretched, but it should retain its slight natural curve with your chin parallel to the floor, neither tucked in nor jutting out.

## A GOLDEN STRING TO BETTER POSTURE

This health tip is borrowed from the Alexander Technique, and it is a way to help you walk taller without injury. Imagine there is a golden string running vertically up your body through your spine, stretching you upwards through the crown of your head and creating space between each vertebra.

### MAKE SLEEP A SIDE ISSUE

People who sleep on their side take an enormous amount of pressure off their spine compared with those who lie on their front or back. Lying face down is the worst position for overnight spine health.

### LOOK AHEAD TO LOOK SHARP

It might be tempting to look at your feet as you walk along, but for the best posture you should focus on an imaginary spot about 3.5m–6m (12ft–20ft) in front of you. If your head is down, this increases strain on the neck and shoulders.

### WALK FASTER, NOT LONGER

It is counterproductive – and potentially harmful to your back – to increase the length of your stride unnaturally. Speed and efficiency in walking are generated by hip flexibility and using quicker, not longer, steps.

### STRETCH YOUR NECK TO RELEASE STRESS

Stand up straight with your back against a wall. Keeping your head level, without looking up or down, jut your neck forward. Then bring your chin straight back as if on railway tracks. Repeat five times to release tense neck muscles.

## pressure points

### GIVE YOURSELF A HELPING HAND

Your LI4 pressure point is located on the top side of the hand, between your thumb and your index finger. To locate it, squeeze the thumb against the base of the index finger. The point you are looking for is located on the highest point of the bulge of the muscle. Press this point for about 30 seconds to induce calmness and for a health-inducing digestive detox. However, you should not try this technique if you are pregnant.

### PUT YOUR BEST FOOT FORWARD

Your L3 pressure point is found on the foot, on the line running between the big toe and the second toe and about three finger widths from the edge in the hollow on the top of the foot. Move your index finger anticlockwise over this point in order to induce relaxation and to unblock any anger and depression.

## CLEAR YOUR KIDNEYS

Your kidney point, which can be used to treat fatigue and lethargy as well as to detox the body through the kidneys, is located on the sole of the foot, just to the side of the ball of the foot under the second or third toe. Press and release several times.

## ENJOY AN EXTRA ENERGY BOOST

Stimulating your stomach point can give you extra energy when you're flagging or tired. It is located just below the knee, on the outside of the shinbone. Press for at least 30 seconds with the pad of your finger or thumb.

## TEND TO NECK TENSION

A tension-relief point, good for reducing pain caused by tension headaches and relieving tired eyes, is found in the occipital hollow, where the bottom of the skull meets the neck on either side of the spine. Use a thumb on either side to compress this area but be very careful not to press too hard.

## ARM YOURSELF AGAINST ANXIETY

A stress-relieving point for reducing anxiety and tension is found at the top centre of the forearm (with palm facing down) in the large section of muscle just underneath the crease of the elbow. Press for several seconds and release several times.

## LISTEN TO YOUR HEART

Your SI19 point is located near the ear, just before the small projection in front of the ear canal. It's in the depression that forms when the mouth is opened. Press for several seconds to release your inner emotions and desires.

## STEP UP TO BOOST METABOLISM

A metabolism-boosting point is found on top of the foot, roughly in line with the middle two toes and directly over the arch. Use two fingers to apply broader pressure here because of the bones and ligaments.

## COMPRESS THE WRIST TO REDUCE THE STRESS

Find the spot between the tendons of the inside of the wrist, three finger widths from the palm. Breathe in, press as you breathe out slowly and repeat several times to reduce stress and strain.

### GET IMMEDIATE IMMUNITY

An immunity-boosting point that is also good for combating fatigue, depression and general feelings of sluggishness is found on the inside of the ankle above the foot between the Achilles tendon and the ankle bone. Press and release several times for 10–20 seconds.

### FORM A FIST TO HELP A HEADACHE

A point for general pain relief (especially of headaches) is found on the back, in line with the kidneys. The best way to stimulate this point is to sit up straight on a chair and form a fist with both hands. Place the fists behind your back so they touch and lie level with the elbow. Lean back gently.

### DO AN ANTISTRESS PRESS

Stimulating the acupressure point that is located in the soft V-shaped area of flesh found between the thumb and forefinger can help reduce stress. Press the pad of your thumb into this area for at least 30 seconds and then repeat the same action on the other hand.

## self-massage

### GET IT OFF YOUR CHEST

In order to reduce tension across the front of the chest area, and to free up your breathing and loosen stress in your neck, place the four fingers of your right hand on the left side of your chest, underneath the clavicle bone. Move the fingers in circular motions, working outward towards the shoulder joint in deeper strokes. Repeat on the other side. Breathe in and out slowly as you massage.

### HEAD OFF TENSION

To reduce tension in the scalp, spread out the fingers and thumbs of both hands and place them on either side of your head with the thumbs towards the back of the neck. Work in small circular motions, and then, after a few seconds, move the hands so they cover a different area.

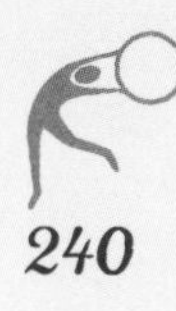



### STICK YOUR NECK OUT

To reduce neck tension, move the four fingers of your right hand in circular motions over the top of your left shoulder, turning your head to the right to stretch the muscles and ligaments at the front of the neck. Repeat on the other side.

### DRAW TENSION FROM YOUR JAW

To relieve tension in your jaw and the sides of your face, place the four fingers of your left hand together on the jaw so the index finger fits into the bony area in front of the earlobe. Using small circular motions, work lightly, being careful not to press too hard.

## sense & sensation

### LISTEN TO YOUR TASTEBUDS

If grapefruit is too bitter for you, you could be a supertaster. Supertasters average 425 tastebuds per square centimetre on the tips of their tongues, compared with 184 for most people.

### EAT BEFORE YOU GET TOO HUNGRY

Hungry people taste salt and sugar more strongly than people who aren't hungry, so to avoid those salt and sugar cravings don't go for long periods without eating – have a healthy snack before you feel ravenous.

### DON'T IGNORE YOUR FEMALE INTUITION

It's far from being a myth. Studies have shown that women who listen to their sixth sense are happier and healthier than those who ignore underlying feelings.

### ADOPT A SENSE OF THE DAY

To make the most of your senses, pick a sense every day and make the most of it by fine-tuning. Concentrate on the everyday sensations you usually ignore to become more attuned to good sensations.

### LOOK AT YOUR FOOD

Without smell, our sense of taste would be next to nothing, but many people don't know that the look of food is important for taste as well. Food that looks good, quite simply, tastes good too.

### BECOME A CHILD EXPLORER

Children explore their environments with all of their senses – taste, smell, touch, sight and sound. So the next time you go somewhere new, don't rely just on sight and sound but think about how your other senses react as well.

### DON'T NEGLECT YOUR MOST IMPORTANT SENSE

One of our senses is far and away the most important of all for health and happiness – so whatever you do and wherever you are, don't forget your sense of humour. People who can see the funny side of difficulties and problems are quicker at bouncing back from adversity.

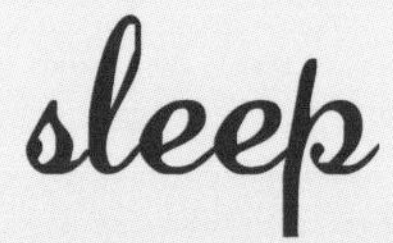

### SLEEP TO SURVIVE

Sleep could be as important as food for survival. Scientists have shown that animals deprived of sleep die within two to three weeks, almost the same length of time as if deprived of food.

### JUICE UP TO DRIFT OFF

Juice together 3 apples, 2 oranges, 1 lemon and 2 handfuls of iceberg lettuce leaves (which contains lactones, calming substances that act as a natural sedative). Drink a glass before bed to help you sleep like a baby.

### WATCH OUT FOR THE BURNOUT

If you feel tired during the day but can't sleep at night, it could be a sign that you're overtraining and not giving your body the rest it needs to thrive. If you don't feel motivated and alert within ten minutes of starting your workout, stop.

### TRYP OFF TO SLEEP

Tryptophan is one of the eight essential amino acids obtained in the diet from protein foods such as milk and meat. It enhances sleepiness and stimulates the production of sleep-inducing hormones in the brain.

### SNACK ON SWEETCORN FOR A SLEEPY NIGHT

Some foods – including sweetcorn, oats, rice, tomatoes and bananas – contain traces of melatonin, which helps regulate sleep.

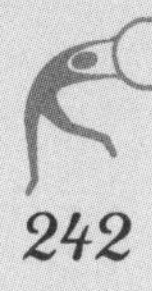



## HOLD YOUR TONGUE

Experts suggest that you try this clever sleep trick to help you drop off: close your eyes and hold your tongue so it's not touching your cheeks or the roof of your mouth, as if you're yawning with your mouth closed. You'll be sleeping like a log in no time.

## BEAT SNORING BY SLEEPING MORE

Sleep deprivation, especially if it's over several weeks, causes the muscles of the throat to sag, which leads to more snoring and less sleep. To stop snoring, aim for at least seven hours of sleep a night.

## SLEEP TO STAY FIT

Cardiovascular function can be reduced by an astounding 11% after cumulative sleep deprivation, which means sleep is essential if you want to stay fit and healthy.

## GO WITH THE FLOW

There's some evidence that reduced blood flow to hands and feet can keep you awake. Keep feet warm by wearing socks in bed or by investing in a hotwater bottle.

## PUT SLEEP FIRST

Lack of sleep impairs your coordination, judgement and immune system, say the experts, so put sleep first for a healthy life and get into good habits by going to bed at about the same time every night. If a particular job or task isn't done by bedtime, just leave it until tomorrow.

## BE A SLEEPING BEAUTY

Overnight, while you are asleep, your skin, hair and nails get a chance to regenerate themselves and deal with any health problems. Reducing the amount of sleep you get will therefore reduce the health of everything about your body, including the way you look.

## BE A HERBAL HIBERNATOR

Certain herbs such as valerian, camomile, hops and lime tree flowers have been shown to have sedative properties and are often taken either internally as a herbal tea or used within herbal pillows to enhance sleep.

## BEWARE OF KNOCKOUT MEDICATIONS

Some medications used to treat insomnia may increase sleep, but if they reduce healing REM sleep you won't get the benefit of sleeping longer. Consult your doctor for advice.

## SOAK AWAY INSOMNIA

A warm bath before bedtime can help you sleep by relaxing muscles and encouraging inactivity, which is essential for sleep. Try using calming aromatherapy oils such as lavender and lowering the lighting for an even sleepier experience.

## DON'T EXERCISE LAST THING AT NIGHT

Because undertaking physical exercise raises internal body temperature, which, in turn, wakes you up, exercising before bedtime is not a good way to tackle insomnia. Instead, try relaxing stretches or an indulgent bath.

## KEEP YOUR SLEEP ON SCHEDULE

According to the experts, going to sleep at about the same time every night helps your body get into a regular sleep rhythm, which will help put a stop to any sleep problems. Similarly, try to get up at the same time every day in order to keep your schedule on track.

## AVOID CAFFEINE AFTER DARK

Caffeine has well-known stimulant effects and drinking it before bed is likely to impair the quality of your sleep. Remember that chocolate contains caffeine, too, so that late-night treat might not in reality be a good idea either.

## DON'T SPEED INTO SLEEP

If you are one of those people who fall asleep the very second their head hits the pillow at night, you could be suffering from the first effects of sleep deprivation. Healthy sleepers take an average of ten minutes to drop off.

## SLEEP TO REGENER-EIGHT

It is estimated that the average person needs eight hours' sleep a night to re-energize body and mind, so don't beat yourself up about that weekend lie-in – your body needs it!

## AIR YOUR SHEETS TO REFRESH YOUR SLEEP

Bacteria, mites and bedbugs thrive in moist conditions, so after you get up in the morning and instead of making the bed immediately, turn back the covers to allow the sheets to breathe for 30 minutes. Airing your bedroom by opening a window will help, too.

## SLEEP LONGER TO LIVE LONGER

Recent studies have shown that people who sleep for less than six hours a night have a much higher mortality rate than those who give themselves just an hour or so longer in bed. So if you want to live longer, stay in bed.

## STAY HIGH CARB FOR HIGH SLEEP

Glucose provides fuel for your brain, which is just as important while you are sleep as when you are awake. Eating foods that are rich in carbohydrates in the evening, especially those that release their sugar content slowly, helps promote long and healthy sleep.

## SINK INTO EGYPTIAN COTTON

Egyptian cotton sheets wick away about 18% more moisture than other types of bedding. This not only leaves your skin healthy and dry, it also prevents moisture problems developing and increases overnight comfort.

## BANISH INSOMNIA WITH ELVIS'S CURE

Elvis's favourite treat, the peanut butter and banana sandwich, could also be the best bedtime snack because of the high levels of sleep-inducing tryptophan it contains. It also releases energy slowly, promoting healthy sleep cycles.

## DON'T NAP AWAY YOUR NIGHT'S SLEEP

Napping can ruin sleep habits, so keep it down to 20 minutes and don't leave it until late – mid-afternoon is the best time.

## SLEEP ON YOUR PROBLEMS

If you're living a stressful life, sleep might be the only chance your brain gets to sort out problems. The unconscious workings of your brain could mean you wake up in the morning with a surprise solution.

### HAND CARE WHILE YOU SLEEP

Not only does lavender hand cream give hands and nails a well-deserved moisture boost, but its scent induces deep sleep.

### BE A COOL SLEEPER

Body temperature should drop naturally at night for the soundest, deepest sleep. Keep your bedroom cooler than the rest of the house and don't use covers you don't need. Research indicates that 16°C (62°F) is most conducive to restful sleep while temperatures above 24°C (71°F) are likely to cause restlessness.

### SLEEP TO STAY SLENDER

A lack of sleep could slow down your metabolism, causing your body to hold onto weight. To stay slim and keep your metabolism optimal, make sure you are getting at least seven hours of good-quality sleep every night.

## workout wisdom

### DRINK UP TO WORK OUT

Because water is essential to maximize metabolism, you won't reap the full benefits from your exercise routine unless you stay hydrated throughout. You can boost your body's performance on workouts simply by keeping topped up with water. Studies have shown that just a 3% loss in body fluid can lead to a 7% reduction in overall physical performance, so drink plenty of water before, during and after your workouts.

### STRETCH IT OUT

Studies have suggested that stretching before undertaking exercise isn't as important as stretching afterwards. Instead, warm up at a slow pace beforehand and devote more time to stretching properly when you have finished.

### GET INTENSE

High-intensity workouts have a greater and longer-lasting effect on increasing your resting metabolic rate, essential for long-term fat burning. Researchers have found that upping the intensity when you work out could help you burn as much as 300 extra calories a day, even at rest.

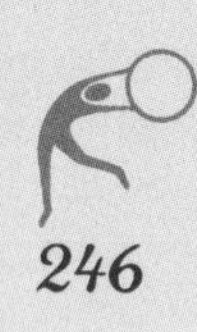



## DO EXERCISE TO AVOID DIABETES

Exercise reduces fat tissue in the body and makes cells more responsive to insulin. Exercising five times a week has been shown to reduce the risk of diabetes by 45%, two to four times a week by 40% and once a week by 25%.

## DON'T STARVE IF YOU WANT TO STAY FIT

People who don't feed their body enough fuel in the form of carbohydrates and proteins can't reach the same exercise intensities as others and therefore don't achieve the same metabolic changes or weight loss with exercise.

## USE FRUIT FORCE

Snacking on healthy fresh or dried fruits, which contain slow-release fructose, teamed with a glass of milk after your exercise routine could improve long-term fitness and performance by rebuilding carbohydrate levels in the body, helping to metabolize fat.

## BELT UP TO CURE SIDE PAIN

If you often suffer side stitches when you exercise, wearing an exercise belt could prevent pain. Raising your arms above your head or pressing the affected area for several minutes could also help.

## BREATHE IN, BREATHE OUT

Keep breath flow steady to nourish your body with oxygen. As a rule, inhale on the easy part of an exercise and exhale on the hard part to keep optimum oxygen levels.

## STEP IT UP IN STYLE

Don't crank up the resistance on the Stairmaster or step machine so high that you have to lean on the arm posts, because this reduces efficiency. Instead, pump with your legs, get your heart rate up and progress slowly as you feel more comfortable with each level.

## EAT MEAT TO BUILD MUSCLE

Meat-eaters who exercise regularly are more likely to build muscle, lose fat and tone up than their vegetarian counterparts, probably as a result of the higher levels of protein in the diet.

## BE A VARIETY PERFORMER

For most of us, doing the same workout routine daily can induce boredom, not only in your head but also in your body, as it adapts to tasks. So vary your workouts and type of exercise to boost mental and physical fitness.

## SCORE A GOAL OF THE MONTH

Set small, realistic goals – don't set yourself up for failure by aiming for unachievable targets. Decide on small goals you can achieve, such as three 30-minute sessions at the gym each week, which make it easier to experience success.

## GIVE YOURSELF A GOLD MEDAL

Reward yourself for your successes. When you don't feel like exercising, remember how good you felt after exercising the last time, and reward yourself with healthy treats such as exercise clothes, new music to work out to or a sports massage.

## PUT YOUR BACK INTO IT

When devising a complete exercise plan, don't forget back exercises – although they might not seem as important as those showy triceps curls or leg squats, a strong back is absolutely key to effective, injury-free training.

## POSTURE-PERFECT WORKOUTS

As you work out, don't forget to engage your core strength muscles in your abdomen, which will keep your trunk strong and steady and help you avoid succumbing to injury, as well as preventing bad exercise habits.

## DON'T CURL UP TO SIT UP

Many people don't really work their abdominals properly during their situp exercise routines. Make sure you are moving the top of your body towards the ceiling, rather than curling it up towards your knees, which doesn't work the muscles as hard.

## CATCH A WAVE TO TONE YOUR THIGHS

If you're not into sweating it out in gyms or taking up a team sport, but want to tone your legs the best way possible, get yourself a surfboard and catch a wave. Surfing is great for toning legs and abdominals as well as honing balance.

## ANYONE FOR TENNIS?

Tennis burns 400 calories an hour and although it might not be such a good cardiovascular exercise as running or swimming, the tactical thinking stimulates your mind as well as your body, giving you a true holistic workout.

## SQUASH UP YOUR BACKSIDE

Played competitively, squash will really firm up your arms and abdominals, as well as giving your system a cardiovascular boost. But it is also one of the best exercises around for toning up those flabby behinds because of all the lunging around court that is involved.

## EXPLODE FOR STRENGTH

Explosive exercises – such as lunging – boost strength much faster than other types of weight training. To test this out, try doing your normal exercises more slowly, but with a high-impact beginning and ending.

## SADDLE UP TO RIDE AWAY SADDLE BAGS

Horse-riding not only tones hips, legs and thighs through a series of leg exercises as you ride, it also increases strength and flexibility in your pelvis, hips and lower back, and works the thigh muscles to reduce fat.

## ADD A FOOT OF TEXTURE

Simply wearing textured insoles inside sports shoes could help prevent knee and ankle injuries by increasing people's awareness of the position of their feet, particularly in fast-response sports like soccer and basketball.

## SLAM DUNK THAT STOMACH FLAB

Basketball might be better known for toning arms and legs than stomachs, but all that twisting and stretching for the basket is, in fact, one of the best ways to get rid of stomach flab, especially if you're shooting hoops.

## PUNCH YOUR FIGHTS OUT

For the ultimate body and brain-boosting workout, invest in a punchbag and a skipping rope. It has been shown that working out like a boxer will not only increase your cardiovascular fitness but also get rid of aggression and allow stress to flow out of the system.

## BOULDER YOUR WAY TO BETTER ARMS

If rock climbing is perhaps just a bit too extreme for you but you'd love the upper-body benefits, then try the safer alternative of bouldering. This is a sport in which you travel along the rockface rather than scaling it upwards. It builds great arm strength and, as a bonus, burns a whopping 360 calories in just 30 minutes.

## BOWL AWAY CALORIES

Next time you're playing a game of baseball, softball, rounders or cricket, volunteer to bowl or pitch – it burns the most calories of any other position on the playing field.

## STEER CLEAR OF A CAFFEINE STITCH

To avoid a painful side stitch while you're exercising, avoid drinking caffeine for at least an hour before you start. Caffeine drinks, particularly if they are carbonated as well, have been shown to increase side-stitch pain.

## WORKOUT BURNOUT

Overtraining can be just as dangerous as under-training. To prevent problems, make sure you have at least one complete rest day a week and give yourself a whole week off every two to three months to stay physically and mentally healthy.

## BANISH THE BANISTERS

Leaning on the banisters or handrail as you climb the stairs robs your legs of a strengthening workout. Keep your arms by your sides to boost strength and balance (and the same goes for the step machine).

## BOOST METABOLISM BY WORKING OUT EARLY

A workout first thing in the morning helps fire the metabolism all day, and when your metabolism is higher, you burn more calories. As a consequence, morning workouts mean you can eat the same amount and still lose weight.

## BE STRETCH EFFECTIVE

Stretches are ineffective unless they are held for a certain time. You should ease into position until you feel the stretch, then hold it for at least 25 seconds. Breathe deeply to help your body move oxygen-rich blood to sore muscles.

### GET RID OF YOUR JELLY BELLY

Belly dancing, because of its constant use of the abdominal and pelvic muscles, is one of the best exercises you can choose to tone up flabby bellies. It's fun, social and sexy, too – what more could you ask of a workout?

### GO STRAIGHT FOR THE WEIGHTS

Experts suggest that weight training should be done before any cardiovascular work in the gym, because it requires fresh energy. Cardiovascular exercise requires less energy and helps flush toxins away from muscles, so it should be saved for the end of a workout session.

### GET MORE FROM YOUR WORKOUT

During exercise that lasts more than 30 minutes, recent research shows that there is better performance, recovery and efficiency in people who drink at 10 to 20-minute intervals throughout the training session.

### DON'T SIT UP

Sipping water little and often while you exercise isn't as effective at rehydrating your body as taking large gulps less often, because larger amounts of water travel through your stomach quicker and are more likely to be absorbed.

### ASTHMA-FRIENDLY SPORTS

More than 10% of Olympic athletes suffer from asthma, so don't let it prevent you exercising. Go for sports near water, where asthma is less of a problem, like swimming, canoeing, sailing and windsurfing.

## time savers

### MAKE IT WORK FOR YOU

If you don't enjoy your job but don't feel you have a choice about giving up for something else, don't fall into the trap of wasting your time. If you have to stay in your job, work hard and try to find a niche within it that suits you.

## GIVE YOURSELF A KISS

Whenever you feel life's getting on top of you, remember the KISS principle – Keep It Simple, Stupid! Problems often crop up because we allow things to become overcomplicated, so keeping it simple is a great way to keep things in perspective. An approach that seems too easy to be true can be simply the best way.

## LEAVE GAPS

When you plan your day, don't fill every minute. Leave about 15–20% for contingencies. Then, if emergencies and interruptions happen, you won't be thrown completely off course.

## A STITCH IN TIME

Don't waste time re-doing jobs you've rushed through and therefore done badly. Take a little extra time to do a proper job and you'll save time in the long run.

## TURN OFF THE TV

If you're the sort of person who just can't find time to do anything in the evening, turning the TV off for an hour each evening will give you 365 hours (equivalent to 9 weeks) of extra time a year to achieve something.

## KEEP IT RELEVANT

Studies have shown that people who keep in mind the "value" of their job are generally more satisfied. For instance, if you have to work overtime for a few weeks, remind yourself that the extra money will allow you to buy that treat you've wanted.

## TREAT YOURSELF

When you complete a task or finish something as planned, give yourself a little treat. It could be something small like 20 minutes' rest with a magazine or something big like an evening out. This will help train your brain to want to finish tasks.

## TAKE 24

Try to make sure that each week you have at least 24 hours when you don't think about work. Use it to see friends, get out of the house, spend time with your family and other things you enjoy. It will help you work better the following week.

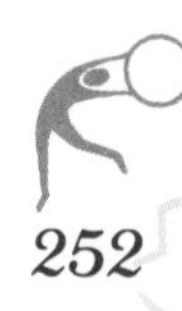



### POP ON THE PASTA

For people with busy lives, pasta is a great choice for meals as it provides a slow-release source of energy to get you through the day. It's also really easy to make. Make it even easier by freezing some of your favourite pasta sauces for an instant meal. Throw in some in-season vegetables and you have a healthy meal.

### BREAK UP BIG TASKS

If you find large tasks intimidating and overwhelming, split them into smaller tasks and do a little at a time. For instance, putting a year's worth of photos in albums might seem daunting, but not if you take a few at a time and spread it over several weeks.

## managing your lifestyle

### TAKE CONTROL

Feeling powerless is a major cause of stress and it's the choices you make that determine whether you're running your life or it's running you. Even where you feel you don't have choices, chances are you do, so make decisions rather than avoiding them.

### DON'T TAKE THEM FOR GRANTED

Many people – particularly men – who work hard and achieve great things take their personal lives and family for granted. To boost home harmony, realize what you have and remember to let your family know how much you appreciate them.

### BE CHOOSY

Everything in your life is not equal, and it's important to see it that way. Re-evaluate the amount of time you spend on tasks and with people, according to how important they are to you.

## KNOW YOUR LIMITS

Don't be drawn into spending longer and longer at work to get your jobs done. Talk to your boss or line manager about the number of extra hours they can reasonably expect of you and stick to your limits.

## WRITE A REVIEW

Every six months or so, review your priorities at work. If your job is not working as well as you had hoped, look at what needs to be changed and how you can make it work so that you feel your career is on track.

## STOP AND THINK

Many people work hard because they find it difficult to stop and relax, or are frightened to. Allow some space into your life where nothing is planned to give your body and brain the chance to unwind.

## CHOOSE CAREFULLY

If you find work takes over your life and it's all about income, think about changing careers for one you find more fulfilling; that way, it won't just be about money.

## SET AN EARLY DEADLINE

If you're the sort of person who only works well when deadlines are near, use tricks to help organize your working life. For instance, set your deadline a few days before the real one to give you a cushion in case anything goes wrong.

## GET A LIFE BALANCE

Keep your lifestyle expectations realistic, and strive for a balance of being happy at work and home. For instance, you may be prepared to sacrifice expensive holidays for fewer hours at work so that you can attend classes and learn a new skill. Deciding what your priorities are will help you make decisions more easily.

## HOME PRIORITY

Some people think work is more important than home life, but most people who overwork have simply fallen into the habit of being that way. Putting the priority back on your home life could help you make decisions that make you feel happier both at home and at work.

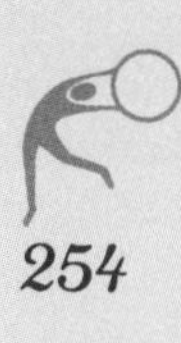



## DON'T OVERCOMPENSATE

If you're working because you feel high achievement makes you a better person, think again about your self-esteem. Try to find things you could do in other areas of your life that would help you feel as good.

## A PARTY OF ONE

Ensure you have at least one evening a week for yourself and your family, when you don't allow work to be thought of or mentioned, and you simply enjoy each other's company.

## JUST SAY NO

If you find it difficult to say no at work, practise in the mirror or with friends or a partner. Get them to ask you the sort of question you would usually find it difficult to say no to and practise your response.

## YOU'RE NUMBER ONE

Don't let your work become the most important thing in your life – make sure you are always number one in the decisions you make. Look after yourself and you'll end up far happier and healthier.

## GET A MANTRA

If you find yourself getting stressed and overwhelmed by work during the day, choose a phrase that reminds you to relax ("slow down, breathe better" or "I can feel the space inside my head"). Then close your eyes and repeat the phrase to yourself when you feel stress levels rising.

## LEARN TO DELEGATE

You'll never be able to do everything on your own, so learn the art of delegation. That means trusting people to complete tasks on their own, not hovering over them and wasting both your time and theirs.

## GET SOME PERSPECTIVE

It's all too easy to lose perspective when you're working too hard, but life is more rewarding when work and personal life are balanced. You'll be surprised at how acknowledging a problem can help you enact a beneficial change.

### TAKE AN INVENTORY

Many people have regular reviews at work, and it's a valuable tool to help you address problems and aspirations. Give yourself a career review every six months and check everything is working towards your goals.

### DON'T GIVE 140%

It's fine to give all of yourself to your job when you're doing it, but make a rule that evenings are to be work free.

## healthy finances

### OWN UP TO DEBT

If you're going to solve your financial problems with your partner, it's important you own up to debt and work together to solve problems. Don't be secretive about your spending habits. Make the time to work out budgets together.

### SHARE THE WEALTH

If you're the wage earner, never use money as a weapon. The way people deal with money in a relationship says a lot about who has the power, the freedom and the control, so make sure you keep it as equal as possible.

### BE A SPENDTHRIFT

A major cause of money worries is over-spending and increasing debt. For a month, don't allow yourself to buy anything that isn't absolutely essential. Be strict and at the end of that period, you'll be amazed at how little you've missed those things you thought were so important.

### BE VIGILANT

Check through your credit history carefully and if there's anything you think is strange, like a loan application you didn't make, you could be a victim of ID fraud. Get in touch with the lender immediately to make sure. Your credit report changes all the time, so it's important to check it regularly to make sure it's up to date and there are no mistakes or problems.

## PRIORITIZE PAYMENTS

If you're worried about paying all your debts, don't just pay the one that shouts loudest. Work out which debts and expenses are your priorities – for instance, mortgage, rent, tax and utilities – and pay them first.

## SHOP SMART

Try to buy things that aren't essential in sales or at discount outlets. Make it your aim never to pay full price for nonessential items and you'll get the feel-good boost of having bagged a bargain as well as saving yourself money.

## SEPARATE YOUR FINANCES

When the financial credit check companies go through your report, they may also check the reports of people with whom you have had financial dealings in the past, like joint accounts or loans, which may impact your credit rating. If you are separated, make sure your finances are, too.

## DON'T BE DISTRACTED

When it comes to choosing a bank account, don't be distracted by "free gifts" and special offers which can often mask lower interest rates or higher fees. Choose the account that works for you best.

## THINK AHEAD

Get a pension as soon as you can, which will help you reduce those worries about what will happen as you get older. The longer you save for, the less you will pay, so sooner is best.

## THE REAL COSTS

Before you sign up for store cards, credit cards and loans you should get out your calculator and work out exactly how much you will be paying back, to make sure you'll be able to afford the repayments.

## LET LENDERS KNOW

If you are struggling with repayments, don't hide your head in the sand. Many companies now have protocols in place to help people who are struggling, including freezing and reducing repayments.

## OPEN YOUR BILLS

Always open your bills and bank statements and read through them, particularly if you are having money problems. Ignoring them won't make problems go away and you're best off knowing the whole picture.

## TALK TO CREDITORS

If you need to stop some repayments, talk to your creditors first rather than just going ahead. If you explain your problems, they are likely to be more understanding.

## DON'T ROB PETER TO PAY PAUL

Avoid falling into the trap of borrowing money or taking out a loan to pay off existing debt. This is likely to lead to many more problems in the long run and will ultimately mean you pay more interest.

## MAKE CONTACT

If you find something in your credit check you disagree with, make sure you contact the relevant lender or authority in writing as soon as possible. Keeping a record of correspondence can help settle issues.

## REGISTER TO VOTE

Money lenders use the electoral register (voter registration) to check that you are who you say you are and that you live at your address as a protection against fraud. Make sure your information is up to date.

## REDUCE YOUR DEBTS

Instead of owing small amounts of money to lots of creditors, try to pay off a few entirely. Not only will this be easier to manage but it will look better on your credit score.

## TELL THE TRUTH

Don't lie or bend the truth in any way on an application form for finances. It might seem like a small thing but it counts as fraud and could leave a permanent black mark on your credit rating.

# finding your vocation

## DO YOUR RESEARCH

Once you've decided on a vocation or career that you think is right for you, do some research to check there isn't anything that puts you off before you take the plunge. Look for things like salary ranges, educational requirements, working hours and conditions.

## GET SOME VALUE

Working out what your values are is an important part of choosing the right career. There is no right or wrong when it comes to values, it's simply what you hold dear. Be honest with yourself.

## THE REAL YOU

If you want to find a good career match you've got to know what makes you tick. Don't listen to what your friends and family think, because the only one who really knows what's in your heart is you.

## MEASURE YOUR EXCITEMENT

A good gauge of what is likely to motivate you in a career is what keeps you awake and interested in general life. Make a list of things you're really into and try to think of a career that would combine them.

## LOCATION LOCATION

If you're trying to choose the right career, think about where you'll work as well as the job. For instance, do you see yourself as an office person or more of an outdoors type? Do you like quiet or bustle?

## WORK ON YOUR SKILLS

Having an interest in a certain career – or even a talent for it – doesn't count if you haven't got the skills to match. Volunteer, take classes and work on honing your skills to suit the job you want.

## DON'T BE EMBARRASSED

If you have strange interests or interests that aren't the same as your family and friends, don't be pressured into doing what they do. Be honest with yourself about what you like and you'll be happier for it.

## UNEARTH YOUR TALENT

Talent is important because it makes us feel good about ourselves. Chances are, you'll probably like the things you're good at. If you don't know what your talents are, ask your nearest and dearest for their thoughts.

## TAKE A TEST DRIVE

If you're thinking of starting a career path or changing careers, why not give it a test drive first? Volunteer or job shadow so you can see what the job is really like.

## BE OPEN-MINDED

When it comes to choosing a career, it isn't just about how well you perform academically. Consider how you relate to others – are you a born leader, well organized or good at putting people at ease? These too are important things to consider.

## CHOOSE THE JOB FOR YOU

Your work is part of your life, not your whole life, but chances are you spend more time at your place of work than at your home. Make sure you choose a job that works for you rather than being pushed into something you don't like.

## FOLLOW TRENDS

If you want to find the right career, it's important to have your finger on the pulse when it comes to new trends and how they alter the jobs on offer in the workplace. This will help you plan a career being mindful of changing technology. Read the jobs pages in the newspapers and talk to other people about what's happening.

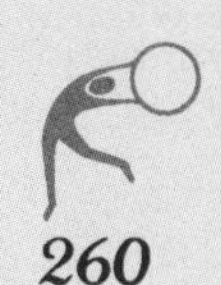



# work it out

## WALK IT OUT

If possible, try to work near where you live. Studies have shown that people whose home-to-work journeys are less than half an hour are significantly less stressed, especially if they can walk to work.

## BRING YOUR FAMILY TO WORK

It has been proven that people who feel relaxed at their desks are more productive. Within reason, make your work environment more appealing with family photos, plants or other decorations. Don't let paperwork build up around you. Clear the clutter and put things into containers.

## SET PRIORITIES

Don't let small, insignificant tasks get in the way of big ones. If you have trouble prioritizing, try writing lists in a colour system, with red for "essential", black for "required" and blue for "optional", and concentrate on red first to make sure you don't lose track of what's important.

## GET GOSSIPING

Don't spend your well-earned tea break talking or thinking about work – your brain will function much better on your return if you give it a complete rest, and studies have shown that gossiping is good for productivity!

## GO PUBLIC

Make sure you forward plan when it comes to your job so you aren't surprised by sudden increases in workload. Think ahead and talk to someone who can help beforehand if you think you're going to struggle rather than waiting until it's all too much.

## MAKE ONE JOURNEY

Try to work out your journey to work so you rely on one mode of transport only. Changing from car to train to bus is the most stressful part of commuting.

### REAP THE REWARD

Whether it's a home or work project, you'll benefit from setting targets. Divide your project into long and short-term goals and give yourself a treat whenever you reach one.

### COOK UP A STORM

Food is really important to maintain brainpower. If you've got a big project coming up at work and are likely to be too tired to cook in the evening, make up a few batches of nutritious food for the freezer so you can make sure your brain stays in tiptop form.

### CUT THE NEGATIVITY

For a whole week, don't allow yourself to say anything negative about anyone else at work. Stopping yourself will make you realize how negative you can be and how much it affects you. Try to find positive things to say about your co-workers.

## office angels

### KNOW YOUR ENERGY

Take a few days thinking about what is your most productive time of day and try to organize your time around them. For instance, if you have a natural dip at 4 pm, maybe that's a good time to do tasks that require a little less brainpower.

### HOLD A MEETING

When there are big decisions to be made, it's always best to meet face to face (or at least by video link if a face-to-face meeting isn't possible) because it's human nature to want to see reactions.

### AN EARLY BIRD

If you often find yourself rushed and flustered when you get to the office, start getting up 15 minutes earlier. The extra time will give you a chance to read through your work notes for the day so that you can start the day feeling well prepared.

### CHOOSE A BAD JOB

Work through your to do list sensibly – don't choose all the jobs you like first and leave the bad jobs till last. Instead, try to alternate an enjoyable job with one you don't feel like doing.

## DON'T PROCRASTINATE

Open your post immediately rather than leaving it in unopened piles. Throw away or recycle anything you don't need to keep and try to file everything else straight away, keeping out only what you need to deal with. Aim to look at each piece of paper only once and don't let it pile up.

## GIVE YOURSELF A BREAK

Did you know that 91 million working days a year are lost to mental ill-health in the UK and in the USA 200 million working days are lost annually? Working till you drop isn't going to do anyone any favours in the long run, so make sure you give yourself regular breaks to stay on top of things.

## MAKE A LIST

Before you leave work at night, make a fresh list for the next day and stick it on your screen or desktop or leave it open on your desk. It will stop you wasting time the next day and help your head stay clear in the evening.

## BE REALISTIC

If you're commuting in the winter, make sure you allow more time as many accidents are caused by people rushing in inclement weather. Planning journeys in advance will make you less stressed.

## A GOOD POSITION

Make sure your chair is comfortable and your lower back is supported, and that you're not too far from your keyboard. Nothing should feel strained or stretched, especially if you stay in the same position for a while.

## CLEAN IT UP

Invest 5 minutes of time in cleaning up your desk before you leave the office – arriving to a clutter-free desk in the morning will help you start the day on the right note.

## TELL THE TIME

Make sure you have a clock on your desk or prominently displayed on your computer. That way, you'll be able to monitor how long it takes you to do things so time doesn't run away with you.

## GET ELECTRONIC

Buy an electronic organizer, or use your phone or BlackBerry, to serve as your diary, address book and calendar. Using it to remember things like birthdays as well as meetings will free up brain space for more efficient working.

## CREATE A SYSTEM

Spend a few hours making sure your filing system is clear and concise and that it works for you. It's stressful not to be able to find essential items when you need them.

## COMMUNICATE WITH STAFF

If you're a manager, don't get so bogged down in trying to assign tasks that you forget to ask your workers what they want – research has shown that people work best if they enjoy their role, so keep in the loop.

## GET MOBILE

Instead of being stuck in the office, buy a laptop so you can move your office with you and maximize flexibility – get one with a built-in fax facility.

## TELEPHONE TENNIS

Return a call once, leaving a message and telling the person when you are available. Make sure you're available when you say you will be and you'll avoid wasting time to-ing and fro-ing with answer messages.

## EAT LIGHT

At lunchtime, make sure you don't overeat and try to avoid too much caffeine and alcohol which might cause a dip in energy in the afternoon. Keep lunch light and energizing with salads, fruit and protein.

## MULTITASK

Jobs that aren't too critical and don't require 100% concentration can be joined together to save time; for instance, deleting junk emails or organizing papers while "on hold" on the phone.

## KEEP IT BRIEF

Try to keep work phone calls brief and to the point. Spend a minute deciding what you want to say beforehand and try not to be distracted.

## SET A STANDARD

To save time when you're sending emails or letters, try to create standard templates you can use so you don't have to worry about starting afresh each time. This will help you free up more office time for other tasks.

## GET OUT AND ABOUT

Your office will work more efficiently if everyone has a lunch break. Try to encourage everyone to go out for at least a 10 or 15 minute break to perk them up and keep them going for the rest of the day.

## BE PREPARED

If possible, try to set out your clothes the night before so you don't rush in the morning. If you take a packed lunch to work, make sure it's already prepared so you can get out of the door quickly.

## SOUND OF SILENCE

In laboratory experiments, it has been shown that mice who were played irritating noises found it harder to concentrate. Make sure your office is free of audible irritations.

## FILE IT AWAY

Make a scheduled time to do your filing every day so papers don't get on top of you. It's an easy job, so right after your lunch break or later in the afternoon is usually a good time to choose.

## PAIN BEFORE PLEASURE

It might be tempting to do all the enjoyable things in your life first, but studies show you'll actually enjoy your leisure time more if you feel you've achieved something beforehand – so work now, play later.

## GET COMPETITIVE

To help keep you all motivated and if you have co-workers who are interested, get them involved in deadline competitions for tasks or see who delivers the best quality product or service within the time.

## CLEAN OUT

Make it a rule to get together every month in the office to clear it of unwanted papers and accumulated junk. Put on some music and go through everything to declutter.

## ASK FOR QUIET

If certain colleagues cause disruption in the office, why not instigate a "quiet" period every day or ask for a "red flag" system where you can ask for calm if you've got important work or preparation to do.

## CLUB THINGS TOGETHER

If your job can be split into different compartments like making sales calls, sending emails, creative thinking time etc, try to lump them together into separate time blocks so you can work more efficiently.

## GIVE PRAISE

Every time someone does something on time at work or at home, make sure you show your appreciation. Workers will be prepared to go that extra mile if they feel that their efforts are noticed and appreciated.

## STAY UP-TO-DATE

If you work from home or have a small office, make sure you concentrate on getting up-to-date equipment like integrated faxes and scanners.

## DON'T MEET UP

Avoid unnecessary meetings, which can be a big drain on your precious time. If something can be resolved without a meeting, do so, but stick strictly to agendas if you do meet up.

## KEEP WORK SEPARATE

If possible, try not to take work home with you and if you must, then try to limit it to one or two pre-planned nights a week. Similarly, make it a rule if at all possible, not to take your home life into the office. Keep phone calls to lunchbreaks if there are things you need to sort out.

## BE AN ENERGIZER

Many of us like to have a good moan, but did you know that lack of energy and motivation is contagious? If you feel energetic, you'll help the people around you feel energetic, too, which makes everyone happier. Make an effort to be positive around your workmates for a week and see the difference.

### TRACK YOUR TIME

Keep a diary detailing what you do for a week and at the end of the week tot up the amount of time you spent on various different tasks. Use it to plan your own time or talk to your manager about changing things if necessary.

### THINK ABOUT IT

If someone asks you to take on more responsibility at work, don't say yes immediately just because you feel flattered. Ask for time to think about it and really stop and evaluate what it would mean to your time management. Will it make your job more stressful and can you really manage to fit it in?

### GET CALLER DISPLAY

Buying a caller display unit is a great way to cut down on phone interruptions because you can see who's calling before you pick up the phone. You can then make a decision about whether to pick it up or leave it to go to answerphone.

### IGNORE THE PHONE

It's all too easy to pick up the phone the instant it rings but if you find you are constantly being interrupted by calls, try to have a time devoted to the telephone and a period during the day when you turn it off or switch it to answerphone and concentrate on your other jobs.

## homeworking

### EAT OUT

It's often tempting to eat lunch in the office if you're working from home, but try to give yourself at least one proper break during the day. Allocate half an hour and try to eat lunch in another room, or even go out for lunch.

### WORK BETTER HOURS

People who work from home are up to 20% more efficient than their office-based colleagues, probably due to the 'social distraction' factor. If you are on a contract or using flexitime to work at home, ask your bosses if your working day can reflect this with longer breaks or shorter hours.

## A TELECOMMUTER

If you find getting to work is taking up too much of your day, see if you can negotiate working from home a few days a week, then use the time you would have spent travelling to exercise, relax or do something else that makes you feel good.

## LOOK AWAY

People who work from home are much less likely to take breaks and look after themselves. Make sure you give your eyes a break from the screen every 15 minutes or so for at least a minute and use it as thinking time.

## SET A RECORD

It's fine to watch TV during break times if you're working from home, but don't let it set your timetables. If there are programmes you want to watch, record them so your work won't suffer.

## GET A LINE

To avoid unnecessary disturbances, get a separate business telephone line for when you're working from home and don't give the number to family and friends.

## BE SELECTIVE

Joining email groups and lists can be tempting, but make sure you police their activity – some groups generate a large number of emails that could be distracting if you're trying to work.

## GET A REVIEW

Just because you work from home, don't lose out on the regular reviews and progress reports you are entitled to if you work in an office. Schedule a regular timeslot with your line manager to keep you in the loop.

## WORK SPACE ONLY

Make sure you have a separate area used only for working, so you can leave paperwork around without the dog dribbling on it and you are still able to walk away at the end of the day and switch off.

## MEET UP

Schedule a meeting or lunch with co-workers to get yourself out of your home office at lunchtime. It will help you catch up on what's happening in the office as well as give you a break from your surroundings.

### GET A SEPARATE ACCOUNT

Email is great for keeping in touch, but it can be a distraction. Think about setting up different accounts for work and leisure, and be strict about using them.

### SAY NO TO FRIENDS

Ironically, it's often not colleagues who cause a problem when you're working from home, but family and friends who think if you're not in the office it's a day off. Let them know you're not available during working hours.

### CUT-OFF HOUR

Just because you are a home or are a remote worker, it doesn't mean you have to become a prisoner of your work. Make sure you stick to your working hours and don't be tempted to carry on into the evening on a regular basis.

### GET A FILTER

Set up filters in your email program to sort and keep track of email (this is particularly important if you can't have separate work and leisure accounts). This way, you'll be more able to separate work and home life.

### DO SOME CHORES

If you work from home, set yourself break times and use those times to achieve something in the house – that way, you'll be less likely to be distracted when your break ends. Try a load of laundry or washing up. And don't forget lunch.

## back to work

### BACK TO WORK

Going back to work after a baby is a big decision. Make sure you've weighed up the pros and cons by writing a list and really thinking about what's best for your family. Some mothers would be miserable without the extra money or adult time, but others would feel guilty or resent the intrusion of work into family life.

## SHARE THE LOAD

Before you decide to go back to work, think about different ways you could make it work better for your family. For instance, some families find that both parents working part-time works better than one full-time and one at home with the children.

## GET REAL

Make your expectations realistic so you allow yourself to succeed. It's impossible to be perfect in every area of life so allow for some failure and for some things to not be done as well as you'd like.

## INVOLVE YOUR FAMILY

Discuss any changes that are due to take place with your family when you sit down together at mealtimes. Let them be involved in deciding how everyone can contribute to make the transition easier. Apart from child care, there are household tasks to reassign.

## ASK FOR ADVICE

If you're going back to work after having children, involve your employer in making the transition easier – do they have flexible hours, courses on time management or subsidized child care which could help you?

## CHANGE CAREER

Going back to work after having children doesn't necessarily mean going back to the same job. Don't be afraid to choose a career that is less demanding on time and nerves if it seems like the best decision for the whole family. Why not visit a career advisor to help you decide?

## ASK A FRIEND

Rather than taking the leap back to work alone, talk to your friends and family who have already made that transition for ideas on how they coped and any possible pitfalls they encountered. Take advantage of hindsight and learn from other people's mistakes.

## PLAN A REST

When you plan out your day do not forget to include rest and recreation time for yourself, and don't treat it as an indulgence. Relaxed, rested people are far better able to cope with life's ups and downs and come out on top.

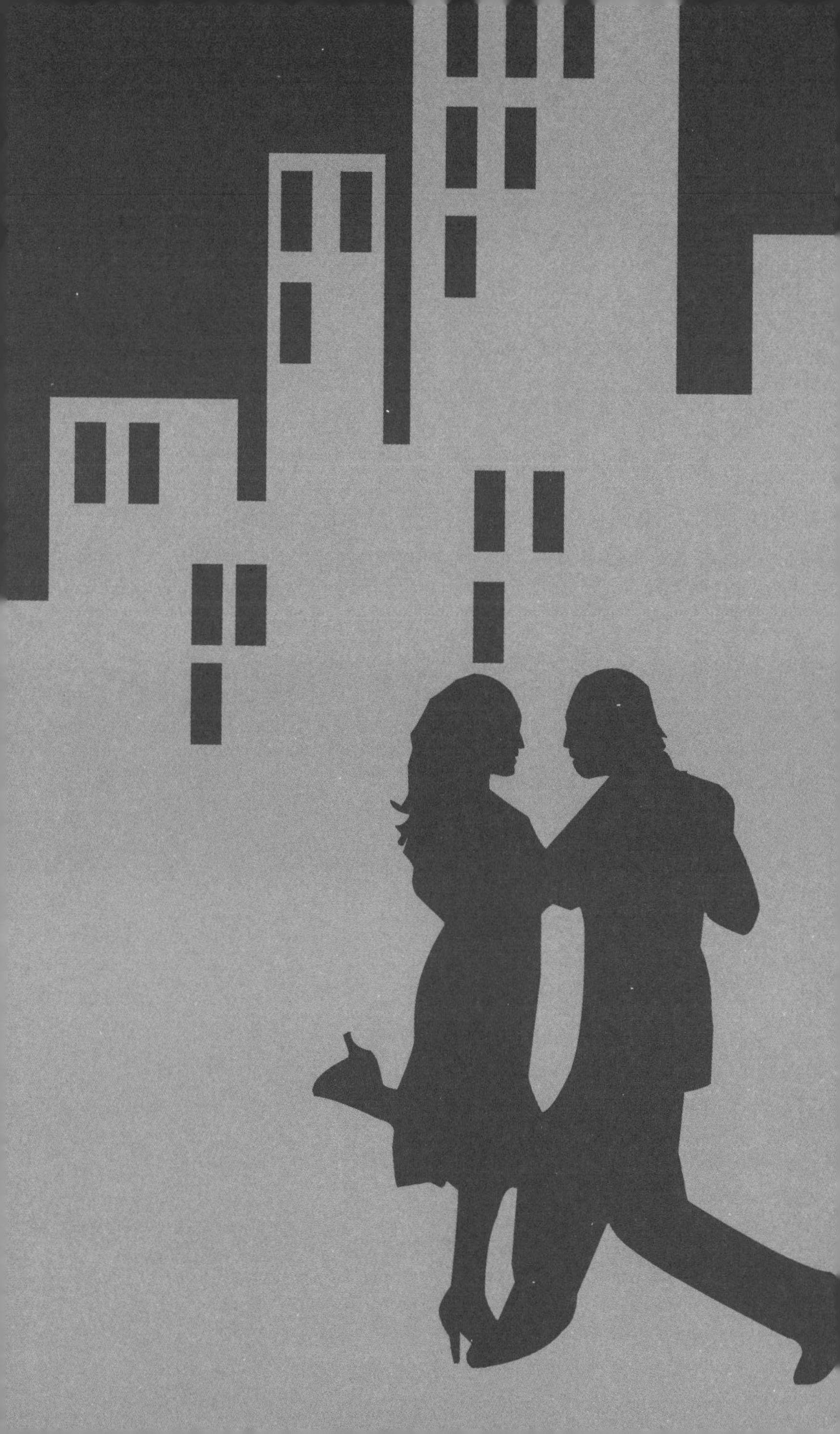

# Staying Healthy

With preventative tips as well as direct health remedies, this section covers everything from combating allergies, arthritis and back pain to colds, flu, fever, first aid, joint problems and female health. In addition there is a section that relates to health issues that occur throughout life, and through various stages of life, from your twenties to your later years.

# allergies

## SMOKE GETS IN YOUR EYES

Keep rooms well ventilated. Fumes that hang in the air, such as those from fresh paint, tar fumes, air pollution, insect sprays and tobacco smoke, can all aggravate allergic symptoms by irritating the sensitive mucous membranes in your eyes, nose and mouth.

## STAY IN TO DRY OUT

To avoid windborne pollen and grass seeds coming into contact with you, sticking to your clothes and causing allergic reactions, dry clothes and bedding inside instead of hanging them out on a clothesline.

## BRING BACK BATHTIME

Remember when the last thing you did before bed was have a bath? Washing your skin and hair in the evening rather than in the morning has been shown to reduce allergic reactions overnight by getting rid of allergens in hair and on skin.

## HUNT FOR HIDDEN DAIRY

If milk doesn't agree with you and makes you sick, you need to be aware of products that contain hidden sources of some of the allergens it contains. Watch out for casein, sodium caseinate, lactoglobulin and nougat on ingredients labels.

## IMAGINE YOURSELF SNEEZE-FREE

Studies have shown that, far from being quackery, taking some time out every day to think away your allergy could reap benefits. Take ten minutes in a quiet spot and create a mental image of yourself without your allergy – symptoms could begin to lessen after a few days.

## A SWEET HEALER

The healing properties of honey are thought to flow from its high proportions of pollen and plant compounds, producing a natural immunity in the body. Bee pollen, royal jelly, honeycomb and unfiltered honey are all believed to help.

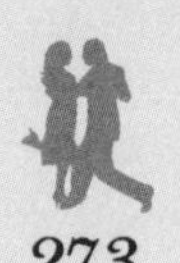



## BREATHE NEW LIFE INTO YOUR THROAT

Mix up an inhalation mixture with hot water and a drop each of lavender, eucalyptus and camomile essential oils to soothe breathing and reduce swelling and inflammation of the nose and throat. To trap steam, cover your head with a towel and bend over to inhale.

## GO FOR GARLIC

Garlic is thought to boost immunity, which could help regulate the body's allergic reaction to pollen grains.

## C FOR YOURSELF

Vitamin C is definitely the wonder vitamin when it comes to your immune system. Make sure you get a generous daily dose of fresh fruit and vegetables or take a supplement to keep your body fit to fight off infections.

## GET STEAMY TO CLEAR YOUR HEAD

Coughing during the night can be eased by hanging a wet towel on or near a radiator to increase humidity in the room overnight, preventing the lungs and throat from drying out and decreasing the chances of damage or infection.

## GIVE IT SOME ELBOW GREASE

Some of the worst allergy irritants, such as formaldehyde, phenol and ammonia, are found in cleaning fluids. Think about using alternatives, such as vinegar, soda crystals, lemon juice, water and a bit of hard work!

## DON'T STAND THE HEAT

A hot, humid house is a breeding ground for mould, mildew and dust mites. Turn down central heating to about 21°C (70°F) and if your house is humid, think about investing in an air-conditioning system or dehumidifier to help clear allergens.

## TREAT YOURSELF TO BREAKFAST IN BED

Habitual sneezing and coughing in the morning are often due to a sensitivity of the body to the cold, so giving your body some time to get used to the temperature change first thing by eating a warm breakfast or drink in bed could help prevent these irritants.

### SOOTHE YOUR STRESS

Emotional stress can worsen responses to allergens, so relaxation techniques may help relieve the symptoms of allergic reactions, especially with breathing problems.

### GET SALTY FOR SINUSES

If your sinuses are causing problems, you might want to try the 3000-year-old yogic practice of sniffing saltwater, which can help fight and prevent sinus infections. Ask a doctor or nurse for advice.

## arthritis

### GO ALKALINE TO NEUTRALIZE ACID PAIN

Acidic foods, like tomato, citrus fruits, fruit juices and red meats, can make the pain of arthritis worse from the build up of acid crystals in the joints. Plump for high-alkaline or neutral foods instead, like green vegetables, eggs, dairy produce and water.

### EASE PAIN WITH PINEAPPLE

Pineapple has been shown to suppress inflammation and boost bone health, thus improving joint pain in arthritis. Its anti-inflammatory properties are thought to be due to its high bromelain content.

### BOTH HANDS FOR LIGHT LIFTING

Using both of your hands rather than just one when lifting frying pans, pouring water from a kettle or jug, and carrying heavy household items eases the stress and strain that is caused by friction on joints and it can as a result reduce the effects of pain and discomfort.

### GET A JELLY GOOD CURE

A daily supplement containing gelatine, which has unique physical and chemical properties that enable it to reverse the effects of arthritis, can help ease arthritis symptoms significantly after three months of taking it.

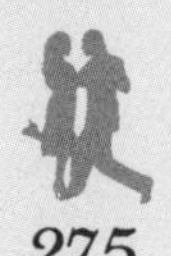



## STEER CLEAR OF SAUCES

Condiments and sauces like mustard, mayonnaise and vinegar can disrupt the pH of the body, turning it acidic and causing more pain to arthritic joints. Use natural yogurt as a garnish or opt for tomato-based sauces.

## GO LARGE FOR A BETTER GRIP

If you suffer from the problems associated with arthritis of the hands, life in the kitchen will be far easier if you choose gadgets and equipment fitted with large handles. Alternatively, wrap tape or foam around skinny handles so they are easier on your hands when you grip them.

## LEVER YOURSELF TO FREEDOM

If you have a weak grip, rather than struggling with hard-to-turn taps (faucets), why not fit levers? These will make your life much easier, as you will have to exert far less strength to turn them on and off. You could also replace doorknobs with levers to help you with doors.

## SOAK AWAY PAIN

Morning baths in warm water, or soaks for feet and hands, can help to ease pain from arthritic joints, which is often worse first thing. A good soak for at least ten minutes will reap maximum benefits.

## GO ELECTRIC FOR TIP-TOP TEETH

An electric toothbrush makes it easier to maintain dental health despite difficulty gripping with arthritic hand joints.

## TAKE UP TAI CHI FOR FLEXIBILITY

The ancient Chinese art of Tai Chi has been shown to reduce both the effects of arthritis and the distress caused by stiff, painful joints. Practising at least two or three times a week is most beneficial.

## STEP OUT AND STRETCH OUT

Regular walking, light weightlifting and stretching can reduce the pain from arthritis by up to a third. Aim for 20–30 minutes of exercise every day, mixing it up for maximum pain relief.

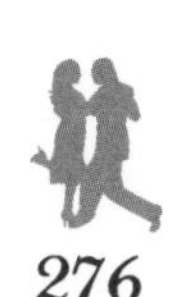



### CURRY FLAVOUR TO STOP SWELLING

Curries that contain high levels of the herb turmeric contain circumin, a natural anti-inflammatory that can help alleviate pain and swelling. If you don't fancy the hot stuff, supplements are also available.

### DROP A SIZE TO BE KNEE-WISE

According to experts, being overweight is such a danger to joints that losing as little as 5kg (11lb) may cut the risk of osteoarthritis of the knee by 50%.

### RUE THE RHUBARB

Rhubarb contains oxalic acid, which inhibits your body's ability to absorb calcium and iron from other foods. It can aggravate arthritis and may even cause an attack if eaten to excess.

### BE SUPER-CAREFUL IN THE SUN

Arthritis can make the skin more sensitive to the sun, so make sure you cover head, shoulders and eyes on bright days.

## back pain

### DESTRESS TO HELP YOUR BACK

Stress causes muscle tension that can lead to pain, especially in the lower back as the postural support muscles are overworked. Experts estimate that almost a fifth of all back pain is due to stress, so relaxation could be the most important prevention.

### HAIL A TAXI TO HEAD OFF INJURY

Choosing comfortable shoes, with a small heel to support the feet, could be key to back health. Each 2.5cm (1in) on the heel doubles the strain on joints and can throw the pelvis off balance, so avoid walking too far in them on those glamorous nights out.

### QUICK-RELEASE YOUR BACK

For a quick back stretch at your desk, place your feet flat on the ground and lean back on your chair so your back arches slightly. Drop your head backwards and then take a few deep breaths.

## DON'T BE AN ARCH VILLAIN

The spine begins to show signs of wear and tear as early as age 35, so from this age onwards it's important to keep it flexible and strong. Lots of people forget that the back doesn't only bend forward – it's important to stretch it into an arched position as well. You can do this by simply leaning backwards to release muscles or try backwards bend yoga postures.

## BEND INTO GOOD POSTURE

Many back problems are caused by adopting a bad lifting posture and by carrying heavy objects incorrectly. The best lifting posture is where the legs, not the back, do the work. So, when lifting, be certain to bend the knees and always carry heavy objects close to the body at waist level.

## BAG A HEALTHY BACK

Carrying your bag on the same shoulder all the time can lead to muscle imbalance and weakness, leading to pain. Resolve to swap shoulders every other day or use a backpack.

## BED DOWN IN COMFORT

Sleeping on your stomach can put the back and neck into various strained positions, causing stiffness and pain when you wake in the morning. To prevent problems developing, lie flat on your back with a pillow under your knees. Or sleep on your side with knees slightly bent and a pillow between your legs.

## LOSE WEIGHT TO LESSEN PAIN

Being overweight forces your body to carry more than its natural weight and, as most people walk at least a mile every day just in normal life, every pound counts. Slimming down could help most overweight people with back problems.

## GO HOT AND COLD TO STOP SWELLING

Using cold packs for five to ten minutes at a time on affected areas will reduce inflammation. If the pain lingers after 24 hours, switch to heat treatment with hot towels or a shower or bath.

## DON'T STOP MOVING

Studies show that people with acute back pain who go about their everyday activities as normally as possible heal better than those who rest, because movement naturally causes the body to pump fluid into the spongy discs that separate and cushion the vertebrae in your back. So don't rest too much unless you have to.

## SIT UP WITH SIT-UPS

It is estimated that strengthening the abdominal muscles could prevent more than 75% of lower-back problems. Regular sit-ups and abdominal exercises can help, as can core strength training with Pilates and yoga classes.

## GIVE YOUR BACK SOME BACK-UP

Use a chair with a proper backrest to prevent pressure on the lower back, or slip a thin cushion or rolled-up jumper (sweater) behind your lower back for correct support.

## BE A SCREEN SIREN

Make sure your computer screen is at the right height for comfortable viewing – you shouldn't need to lean towards or away from your screen, for example, and it should be level with your eyes. In addition, your arms should rest lightly on the desk's surface as you use the keyboard.

## IT'S HIP TO STRETCH

Many back problems stem from the hips. Stretch out your hip flexor muscles by lying on the floor with one leg flat and the other bent at the knee. Then slowly pull the bent leg towards your chest while pressing your whole back to the floor. Hold this position for 30 seconds.

## SITTING PRETTY

When sitting at a desk for long periods of time, rest your feet flat on the floor or use a foot support to prevent the weight of the lower legs being supported by the front of the thighs.

## STRAIGHTEN THOSE LEGS

Bear in mind that you shouldn't cross your legs, which can cause the pelvis and hips to tilt and strain, or have your thighs pressing against your chair seat too firmly, as this puts pressure on the veins on the underside of your thighs.

## HAVE A SIESTA

The pressure on the back is more than two and a half times greater when sitting than when you are standing, and a massive ten times greater when you are sitting rather than lying down. In light of this, a ten-minute nap or lie-down in the afternoon could deliver enormous back benefits.

## QUIT SMOKING FOR HEALTHIER DISCS

Smokers are more likely to suffer back pain that non-smokers because nicotine restricts the flow of blood to the intervertebral discs that cushion the spine. To ease the strain and any discomfort in your back, get down on your hands and knees, hands palm down in line with shoulders, looking at the floor. Slowly push your back up into an upward curve, hold this for five seconds and then release. Repeat this ten times.

## DON'T EVEN THINK ABOUT IT

It would now appear that the old wives' tale is right after all – the more you think about your pain, the worse it will feel. Researchers have found that the people who don't pay any attention to their pain seem to suffer less.

## TOP UP ON CALCIUM

Calcium is essential for keeping the bones of the spine firm and flexible. There are plenty of sources besides milk, including yogurt, broccoli, kale, figs, almonds and calcium supplements.

## TILT YOUR PELVIS TO TREAT YOUR BACK

Try this pelvic exercise to ease any stress you might be feeling in the lower back region. Lie flat on your back with your legs bent and feet flat on the floor. Press your lower back to the floor by tightening the abdominal muscles; hold for ten seconds and then release the position. Repeat five times, breathing normally throughout.

## PACK SOME HEAT TO DULL PAIN

To relieve chronic pain and stiffness in your back, try heated water therapies such as swimming pools, whirlpools, warm showers and steam rooms. Alternatively, apply warm compresses, hot towels or microwaveable heat packs to the area.

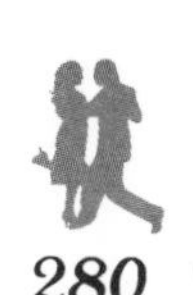



### SWIM INTO HEALTH

Swimming is an excellent exercise for healthy backs because it avoids the strain of impact sports and allows the body to realign itself while supported by the water.

### CURTAIL YOUR CAFFEINE

While you may be convinced that you really need the extra burst of energy that coffee provides in the morning, try to resist the temptation to have those second and third cups. Recent studies show that the extra caffeine can actually weaken bones.

## beating cancer

### AWARE IT WELL

Being aware of changes in your body is a surefire way to catch cancer early, boosting chances of effective treatment. Know how your skin looks and feels to track changes.

### SWEAT IT AWAY

Studies have shown that regular physical exercise prompts a series of changes within the body that actively fight cancer. The risk of colon, breast, prostate and other cancers lessens with regular activity.

### A GREAT WHEY TO BEAT BREAST CANCER

Whey – this is the watery part of milk that remains when the curds have been separated – could help protect against breast cancer by reducing the hormone oestrogen. Experts also believe that soy sauce could have a similar effect.

### SPROUT A DOUBLE CANCER CURE

Green leafy vegetables contain a combination of two components that are 13 times more powerful at fighting cancer together than alone. Selenium and sulphoraphane are found in high levels in Brussels sprouts, broccoli and cabbage.

### COUNT CALCIUM TO FIGHT CANCER

Low-fat diets that limit intake of dairy products could be exposing slimmers to colon cancer by reducing their calcium intake to dangerously low levels. Studies suggest that even small increases in calcium can cut the risk by half.

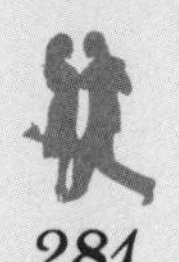



## GET A PIZZA FOR ANTICANCER ACTION

Pizzas aren't all bad, and the more tomato sauce they have on top, the better. The powerful antioxidant lycopene, which makes tomatoes red, has protective effects against cancer. Cooked tomatoes are best.

## GO GREEN TO PROTECT YOURSELF

The polyphenols and catechins in green tea have powerful antioxidative and anticancer effects when taken regularly. Aim for at least one cup a day.

## VEG OUT ON FRUIT

Fresh fruit and vegetables are such powerful anticancer agents that they can even lower the risk of lung cancer in heavy smokers.

## PEACHY KEEN

Peaches, sweet potatoes and apricots contain high levels of betacarotene, which cannot only prevent cancer cells from growing but can even kill them off.

## BE A LEMON TO FIGHT DISEASE

Citrus fruits, such as grapefruit, lemon and orange, are powerful anticancer agents because they contain a collection of all the natural substances known to ward off cancer cells.

## GET SMELLY TO GET HEALTHY

Pungent foods like onion and garlic not only have a powerful effect on cancer tumours but also work to boost the function of the immune system.

## UNDERCOOK FOR GOOD HEALTH

Charring food during roasting, grilling and barbecueing can produce carcinogens in the burned areas. The healthiest food is cooked through but not burned.

## EAT UP A RAINBOW

Everyone seems to recognize that the red-coloured fruits and vegetables are good for us, but don't forget your other colours, too. For example, a low intake of green and yellow-coloured vegetables has been linked to the development of cervical and breast cancers.

## SPOON OUT SPINACH

Spinach contains gluthione, a powerful anticancer agent. Gluthione is found in lower levels in other green leafy vegetables, too.

## BE A GOOD BEAN

Eating beans, including chickpeas, kidney beans and lentils, on a regular basis – say, one portion every week – could cut the risk of death from cancer by nearly half. This is because beans contain various anticancer agents.

## TRAIN YOUR TASTEBUDS

Sugar is a major risk factor for cancer. Instead of choosing high-sugar options, train your tastebuds by gradually reducing sugar in your diet or swapping it for healthy alternatives, such as apple juice, date sugar and rice syrup.

## MILK PROTECTS YOUR BELLY

Large quantities of high-fat milk have been shown to increase chances of bowel and colon cancer, but low-fat milk can actually protect the digestive system from disease.

## PICK YOUR WAY TO A CURE

Blackberries and raspberries are great anticancer agents because of their high levels of antioxidants. The fresher the better, so pick your own for best results.

## KEEP IT FRESH

Aflatoxins, thought to be linked to liver cancers, can develop in peanuts, corn and pepper when stored for a long time. If in doubt, use only fresh ingredients.

## CRESS YOUR ANTICANCER BUTTONS

Watercress contains a cancer-fighting substance called phenethyl isothiocyanate, thought to act against tumours, particularly in lung cancer.

## DON'T GET IN A PICKLE

Some pickles, dried meats and fish contain high levels of preservative nitrites, and these may be linked to stomach cancer. Try making your own chutneys or look closely at labels to see what has been included.

# breathing problems

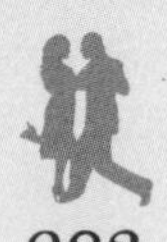



## TALK THE TALK

A good way to keep your breathing calm and regular is to have a conversation with someone or to read out loud. Speech naturally regulates breathing, thus putting a stop to the short and shallow breaths that can lead to problems.

## BREATHE NATURALLY

More than a fifth of all adults with asthma have some sensitivity to aspirin, and many also have problems with other painkillers such as ibuprofen. Be careful what you take if you have breathing problems.

## TAKE A DEEP BREATH

Taking a few deep breaths really does help you stay calm and in control, by stopping the release of the stress hormones adrenaline and cortisol into the blood.

## STRIKE A POSE

Yoga has been shown to help breathing problems and asthma by reducing tension in the breathing muscles and expanding the ribs to allow more air inside the lungs. Aim for three sessions a week to reap the health rewards.

## DON'T SAY LOW, SAY NO

Studies reveal that the risk of contracting lung cancer is no different in people who smoke medium-tar cigarettes, low-tar cigarettes or very low-tar cigarettes, so instead of opting for a low-tar version of your favourite brand, experts recommend that giving up entirely is the only way to protect your lungs.

## VITALIZE LUNGS WITH VITAMINS

A lack of vitamins C and E, betacarotene and selenium (found in lentils, avocados and brazil nuts) in the diet can harm the lungs so much that it's the equivalent of smoking a pack of 20 cigarettes a day for ten years.

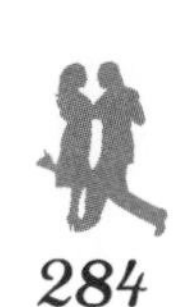



### EAT ONION TO PREVENT CANCER

Eating lots of onion, apple and yellow grapefruit regularly could help protect your body against developing lung cancer by destroying squamous cell carcinoma, which is a specific type of the disease. Combine cooked onion with raw apple and grapefruit for the most potent anticancer effect.

### BREATHE EASY WITH BUTEYKO

The Buteyko technique – a method of breathing correction and concentration – has been found to reduce and cure asthma in even serious cases. Ask your doctor for advice or visit www.buteyko.com.

### POOL YOUR RESOURCES

Swimming is the no. 1 activity for healthy lungs because they're forced to work to their optimal potential as you exercise and restrict breathing. But you've got to put your head underwater to benefit.

## colds & flu

### LISTEN TO YOUR ELDERS

Elderberry flowers contain flavonoids and tannins, substances that reduce fever and promote sweating. The berries are rich in vitamin C, which may prevent flu infection, while other compounds bind to the flu virus and prevent it from penetrating cell walls.

### THINK ZINC FOR SORE THROATS

Zinc gluconate lozenges may shorten colds by an average of three days as well as alleviate sore throats, nasal congestion, coughing, headaches and hoarseness.

### TAKE A BREAK IF YOU'RE FEELING LOW

Extreme amounts of exercise increase the body's production of harmful free radicals, which heighten your risk of succumbing to colds and viruses and can generally cause you to feel run down.

## DON'T OVERLOAD ON WATER

Many people's first reaction when they come down with a respiratory infection is to drink copious amounts of water. However, some experts now believe that overdrinking could worsen the problem by leading to salt loss and fluid overload. Aim for 2 litres (3½ pints) a day.

## WASH AWAY GERMS

Cold and flu viruses access your body through broken skin or the mucous membranes in your eyes and nose. Most people touch their face without realizing it, so wash your hands regularly to avoid passing on the virus.

## STEAM-CLEAN YOUR NOSE

The steam from boiling water can help your system fight off infections, possibly by killing any viruses that have newly alighted in the mucous membranes of your nose. To stay healthy, get down to your local sauna or steam room or invest in a facial steamer for home use.

## GET BY WITH A LITTLE HELP FROM YOUR FRIENDS

Studies show that the more friends you have, the less likely you are to succumb to a cold. This is because you will handle stress better, making you less likely to fall foul of viruses.

## STOP GARGLING TO HELP YOUR SORE THROAT

Gargling when you've got a sore throat is the equivalent of rubbing your eyes when they're sore. Instead, drink soothing warm – but not hot – liquids with a spoonful of honey to help your throat heal.

## CUT PAINKILLERS FOR AN EARLY CURE

If you can handle it, cutting back on taking painkillers regularly when you have a cold may help you recover a day earlier by allowing the virus to run its course.

## CHEERS FOR IMMUNITY

Experts believe wine could be a powerful ally against the common cold by boosting immunity to the hundreds of viruses that cause it. Studies have found that people who drink moderately have a lower risk of catching colds.

## STICK YOUR TONGUE OUT AT COLDS

Pour hot water into a bowl and breathe in, sticking your tongue out as you do so. This opens the throat and allows more steam through to prevent membranes drying out.

## SCHEDULE SOME SHUT-EYE

Sleeping helps your body as well as your brain, so give your immune system a helping hand in virus season by aiming to sleep for seven to eight hours a night.

## SNIFF AWAY SYMPTOMS

Aromatherapy oils of black pepper, eucalyptus, hyssop, pine and sweet thyme can help get rid of coughs, colds and symptoms of congestion. Use with steam to alleviate symptoms further.

## MAKE TIME FOR TEA

Regular tea drinking could boost your immune system. Black, green and oolong teas all contain the bacteria-fighting chemical L-theanine, which can protect against colds.

## AVOID THE FALLOUT

A sneeze can travel at 160kph (100mph) and is a very common way for colds and flu to spread. Look for the telltale warning signs of an erupting sneeze and make sure you get out of the way of the spray.

## SOUP IT UP

Chicken soup helps the cilia (tiny hairs) of the nose and bronchial passages move quickly so they can defend the respiratory system against contagions, and it contains substances that help the immune system fight off attack.

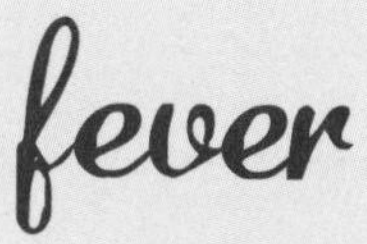


## COVER UP IN MODERATION

If you have a fever, don't cover up under too many blankets or take a hot shower, which may raise your temperature higher. Instead, try to keep to a normal covering.

### KNOW YOUR BODY'S LIMITS

Normal body temperature is 37°C (98.6°F). Contact your doctor for temperatures above 38.5°C (101°F) that last more than a day and seek emergency attention for temperatures of 40°C (104°F) or more.

### DON'T OD ON VITAMIN C

When you get a fever, the tendency is to reach for vitamin C, but be careful not to go overboard. Too much can lead to diarrhoea and kidney stones.

### SPURN PILLS FOR SPEEDY RECOVERY

Lowering temperatures with drugs might help in the short term but research has shown that the body may recover better if mild temperatures are left untreated.

### CUT OUT MEAT TO CUT THE HEAT

Reducing iron if you have a temperature could help fight infection, so avoid iron-rich foods until you're on the mend, then stock up your levels as you recover.

### MAKE YOUR TEMPERATURE TEPID

To ease the discomfort of a fever, don't use cold water, which can shock the skin into holding onto heat. Instead, get into a bath that feels the same as body temperature or dab yourself with a tepid flannel.

## first aid

### LAVENDER CURES

Lavender oil works well on cuts, wounds, dermatitis, eczema, nappy (diaper) rash, pimples, insect bites and burns, while lavender or camomile essential oils can be added to a bath to soothe minor sunburn.

### BE INFECTION-FREE WITH TEA TREE

Cleansing, antiseptic tea tree oil can be applied directly to skin in order to help keep minor scrapes and wounds clean, and it has been shown to be a more powerful antibiotic than many modern drugs. Keep some handy in your medicine cabinet for day-to-day use.

## DON'T GET STUNG WITH AFTER-PAIN

If you are stung by a bee, carefully grasp and pull out the stinger as fast as you can. The less venom that enters your body, the smaller and less painful the resulting welt will be. Ice the area immediately to reduce the swelling.

## A NATURAL ALTERNATIVE TO ANTIBIOTICS

Eucalyptus oil has long been prized for its healing abilities, but recent research studies have shown that it could possibly be even more effective at fighting bacterial infections than some antibiotics.

## TELL THE TOOTH ABOUT MILK

Teeth that have been knocked out, perhaps in a sporting activity or as the result of a fight or accident, can be successfully replanted up to 24 hours later – but only if the teeth have been stored in whole milk. Drop the teeth immediately into some cold whole milk and get to a dentist as soon as you possibly can.

## LEAN FORWARDS FOR NOSEBLEEDS

For nosebleeds, the age-old remedy of tilting the head back can actually increase blood flow. Instead, tilt the head slightly forward and pinch the soft part of the nose. When the bleeding stops, don't blow your nose for at least four hours.

## DON'T FEEL THE BURN

Douse minor burns immediately with cold water for at least ten minutes. Cover major burns with clingfilm (plastic wrap), apply cold water or ice over the top and call for medical attention at once.

## KEEP BERRY COOL

On hot summer days, when heatstroke is a possible hazard, enhance the body's natural cooling system with infusions of raspberry and peppermint tea.

## FIGHT BITES WITH CITRONELLA

The aromas of tea tree, eucalyptus and citronella have been shown to repel mosquitoes and other biting insects. Apply the oils to exposed areas of the skin for a natural repellant to help avoid getting bitten.

### SAY ALOE TO CALMER SKIN

Aloe vera has soothing properties that stop the inflammation and redness of skin rashes, including prickly heat. Apply liberally for best results.

### SOOTHE SPOTS WITH CALENDULA

Calendula oil or ointment is another great helper for skin problems. It soothes and draws out heat, making it useful for bites, stings, blisters and other skin ailments.

## headaches

### TRY TEMPLE MASSAGE

Massaging the temples in a circular motion with aromatherapy oils helps ease the pain of migraine and tension headaches, as well as reducing stuffiness and eye pain.

### HOOK A HEADACHE CURE

Omega-3 essential fatty acids (EFAs), found in oily fish such as tuna and salmon, can lower the production of hormones that cause inflammation and pain, so eating fish regularly could help stop those migraines once and for all.

### PUT JAW PAIN IN LINE

Many headaches are due to stress and tension in the muscles of the jaw. Check if your jaw might be to blame by sitting in front of a mirror and opening and closing your mouth slowly in a straight line. Many people find that their jaws are way off line at the beginning of the exercise.

### WATER DOWN THE TENDERNESS

Give yourself a pain-relieving massage by standing in the shower with the water stream directed to the back of your neck, then slowly turning to look behind you. This removes lactic acid from the muscles and makes the blood vessels less "irritable".

### FEAST ON FEVERFEW

Feverfew contains niacin (a B vitamin) and iron, and provides nutrition to the central nervous system and alleviates migraines. At the onset of a headache, try a sandwich of feverfew leaves or brew up a warm tea.

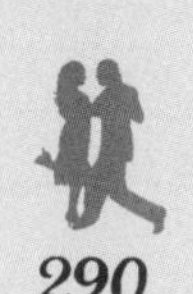



## AVOID THE HOT AND COLD OF IT

Extreme chilling or warming of the neck can bring on headaches by altering blood flow to the head, which replicates the migraine mechanism. Wear a scarf if you're moving between different temperatures.

## PILL YOURSELF TOGETHER

Headache sufferers who take lots of pain-killers could be giving themselves more pain with rebound headaches as they withdraw from their regular dose. If you think this might be you, see your doctor.

## INDULGE IN A SPOT OF COFFEE THERAPY

Coffee can help cure headaches because of the injection of caffeine it gives the body (but take care not to overdo the caffeine – many over-the-counter headache remedies already contain a healing dose).

## HOLD THE HOT DOGS

Some people are very sensitive to the nitrites that are used as a preservative in a range of processed meats, especially hot dogs, burgers and cold cuts. Avoid these foods and, if your headaches disappear, stay off them.

## SNIFF AN APPLE A DAY

Apples could keep the doctor away after all. Research studies have shown that the scent of green apples can reduce the severity of migraines, so the next time you feel a headache coming on, reach for the fruit bowl and inhale deeply.

## GO BANANAS

If your headaches tend to come on in the late mornings, late afternoons or after a long lie-in, they might be due to low blood sugar (hypoglycaemia). These headaches can be helped by eating foods that release sugar slowly, such as bananas, wholegrains and oats.

## CHANGE YOUR BRA TO CURE YOUR HEAD

Overtight bra straps can dig into the shoulder and put pressure on the cervical nerve, causing frequent headaches. Full-breasted women are most likely to suffer from this, but all women are at risk. Buy bras with wide straps and check that your bra fits correctly around the chest.

### BITE THE BULLET

Poor tooth or jaw alignment has been found to be the cause of some chronic headaches. A few sessions in the dentist's chair could clear your head for good.

### COME DOWN FROM ON HIGH

Headaches that usually occur only when you're angry, during vigorous exercise, and/or right before sexual orgasm could be down to high blood pressure, especially if accompanied by redness or throbbing. See your doctor if this sounds familiar.

### PAIN BETWEEN THE EYES

Less than perfect eyesight can trigger headaches because the eye and other muscles squeeze in order to focus. If your headaches come on after reading or working at a computer screen, make sure you give your eyes a rest every ten minutes by focusing on a distant object for at least 60 seconds. Make a point of having regular eye examinations, too.

## heart disease

### GIVE YOURSELF A PERFECT TEN

It's just about safe to be 4.5kg (10lb) too heavy, but no more than this, according to heart experts, who have found that even an excess of 5kg (11lb) can significantly increase the risk of heart disease.

### EARN SOME FAT PROFITS

Not all fat is bad. Beneficial essential fatty acids (EFAs), such as the omega-3 type found in fish, olives and flaxseed, have been shown to reduce the risk of heart disease. Instead of banning fat entirely from your diet, substitute good fats for the heart.

### STEER CLEAR OF HYDROGENATED OILS

Just a few grams of omega-3 fatty acids a day can prevent an irregular heart beat, decrease inflammation and promote blood flow. Choose olive oil and fish oils instead of cooking oils, because the hydrogenation process they go through destroys omega-3.

### EGGS ON THE MENU AGAIN

Eggs contain heart-protective nutrients including antioxidants, folate, other B vitamins and unsaturated fat that can counteract the effects of saturated fat and cholesterol.

### NUTS FOR A HEALTHY HEART

Nuts are rich in unsaturated fats and vitamin E, which have been linked to a reduced risk of heart disease in nut eaters, who are a third less likely to suffer such problems than other people.

### SAY ALOE TO A HEALTHY HEART

A diet that is supplemented with aloe vera and psyllium husks could set you on the road to having better heart health by reducing the amount of cholesterol in your system and improving the balance of good and bad cholesterol.

### GET HEARTY WITH VITAMIN E

Acting as a mild anticoagulant, vitamin E reduces the risk of blood clots and the oxidation of cholesterol, inhibiting production of fatty deposits that can block blood vessels and cause the onset of heart problems.

### GIVE ME MORE THAN FIVE

Don't stop at the recommended five portions of fruit and vegetables every day. Eating more could give you an extra health boost, with every additional serving estimated to lower the risk of heart disease by 4%. One serving is an apple or orange, a large spoonful of vegetables or a handful of grapes, cherries or chopped fruit.

### GARLIC BREATH IS HEALTHY BREATH

Garlic and onions, along with other members of the onion family like leeks and chives, have been shown to halve the risk of cancer if eaten regularly.

## joint problems

### GET WITH THE PROGRAMME

Exercise reduces pain. In one study, patients with osteoarthritis of the knee were able to reduce the amount of pain medication they took after participating in an eight-week walking programme.

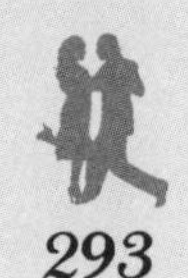



## KEEP IT SLOW TO REMAIN PAIN-FREE

Muscles adapt quickly to new exercises or movements, but joints, ligaments and tendons take longer. Ease yourself into new activities over a course of weeks or months to avoid the risk of injury.

## SOOTHE PAIN WITH GINGER

In a recent trial, 63% of patients taking ginger reported a reduction in knee pain while standing, compared with 50% of those who took the placebo. Those taking ginger also reported less pain after walking a distance of 15m (50ft).

## OIL YOUR JOINTS WITH BORAGE

Arthritis sufferers who have pain, joint tenderness, swelling and soreness, particularly first thing in the morning, could relieve their symptoms significantly by taking borage-oil capsules, a supplement made from the garden herb.

## GIVE BONES A D-DAY

Calcium isn't all we need to keep bones healthy and strong and guard against osteoporosis as we get older. Studies have shown that vitamin D in association with calcium boosts the body's ability to make the most of both substances to increase bone health and strength.

## WARM UP TO AVOID INJURY

Gently warming up your body before undertaking exercise can be likened to warming your car up on a winter's morning before driving off. To keep your body running smoothly, start the session slowly and get up to speed only after your muscles and joints have had at least five minutes of preparation.

## OPT FOR OLIVES FOR HEALTHY JOINTS

People who eat the most olive oil and cooked vegetables are about 75% less likely to develop rheumatoid arthritis than those who eat the fewest servings, so don't beat yourself up about having that extra oil.

## GET OFF YOUR HIGH HEELS

Heels force the thigh muscles to work harder, putting extra strain on the knee joint and tendons, so if you want bunion-free, perfect feet, it's best to go flat.

## GALVANIZE SORE JOINTS WITH GLUCOSAMINE

Truly the wonder drug where the body's joints are concerned, glucosamine occurs naturally in the body. In studies it has been shown, time after time, to strengthen joints, reduce pain, prevent injury and help protect against the degeneration that comes with ageing. Glucosamine is even more effective when taken with chondroitin, a closely related substance that prevents body enzymes from degrading joint cartilage.

## STEP OUT TO EASE STIFFNESS

Exercise, tailored to the individual's abilities, is well known to ease joint stiffness. People suffering from rheumatoid arthritis have cut the amount of time they feel stiff each morning by an average of 68 minutes after just six weeks of regular exercise and physical therapy. Physical exercise actually combats fatigue and sufferers report that they feel less tired after they begin a regular exercise programme.

## DRINK UP TO STOP STIFFNESS

Dehydration is a major cause of post-exercise muscle soreness. Drinking water regularly while you work out should be sufficient to keep levels high enough to combat pain.

## REDUCE PAIN WITH VITAMIN C

Vitamin C and bioflavonoids may help offset the damage that muscles endure during exercise. Taken regularly, these nutrients reduce the incidence of sports injuries and shorten the time it takes to recover from a muscle injury.

## WISE UP TO WARMING UP

Prepare yourself for your workout by moving a little first to get the blood flowing. This will help supply the muscles with oxygenated blood, which will prevent injuries and reduce lactic acid buildup in muscle fibres.

## A PINEAPPLE PICK-UP

Bromelain, which is a fruit extract taken from the pineapple, has potent anti-inflammatory properties in the body that can help to reduce muscle soreness brought about by inflammation. And the fruit gives you a good dose of vitamins that help healing, too.

## STROKE AWAY SORENESS

Massage can help reduce the pain that results from overexercised muscles by stimulating the blood flow in the affected areas, helping lymphatic drainage and promoting tissue repair. Visit a sports masseur or do it yourself with long, gentle strokes towards the heart.

## BUILD UP SLOWLY

The greatest incidence of muscle soreness happens in untrained people. Avoid this by gradually increasing exercise intensity over five or six sessions so the untrained muscles can progressively adapt.

## STAY PAIN-FREE WITH VITAMIN E

Recent research studies have shown that taking daily vitamin E supplements helps reduce muscle soreness when taken for at least a week before a strenuous exercise session. Get your daily dose naturally from vitamin-rich fruit and vegetables, or take a vitamin supplement.

## WIND DOWN SLOWLY

Warm down for a few minutes after strenuous exercise sessions, lowering your heart rate gradually back to its normal level with a low-intensity routine. Cool down after every workout with long, static stretches.

## REMEMBER THE RICE RULE

RICE stands for rest, ice, compression and elevation, and is a great way to reduce soreness. Rest allows healing, ice and compression stave off inflammation and bruising, and elevation (raising the affected area above the heart) drains excess fluid.

## DRINK SMOOTHIES TO HEAL MUSCLE TEARS

Combine calcium-rich milk with potassium-packed banana for a smoothie to treat muscles, cramps and soreness after exercise. Calcium and potassium help muscles heal microtears that can cause pain.

# nausea



## ROOT OUT SICKNESS

Ginger root, taken as powder or tea, works directly in the gastrointestinal tract by interfering with the feedback mechanisms that send sickness messages to the brain.

## PRESS AWAY DISCOMFORT

Acupressure wrist bands, which attach around the forearm and press against certain antisickness acupressure points, have been shown to help prevent motion sickness and nausea.

## CRUNCH ON CRACKERS

Eat high-carbohydrate foods such as dry crackers and toast if you're troubled by nausea. They move through the stomach quickly and may be helpful if eaten soon after you wake up in the morning.

## INFUSE AN ANTISICKNESS TEA

Catnip, raspberry leaf, mint, fennel and, of course, ginger, all make great herbal infusions to help prevent nausea and sickness. Check the labels carefully if you are using them to treat morning sickness, however, as raspberry leaf should be avoided in early pregnancy.

## OUT OF THE KITCHEN

If food smells nauseate you, stay out of the kitchen while meals are prepared – even leave the house, if necessary. Cold foods tend to have less odour, so try eating chicken or salad sandwiches, chilled soups, yogurt and fruit.

## CHEW IT OVER

Nausea can be caused by indigestion, but this can be prevented by adequate chewing of food. Many people gulp down food in large lumps; these are difficult to digest and so can cause trapped wind and general gut discomfort.

## BE WARY OF DAIRY

With the exception of yogurt, dairy products should be avoided if you've been vomiting until the problem is quite resolved. Orange juice, grapefruit juice and fried, spicy or fatty foods should also be avoided completely in favour of dry foods and plain water.

### BECOME AN OLD SOAK

Soaking beans in water can help turn their indigestible, wind and nausea-inducing components into easier-to-digest substances. For the best results, soak them thoroughly and change the water at least once while cooking them.

### FIBRE PROVIDERS

For a healthy digestive system, we should aim for an intake of around 20–35g (1–1½oz) of fibre a day, which is equivalent to a couple of pieces of wholemeal bread or a bowl of muesli. Other good dietary sources are vegetables and oats.

### HUNT OUT HIDDEN CAUSES

One of the major hidden causes of nausea is depression, especially if the nausea and sickness inexplicably last longer than a few days. Make sure that you're giving yourself enough downtime and employ relaxation techniques to ease tension.

### DON'T DO FAST FOOD

Meals that are eaten in front of the television, at your desk or on the move are more likely to cause nausea and sickness. As an alternative, give yourself some quiet time in a comfortable seat to enjoy chewing and tasting every morsel of your slow food.

### PRESS YOUR ANTISICKNESS BUTTON

The acupressure point P6 is thought to relieve nausea and travel sickness. It is located between the tendons on the inside arm, three finger widths above the wrist crease. Press lightly for 30 seconds whenever you need relief.

## neck stiffness

### TAKE A SIDEWAYS APPROACH

Inhale and then, as you exhale, slowly lower your right ear towards your right shoulder (it won't reach so don't force it) until there is a gentle stretch along the top of the left shoulder and neck. Take several slow deep breaths. Inhale and raise your head back up. Repeat on the other side.

## FLEX YOUR NECK

For neck pain and stiffness that have been caused by muscle tightening, gently move the neck to the outer ranges of its movement while sitting in a comfortable chair. This will help release muscle spasms and reduce the associated pain.

## STRETCH AWAY STIFFNESS

For stiffness, inhale and then, as you exhale, slowly start to lower your chin to your chest, giving yourself a long, gentle stretch along the back of the neck. Take several slow, deep breaths with the chin down and then lift your head back up again on an inhale.

## ROLL AWAY RIGIDITY

Lower one ear towards your shoulder, then roll your chin down towards the chest, across the chest and up the other side. Inhale and then, as you exhale, roll your chin down across the chest and up the other side.

## MASSAGE PROBLEMS AWAY

Applying warmth and gentle massage to sore and stiff necks can help reduce pain and increase healing blood flow.

## SHRUG OFF NECK PROBLEMS

Inhale and raise your shoulders up to your ears, pulling them up as high as they'll go. Then let go with an 'ahhh' and drop your shoulders slowly back down. Repeat several times to ease muscle tension.

## STAY IN THE SWIM

The best exercise to ease a stiff neck is swimming on your back. The water supports the head without straining the neck, allowing muscles to be used and stretched without discomfort.

## FORM A SHOULDER CIRCLE

Raise your shoulders up, rotate them back and down, then forwards and up again. Repeat several times, then go in the opposite direction.

## BE ALERT FOR SYMPTOMS

If your neck pain is ever accompanied by a fever, nausea, swelling or feelings of being generally unwell, you should consult your doctor immediately – the neck pain could be a signpost for several different medical conditions.

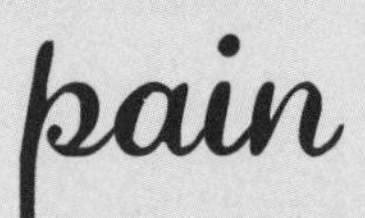

# pain

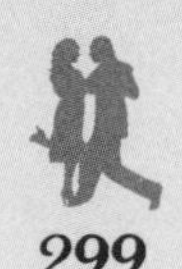





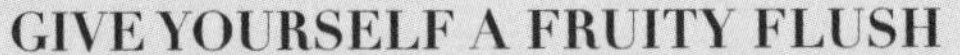

## GIVE YOURSELF A FRUITY FLUSH

Many forms of chronic pain are made worse by indigestion and constipation. A diet rich in fruit and vegetables loosens stools and prevents pain.

## LAUGH IT OFF

Laughing – even when you feel like crying from agony – can relax muscles, relieve pain and even boost your immune system. So, the next time you feel a twinge, get the giggles.

## RING THE EARACHE CHANGES

The pain of tinnitus – which is often characterized by a constant ringing sound in the ears – can be reduced by taking vitamin B6, found in fruit, vegetables and many supplements.

## SAY BYE-BYE TO RSI

An estimated one in 50 people suffer some form of RSI (Repetitive Strain Injury), which is caused by repetitive overuse of the soft tissue muscles of the neck, back, shoulders, arms and hands. Most of these injuries could be avoided altogether simply by taking short, regular breaks throughout the day.

## GET ACTIVE TO GET PAIN-FREE

The last thing you might feel like doing if you're suffering pain is exercise, but gentle activity can actually reduce pain by boosting seratonin levels in the body, which increases the flexibility of blood vessels and reduces pain perception in the brain.

## BLINK AWAY PAIN

Don't become so transfixed on the screen that you forget to blink. Blinking while watching television or looking at a computer screen will stop your eyes from becoming dry and reduce eye problems and pain as a result.

## THINK YOURSELF SOFT

Focus on the part of your body that is feeling tense or is generating pain. What image comes to mind? Perhaps you see a rock or a tight knot. This represents receptive imagery. Try turning it into something soft, such as clay, or change the colour you perceive it to be, and feel your pain begin to dissolve away.

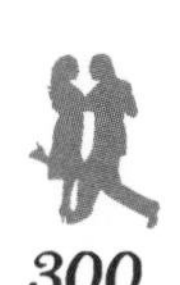



## REACH OUT FOR HEALING HANDS

Massage decreases stress hormones, which can be a contributing factor to pain. It also seems to increase levels of endorphins, which are natural painkillers.

## GO ALL-NATURAL

MSM (methyl-sulphonyl-methane) is an organic form of sulphur that has been shown to alleviate pain without producing side effects. It is found naturally in fruits, vegetables, meat, milk and seafood and seems to be particularly effective at easing muscle cramps.

## DON'T SKIP MEALS IF YOU WANT TO SKIP PAIN

Skipping meals can result in increased pain, possibly because of fluctuations in blood sugar levels in the body brought on by long periods without nourishment. Always take a healthy snack along with you if you know you will be too busy to make time for a proper meal.

## MAGNIFY MAGNESIUM

Soya beans, wholegrains, nuts, seeds, vegetables and fish all contain magnesium, which is an effective muscle relaxant shown to reduce tension pain. Lack of magnesium has been linked to depression, muscle soreness and general pain.

## BLOW HOT AND COLD

Warmth can relieve pain by relaxing muscles. In contrast, cold relieves pain by reducing inflammation. Alternating between the two can help many types of muscle pain.

## INVEST IN SOME SERIOUS SHADES

To prevent eye pain and potential damage, don't skimp on proper eye protection – get a good pair of optical-grade, polarized sunglasses that don't have the distortion associated with some types of cheap lenses. Polarization is essential for cutting glare and reducing eyestrain.

## PEPPER YOURSELF WITH A CURE

Cayenne pepper contains a substance called capsaicin, which stimulates the brain to secrete endorphins, peptides that help block pain signals and reduce chronic pain, such as that from arthritis and bad backs. Sprinkle the cayenne pepper in hot water for a cure with a kick.

## SOOTHE SKIN WITH CALENDULA

Calendula is an excellent herb for reducing the pain of most skin disorders, including nappy (diaper) rash, sunburns, bruises, and insect stings and bites. The herb has a calming, soothing effect on irritated skin by reducing inflammation and combating any associated infection, and there are topical skin ointments and creams available.

## CHECK THE DATE

If soreness and pain are worse at certain times of the month, then what you're feeling could be down to your menstrual cycle. Hormonal changes mean that many women are more susceptible to pain in the week before their period starts.

## BE A PAIN-FREE WATER BABY

Even mild dehydration can trigger pain, so drinking lots of fluids is essential for pain-free living. The head is especially affected, but muscle pain, cramps and eyestrain can be caused by dehydration, too.

## CATCH UP ON YOUR ZZZZZS

Here is one of the easiest tips for you to try – a good night's sleep is essential for a pain-free life. This is because sleep deprivation causes an increased perception of pain. So aim for at least seven hours a night to stay free of pain.

## FIGHT INFLAMMATION WITH FOOD

Some types of food have natural anti-inflammatory properties that can reduce swelling and, therefore, alleviate pain. The best options for you to try are avocado, banana, berries, cabbage, cucumber, fig, mango and melon.

## STEER CLEAR OF TRIGGERS

Some types of foods may actually increase the perception of pain, possibly because of their capacity for raising acid levels in the body. So, if you are suffering from persistent pain, cut down on alcohol, coffee, citrus fruits, onions, chocolate, sugar and salt.

# stomach problems

### GO FOR A WALK

Exercise helps move gas through the digestive tract. That's why experts suggest that you take a short walk after eating instead of taking a nap. Mint tea can also aid digestion.

### SETTLE THE STOMACH WITH MILK

Artichokes and milk products can help indigestion caused by too much stomach acid by lining the inside of the stomach after overeating or excessively rich food.

### SWAP THE FRIES

French fries, red meat, sugar and refined grains in foods can increase the risk of colon cancer in women who eat them regularly. Replacing these foods with healthier alternatives like wholegrains, boiled or baked potatoes and low-sugar options could help cut your risk of colon cancer by half.

### GO FOR PEPPER INSTEAD OF MILK TO CURE ULCER PAIN

Calcium in milk could make ulcer pain worse instead of better. To cure ulcers, steer clear of alcohol and spicy foods except capsaicin, a pepper derivative that seems to help ulcer pain.

### RUB AWAY THE BLOAT

Try stroking gently from your right hip up towards your ribs, across the bottom of your ribcage and down towards your left hip. Repeat several times to encourage the movement of trapped wind.

# tired all the time

### ASK THE EXPERTS

If you feel tired all the time (known as TATT) for longer than two weeks, despite increasing exercise levels, eating a healthy diet and improving your quality of sleep, you must see your doctor. Tiredness is an early symptom of many illnesses, including thyroid problems and multiple sclerosis.

## TRASH THE CRASH DIET

Low-calorie consumption is a major cause of fatigue in women today. Those who diet frequently may not have enough fuel to sustain their body's optimal efficiency level, leading to tiredness and fatigue.

## DON'T COUNT ON CAFFEINE

Caffeine mimics the effects of stress hormones in the body. A person who weighs 70kg (11st/154lb) and drinks more than six caffeine drinks per day (for example, six cups of coffee or cola) can develop caffeine 'poisoning', with symptoms of restlessness, irritability, headache, insomnia and tiredness.

## DO A SLEEP SURVEY

Lack of sleep or bad-quality sleep is a prime cause of tiredness. Keep track of the hours you sleep and note irregularities. Make sure your room is dark and quiet and don't carry stresses to bed with you.

## DON'T DISMISS DEPRESSION

One of the major symptoms of depression is extreme tiredness, so if you feel fatigued all the time you might want to consider depression as an underlying cause. Consult your doctor if you need advice.

## CAN TIREDNESS WITH SARDINES

Tiredness can be a result of low iron, which also leads to cracked lips, cold hands and feet, poor memory, headaches, poor resistance to infection and pallor in the face and inner eyelids. Eat iron-rich sardines to boost energy.

## KEEP ZIPPING ALONG

Fatigue is one of the first symptoms of dehydration.Increase your daily intake of water by drinking a glass with each meal and sipping throughout the day.

## B WISE TO ENERGIZE

Adequate supplies of vitamins and minerals are essential for healthy metabolism. If these become in short supply for any reason, you will soon experience persistent tiredness. The B group of vitamins is especially important, as it's needed to produce energy.

## DON'T LET HORMONES WEAR YOU OUT

Low oestrogen levels can cause tiredness, especially when hormone levels drop in the week before your period or during the menopause, when tiredness can be overwhelming. Some studies have shown that regular carbohydrate snacks can help prevent this feeling.

## STUB OUT THE CIGGY

Smoking affects everything to do with your body, increasing dehydration and stress levels and generating a whole range of metabolic problems. Heavy smokers often feel tired due to a lack of oxygen in their bloodstream.

## MAKE A MENTAL NOTE

If you are worrying that you haven't completed some chore or important task, make a mental note that you are going to do it and when, which will help your brain stop worrying about it.

## GET YOUR TIMING RIGHT

Organizing your life better can help you build in more opportunities for relaxation. Aim to balance all the aspects of your life, scheduling in time for your domestic chores and job as well as your social activities.

## LEAP INTO ACTION

Lack of exercise is one of the key causes of low energy and feelings of constant tiredness. Inactivity can also encourage weight gain and this in turn is likely to make you feel depressed.

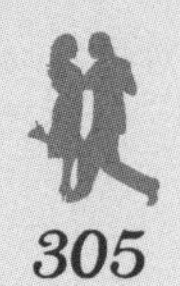

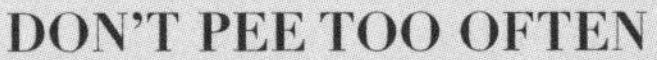

# waterworks

## DON'T PEE TOO OFTEN

Going to the toilet too frequently can weaken your bladder by causing muscle fatigue, while women who crouch over the toilet are less likely to empty their bladders fully and are at risk of infection.

## GET IT DOWN TO A TEA

Drinking tea made from raspberry leaves has been shown to reduce the pain and duration of urinary tract infections, and it is especially effective if taken regularly as problems begin.

## DON'T FORCE IT

If you feel the need to go to the toilet but once you get there you're as dry as a bone, you could have a urinary tract infection. Consult your doctor straight away in order to prevent the problem spreading to the bladder and kidneys and becoming even more serious.

## JACK IN THE PACK

Smoking increases the risk of urinary tract conditions as well as raises blood pressure and stimulates coughing, which can add to problems with bladder control. It also increases the risk of bladder cancer, a risk that can stay with you for years after you have quit smoking.

## GET THE ALL-CLEAR

Aim to drink enough water to make your urine pale yellow and clear. Dark yellow or cloudy urine is a sign that you aren't consuming enough fluid, so drink up.

## STAY OFF STRONG STIMULANTS

Coffee, alcohol, spicy foods, citrus fruits and chocolate can all aggravate bladder problems, making urine more concentrated and so forcing the body to expend water in order to detoxify itself.

## SIT DOWN AFTER SEX

During sexual intercourse, bacteria may enter the urethra. By going to the toilet straight afterwards, you help wash out the invaders right away and avoid infections.

### WIPE AWAY PROBLEMS
Keep infections at bay by cleaning the vaginal area with a front-to-back motion, which helps prevent the spread of bacteria from the anus.

### HALT THE FLOW TO STAY STRONG BELOW
When you pee, practise stopping and starting the flow using your pelvic floor muscles to keep them tight and strong, Don't overdo it, though – three times a day is enough to help build muscle strength.

### AVOID THE FIZZ
Fizzy water can exacerbate some urinary tract conditions, so if you want to stay pain-free, have plenty of still, clear water to flush out the problems.

### CHOOSE CRANBERRIES FOR CYSTITIS
Women have known this for years, but drinking cranberry juice regularly can help ease the symptoms of cystitis, possibly because it alters the acidity levels of the urine.

### EAT TO CURE URINARY INFECTIONS
Health-inducing blueberries are rich in the bacteria-killing anthocyanosides, which will also see off the dreaded E. coli infections by preventing the infectious bacteria from clinging to the cells that line the urinary tract and bladder.

## periods

### JOG AWAY PAIN
Taking regular exercise – for example, aerobics or jogging – can help reduce the symptoms of PMS (PMT). However, you should exercise on a regular basis, not just when the symptoms occur, if you want to enjoy the full health benefits.

### STAY CHASTE TO CHASE PAIN AWAY
Chasteberry, which is also known as vitex agnus-castus, regulates female hormonal imbalances in the body by working on the pituitary gland in the brain, helping with PMS (PMT) irritability, breast pain and water retention.

## TAKE YOUR FINGER OFF THE STRESS TRIGGER

Pinpointing and avoiding any emotional triggers or stresses that make the symptoms of PMS (PMT) worse, and discussing these with your partner or a friend and asking for their support, can be useful ways to avoid problems.

## JUST B HAPPY

Some women have found that taking vitamin B (particularly B6) is helpful in reducing PMS (PMT) symptoms, but there is only limited scientific evidence that this works, and high doses can cause damage to the nervous system.

## SMOOTHIE AWAY SYMPTOMS

Studies suggest that daily doses of magnesium and calcium taken during the time PMS (PMT) symptoms occur could have a cocktail of effects – helping reduce mood swings, muscle pains and fluid retention. Get both minerals at once in a soothing banana smoothie, made with either milk or yogurt.

## EXPERIMENT WITH EPO

Some women find that taking evening primrose oil helps relieve breast discomfort. Long-term treatment (more than three months) may be required before any effect is noticed, however.

## SECURE A FISHY CURE

Fish fats help to relieve the symptoms of premenstrual disorders, including breast pain, PMT, bloating, depression and irritability. Choose oily fish such as mackerel, herring, sardines and salmon for the best effects.

## IRON OUT PMT PROBLEMS

Heavy menstrual blood flow can deplete your body's iron stores, which can in turn cause further bleeding. Women who increase the iron in their diets are likely to suffer less heavy and painful periods. Sources include lean red meat, sardines, egg yolk, dried figs and dark green leafy vegetables like spinach.

## YOU CAN BE TOO THIN

When it comes to weight loss, your periods prove it is possible to be too thin. Beware of dieting so much that your menstrual cycle is affected, as too much weight loss can make periods stop and affect fertility.

## PLANT THE SEEDS OF A CURE

Blackcurrant seeds, evening primrose seeds and borage seeds are all high in gamma linolenic acid (GLA), which helps regulate fluid retention and hormone release, helping minimize symptoms of PMS (PMT) and period problems.

## SEND PMT CRAMPS BALMY

Lemonbalm is often used for menstrual problems as it has a calming and regulating effect in the menstrual cycle. It helps ease menstrual cramps and treats irregularities.

## BEEF UP TO REDUCE CRAMPS

Supplementing the diet with zinc, found in high proportions in red meats like beef and lamb, has been found to reduce cramps, bloating and other PMS (PMT) symptoms.

## STRENGTHEN WITH VITAMIN C

Taking vitamin C and bioflavonoids may strengthen uterine blood vessels and make them less susceptible to damage, so reducing the severity and length of bleeding during periods.

## MANAGE WITH MARJORAM

Essential oil of marjoram has been shown to increase warmth and comfort if used to massage the abdomen during menstruation or in a burner to encourage pain-free sleep.

## CURB PAIN WITH A HERB

Eating the common garden herb feverfew can lessen cramping, headaches, neck and shoulder pain and muscle soreness during menstruation by acting as a natural painkiller. Make yourself a sandwich or salad garnished with feverfew or a herbal tea from the leaves.

## GIVE THE G-STRING THE BOOT

Swapping your G-string or thong for bigger underwear could help banish such thong-related problems as folliculitis, thrush, redness and soreness. Choose thicker varieties of underwear made in natural, breathable fabrics such as cotton, or go commando during exercise, when they cause most friction problems.

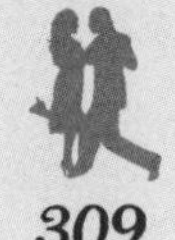



### SWAP FATS TO PREVENT WATER RETENTION

Low-fat diets could not only reduce water retention in the week before your period commences but also lessen the severity of the period itself. Fish oils are a great choice because they will also work to reduce PMS (PMT) symptoms.

### MASSAGE AWAY THE PAIN

Place your hands on your hips with the thumbs on the lower back at hip level, either side of the spine, and move the thumbs in small, light circular motions. Be gentle to avoid pain or discomfort.

## teenagers

### GET A MENTOR

Your teenage years are really important in shaping what kind of adult you are going to become. Identify an adult you can treat as a mentor or role model in your life and go to for advice.

### BURN THE CANDLE

Studies have shown that teenagers actually have different body clocks to people of other ages, being pre-programmed to stay up later and get up later too, so make sure you get enough rest if you want to be able to concentrate at school or college. Aim for eight or nine hours a night.

### BE POSITIVE

It's really easy as a teenager to assume the world doesn't understand you, but take a minute to think about things from another point of view. Every time you feel angry at someone, try to think something positive about them.

### ONLINE IS EASIER

You don't have to meet people face to face to discuss things. Many teenagers find talking about their feelings and emotions easier in online chat rooms where they can be anonymous.

### STI ALERT

Many teenagers feel they're invincible but when it comes to sexually transmitted infections, it really could be you. If you think something is wrong, see your doctor or clinic immediately.

### CHOOSE YOUR ACTIVITIES

Instead of going along with friends who choose to do things you either don't like or aren't good at, try to opt for activities you enjoy and are good at as this will boost your self-esteem. Getting deeply involved in an activity, such as painting, dancing or music, can be therapeutic as well as satisfying.

### BLOG IT

Create your own blog where you can work through thoughts and feelings, as well as improving your communication skills. It might help you to see your problems differently and to come up with solutions.

### BE SAFE

If you go online, make sure you are careful about what information you give. Online predators are a reality so take care if someone asks for personal information and never meet an online friend alone.

### UNDERSTANDING DIVORCE

Lots of teenagers have to deal with their parents divorcing, but rest assured it's not your fault and it doesn't mean your parents don't love you. It can be a traumatic time, but being honest with both parents will help.

### TALK IT THROUGH

Anger and resentment at a situation you can't control, like your parents splitting up, can cause you to feel frustrated with the rest of your life and even to start pushing friends away. Try to face up to your feelings rather than bottling them up. Find a friend or relative you can talk to – it can be a great release to get it off your chest.

### STAY HYDRATED

Teenagers are prone to dehydration and it can affect not only your energy levels but also your ability to hit the books. Make sure you drink lots of water or clear fluids, and try to cut back on tea, coffee and fizzy drinks.

### USE YOUR HEAD

Don't forget that your mental health is just as important as your physical health so aim to spend as much time looking after your mind as you do your body.

## COVER UP

When it comes to STIs, condoms are really the only form of contraception that will give you protection. And if you have unprotected sex, don't forget it's like sleeping with everyone your partner has ever slept with.

## KEEP IT QUIET

If your parents don't know you're sexually active, don't let that stop you seeking advice on sexual health. Everyone has the right to confidential treatment and it's important to get checked out.

## BALANCE RESPONSIBILITIES

Being a teenager is tough – you're almost an adult but often parents won't give you the freedom you desire. Try to make a deal with them that meets them halfway to prove to them that you can take responsibility.

## STAY TRUE TO YOURSELF

For teenagers embarking on their first romances, it can be hard to say no to sexual requests. Never do anything you don't feel comfortable with until you're ready.

## YOU'RE NOT THE ONLY ONE

When chatting to your mates about sex and experience, remember that not everybody tells the truth when it comes to sex. In fact, most teenagers don't; chances are that they're just as confused as you are.

## DON'T PILE ON THE PRESSURE

Be realistic about what you can expect from your exam results. Not everyone can get top grades or make it into the university of their choice, but everyone can do the best they can, so make that your goal.

## TAKE YOUR TIME

Once the law says you're ready for adulthood it might be tempting to go all out and do as much as you can, but there's no rule saying that you have to be super-independent. Give yourself a little time to adjust to coming of age.

### CHOOSE FOR YOURSELF

Don't let other people pressure you into making career or life decisions because of what they expect. Look at your strengths, weaknesses and desires, and choose a life path accordingly.

### NO NEED FOR DIRECTION

There's increasing pressure on young people to know exactly what they want to do for the rest of their lives. Don't pressure yourself to choose a career too early if you're not sure; just keep your options open.

### ONE STEP AT A TIME

Don't forget that your parents have looked after you since you were a tiny baby, so it's no surprise that your newfound independence can be difficult for them. Try taking small steps towards it rather than jumping away from them.

### GET ACTIVE

With so many other distractions, many teenagers stop exercising but studies show it's important to keep active, not only to help your body stay strong (because it's still developing) but to boost concentration, too.

### THINK AHEAD

If you're not sure about career or college choices, don't stress about it by yourself; open up to someone you trust and talk about what's worrying you. Friends may brag they know exactly what they want to do, but they might not be being honest.

## twenties

### BE SAFE

The top three causes of death for people in their twenties are accidents, especially car accidents, murder and suicide. Help reduce your risk by being vigilant about your personal safety and avoiding dangerous situations.

### MAKE FRIENDS

Studies have also shown that people with a strong friendship network live longer, healthier lives. The friends you make in your twenties stay around forever, so make time to get out there.

## QUIT THE WEED

While the risks to your health caused by smoking in your twenties aren't enormous, you're setting yourself up for problems in years to come. Now is the time to quit.

## DON'T OVERDO IT

Your twenties is the time when you have most energy and you will be at your fittest, but make sure you avoid over-exercising. This can not only lead to injury, but can actually have detrimental effects on your body's internal systems, such as liver function and digestion. If you are in any doubt, ask a professional for advice.

## START LIFTING WEIGHTS

Although your body doesn't start to gradually lose muscle mass until you're in your thirties, it's important to start lifting weights in your twenties in order to help your muscles stay strong for longer.

## KNOW YOUR NEEDS

Your twenties are a great time to learn how to deal with relationships – both with partners and friends – to work out what you really want from your nearest and dearest and what they need from you in return.

## BE POSITIVE

Studies show that having a positive perception about ageing can add as much as seven years to your life. Ageing is not an inevitable decline in function and ability, and if you adopt healthy behaviours, attitudes and habits while you are young, you can expect to lead a happier, healthier and longer life.

## EXERCISE FOR THE FUTURE

Use your twenties – when other responsibilities are likely to be fewer – to establish an exercise routine you can keep up as you get older. Work out what activities you like and get a routine that fits your lifestyle. The physical decline that doesn't usually start until you reach your thirties or forties can start in the twenties for people who shun exercise.

# thirties

## WORK AT IT

It is estimated that a quarter of thirty-somethings in relationships are unhappy with the state of the relationship. If you feel your relationship needs a boost, talk to your partner and seek professional help if necessary.

## DON'T HOLD BACK

Research has shown that almost a quarter of people in their thirties who want to change career don't because of a lack of confidence. Your thirties are a great time to make changes, so grab the chance with both hands.

## AVOID A CRISIS

Forget mid-life crises, there's a growing phenomenon of crises in people in their thirties. Remember the three Fs – fun, fulfilment and freedom.

## DITCH THE BAGGAGE

If you're carrying around old resentments and issues from earlier in your life, which are having a negative impact on your life now, deal with them once and for all. If necessary, seek professional help.

## THE FAMILY TRAP

One of the reasons people stay in failing relationships in their thirties is that they are worried time is running out for raising a family. Remember that any relationship weaknesses will be magnified by having children, and many couples aren't starting their families until later these days.

## BE GOOD TO YOURSELF

Your thirties are often filled with family responsibilities and long working hours, but don't neglect your own health as this is the decade that age-related health problems can start to occur.

## KNOW YOUR CORE VALUES

By the time you reach your thirties, chances are you will know what's really valuable to you. Understanding what's most important to you in life enables you to prioritize.

### BOOST YOUR CONFIDENCE

Surveys have shown that three-quarters of people in their thirties wish they were more confident. Hold a confidence-boosting evening with your friends where you tell each other your best characteristics.

### THROW AWAY THE SCRIPT

All of us have certain roles – at work, home, with family and friends. Your thirties is the time to realize what boxes you fit into in your relationships and start to get rid of roles you're not comfortable with.

### TAKE A LONG VIEW

By the time you've reached your thirties, it's likely that you'll have decided upon a career. To avoid your life becoming narrowly focused, create a 'big vision' to give yourself a sense of direction and purpose.

### TAKE RESPONSIBILITY

If you're still relying on other people to get you through life, or blaming them for your problems, your thirties is the time to finally take responsibility and become accountable for what goes on in your life.

### HAVE SEX

Self-esteem and body image is better in people over 30 who have sex – they are likely to have greater emotional wellbeing, especially in long-term relationships, which foster togetherness.

## *forties*

### HORMONE PILL

Your body's levels of progesterone begin to decline in preparation for menopause, which can cause increased pre-menstrual symptoms. Hormone pills are effective, so seek help if your periods suddenly become worse.

### SPOT STRESS

It's not just teenagers who suffer from acne – if you find your skin becomes prone to breakouts in your forties it's most likely because of stress. Learning some breathing techniques, meditation or exercising can all help treat the root cause.

## LOOK AFTER MUSCLES

More time needs to be spent warming up and cooling down before exercise in your forties, as muscles are weaker and more prone to strain. Aim for 5–10 minutes before and 10–20 after.

## TAKE A LOAD OFF

Almost a third of forty-somethings work full time and most are still working long hours, with many citing "too heavy a work load" as one of the major causes of stress in their life. Talk to your managers if it's problematic.

## DITCH THE YO-YO

If you've been a yo-yo dieter in your life, your forties is the time to take extra care with your vitamin intake as the regular periods of 'starvation' your body has undergone may have had a lasting effect on metabolism.

## BE SUPPORTIVE

By the time you reach your forties the chances are you've started – or are about to start – experiencing problems with ageing parents, which can be a significant source of stress. Discuss responsibilities with siblings beforehand to help reduce the load.

## MAKE YOURSELF HAPPY

Research shows that people in their forties are more stressed than any other age group, so it's even more important to take action to reduce stress, like making sure you have quality time alone and with your loved ones, doing things that make you happy.

## DON'T DIET

Habitual dieters who snack on high-sugar foods when hungry tend to have a higher blood-sugar level than others, which the body deals with by drawing calcium from the bones. Make sure your calcium intake is high and take supplements if necessary, to avoid osteoporosis.

## MINERAL RICH

People in their forties should aim for a diet rich in iron, magnesium, calcium and zinc, all of which can help your body fight the signs and symptoms of ageing.

## CUT THE CARBS

In your forties, cut down on simple carbohydrates such as bread, pasta and potatoes in favour of fresh fruit and vegetables that contain the minerals and nutrients needed for a healthy body, particularly calcium.

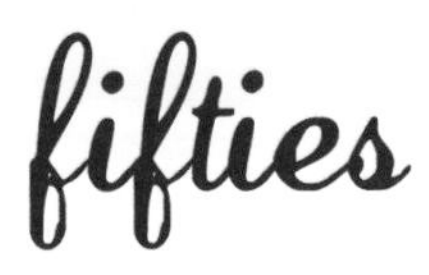

## ENJOY IT

Medical researchers have established that women may derive more pleasure from sex as they grow older because they no longer have anxieties about contraception, but you should still use condoms if you're sleeping with someone new to protect against disease.

## NO NEED TO WIND DOWN

Instead of seeing your fifties as a time for winding down and preparing for getting older, try to see it as a time of personal opportunity where you know yourself well and have time to enjoy life. Take the time to organize travel or social activities that keep you having new experiences.

## HAVE A DAILY PLAN

Don't put off until tomorrow what you can do today. Many people say what helps them to feel good is waking up in the morning and knowing what is planned for the day.

## DON'T BE RIGID

One of the best ways to stay positive is to have a day plan, but don't let your plans rule you – variety is the spice of life so if an unexpected offer comes up or it's sunny and you want to get outside, don't be afraid to ditch the plan.

## MAKE A LIFESTYLE CHOICE

As you get older, it's even more important to start making choices that impact on your life. For instance, why not save the money you normally spend on taxis, cigarettes or wine? Then you can use the extra money to get something that will make a real difference to your life – like a cleaner!

## GIVE SOME CARE

Most women, and many men, in their fifties take on a caring role for family members but be careful not to let this define you. Make sure you carve out time for yourself as well as helping others.

## BALANCE YOUR MONEY

The basic rule to keep in mind in your fifties when you're planning for your financial future is that you don't want to run out of money before you run out of years.

## SPEAK OUT

Many people feel they become invisible as they age and are too afraid to speak out against discrimination. Make it a rule to challenge discrimination if it happens to you.

## BALANCE IT OUT

Reduced activity naturally leads to reduced balance. Keep yours in tune with martial arts like tai chi or yoga, which will keep you strong and supple as well as in balance.

## EARLY SIGNS

Your fifties is when the first signs of many diseases like heart disease and cancers start to appear. It's the best time to start medical screening so you can catch problems early.

## REDEFINE YOUR TERMS

Instead of thinking of 'ageing' as a mental and physical deterioration (the most common reaction), try to think of it positively. Use words like 'maturing' if 'ageing' frightens you.

## GET MENTALLY EMPOWERED

If you are worried about becoming forgetful or losing your mental sharpness, try a supplement formulated for the over-fifties that boosts mental agility. These usually contain a cocktail of B-complex vitamins, omega 3 and omega 6 fatty acids, ginkgo biloba and taurine.

## CHANGE THINGS AROUND

Women over 50 are actually more likely to have a higher sex drive than men, with sex being more important to them than their partners. Keep him interested by not sticking to the same old routine. Sex is also more closely linked to wellbeing for people in their fifties than for any other age group.

## BEAR WEIGHT FOR GOOD BONES

It's really important to make sure at least one of your weekly activities is load-bearing, like running, lifting weights or yoga, as this will help prevent osteoporosis. Make sure you are tested regularly for bone density, too, and follow any advice if a problem is found. The earlier it's detected, the better the results with treatment.

## GET SOME CALCIUM

Losing bone mass is a problem widely experienced by older women, but making sure you have enough calcium in your fifties could help your bones stay stronger for longer. Take a supplement and eat dairy produce, green vegetables and fish.

## CUT OUT SODIUM

Everyone in their fifties should watch their intake of high-sodium foods and fizzy drinks, which can reduce bone mass.

## CONSIDER DOWNSIZING

By your fifties, it's likely that your home has a lot of equity so it may be time to think about downsizing, which will free up some money to make your retirement years more comfortable.

## TWEAK YOUR MONEY

If you have planned well financially for your old age, don't rest on your laurels. Instead, make sure you pay regular attention to your finances and work out the best way to make them work for you.

### PLAN AHEAD

The whole attitude behind financial planning begins to change by the time you reach your fifties. Ten years earlier, retirement seemed very far away but now it seems imminent. Start thinking long-term now if you haven't already.

### START NOW

Instead of waiting until you're older to think about how to stay happy and healthy, start now – it's a great time to join bridge or social clubs that will help you develop a long-lasting network of friends.

### SWAP TO GENTLER SPORTS

If you're quite active you may need to slow the pace slightly. Golf, tennis and swimming can see you into an active old age.

### RECONSIDER INSURANCE

When you had a growing family, your life insurance requirements were large but you may be able to cut your insurance and switch the premiums to investments. Talk to an independent financial advisor.

### SHIFT YOUR SAVINGS

While you may have been bold with your savings and investments when you were younger, now is not the time to take risks. Switch savings to less volatile investments like bonds, but avoid putting all your eggs in one basket.

## sixties

### DRINK UP

Older people are more prone to dehydration and should drink more water than when they were younger, not less. Drinking at least eight glasses a day will help to keep your body organs functioning optimally and keep skin looking younger as well.

### WATCH THE SUGAR

As you get older, your body is more prone to sugar highs and lows and less able to deal with high-sugar foods. It's important to include lots of fibre and wholegrain in your diet.

## FIGHT ALZHEIMER'S

Vitamins C and E are thought to help lower the risk of Alzheimer's disease, and making sure your fresh foods are of good quality and eating them in raw or lightly cooked form rather than overcooked maximizes health giving effects.

## TRY SOMETHING NEW

It's never too late to be a student, so make it a rule to learn something new every day. Even if it's something you read in the paper or hear on the news, making an effort to retain new information will help keep your brain feeling young.

## TAKE A BREAK

Many retired people find volunteering is a great way to meet new people and keep themselves busy. But if you volunteer, make sure you don't work yourself into the ground – take regular breaks and ask for help if you need it.

## EAT UP

In your sixties, your appetite begins to wane and foods seem less appealing as your metabolism slows down. Staying active can help limit this decline so that you won't gain weight even with a little extra food.

## IF YOU DON'T USE IT, YOU LOSE IT

Your taste buds will be less sharp at 60 than they used to be, but to keep them going strong for as long as possible it's important to keep trying different foods and tastes.

## EAT OFTEN

Because your appetite is likely to have reduced, even if you are still active, it might be easier to eat four or five smaller meals a day, rather than three large ones, to help keep your blood sugar levels constant.

## GET A COMPANION

If you are living on your own, consider getting a pet. A cat is a good low-maintenance pet but if you are active, consider a dog. Older pets have less energy, which means they are not nearly as demanding as younger animals. They will provide companionship and give you a sense of purpose.

## DON'T SLOW DOWN

Don't think that because you are in your sixties you have to slow down your activity to a gentler pace – as long as you are healthy, vigorous exercise is a great way to keep your body looking and feeling young.

## THINK WHOLEGRAIN

Make sure you include wholegrains like barley, brown rice, wholemeal bread and quinoa in your diet because they contain lots of fibre which will help keep your digestive tract in top form.

## TAKE A PROBIOTIC

About 90% of the bacteria in the gut of a newborn infant are 'friendly', but this drops to 10–15% in the average adult and after the age of 60, they could be a thousand times less. Taking a probiotic could help.

## MOISTURIZE

Your skin will now be telling the effects of how well you looked after it in previous decades, but all post-menopausal women need to moisturize as the lack of oestrogen means the skin is dryer.

## AVOID THE SUN

In your sixties, pigmentation marks can start to show, with some areas being lighter or darker than others, sometimes in large patches. It's best to avoid the sun altogether, or make sure you're covered up with an spf 30+ sunscreen.

## JOIN A GYM

Keeping going when your body is weaker may require more willpower. Joining a gym can help not only with programmes but also with a social scene to help you stay focused.

## KEEP UP THE ACTIVITY

The levels of DHEA growth hormone drop dramatically by the time you reach your sixties, meaning keeping muscle is harder. Sixty-somethings who don't exercise are ill more often, lose more mobility, have more trouble sleeping and lose coordination much more quickly – so get active.

### WEIGHT LIFT

Lifting weights, or other load-bearing exercise like running and team sports, helps put a stop to muscle wastage and bone density decline, which is especially important for post-menopausal women.

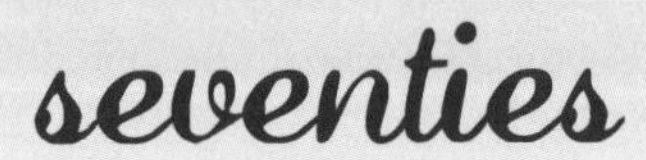


### BE SAFE AT HOME

As you get older you are more prone to falls and accidents, so take a few minutes to check your home for possible hazards, such as dimly lit stairs and hallways. Also avoid standing on chairs and stools to reach high places or light bulbs.

### KEEP FEET HEALTHY

Foot pain and other problems with feet can contribute to an increased risk of falls so make sure you see a chiropodist regularly. It's also important to wear the correct type of shoes as you get older.

### MAKE A CALL

If someone comes to your door claiming to be from a utilities company, don't be afraid to make a call to that company to check their ID. Make sure you get the number from a separate source, like your own bill or directory – genuine callers will not mind waiting.

### IT'S A BALANCING ACT

Exercising regularly, particularly making sure that you concentrate on types of activity which help balance and strength like pilates, tai chi and yoga, is the best defence against falls.

### DON'T BE DIZZY

Some medicines can make you dizzy and increase your risk of falling and hurting yourself. If you suffer dizziness as a side effect of your medication, talk to your doctor for advice.

## FRESH AIR FOR EYES

When our bodies come into contact with natural sunlight they are stimulated to produce vitamin D, which helps keep bones healthy and strong. Aim for half an hour of fresh air a day.

## AVOID LARGE BILLS

The aim with all your spending should be to spread bill payments over the year so that your outgoings match your income in amount and frequency.

## KNOW THE SIGNS OF DEHYDRATION

If you're suffering from any of the following, drink fluids immediately: thirst, dry mouth and skin, or cracked lips; dark-coloured urine; feeling tired, confused or having a headache.

## SEE YOUR DOCTOR

You should always see a doctor for an assessment following a fall, even if you don't think you were badly hurt. If you have regular falls, they can help by running a falls risk assessment.

## USE RESEARCH

If you have to buy something new and aren't sure you're being sold the right thing, seek independent advice from a consumer protection association that will give impartial advice first.

## DON'T KEEP CASH

One of the reasons criminals target older people in their homes is because they are likely to keep cash in large amounts. Keep your money in a bank or at the post office instead for safety and peace of mind.

## COMPARE QUOTES

When you need to have work done, get at least two or three separate quotes from different tradespeople, and don't be pressured into parting with money in advance.

## GET AN EYE TEST

Have your eyes tested regularly. Not only is it important to get your eyes checked so that you are not straining them and causing further damage, eye tests can also help pick up on other problems such as diabetes.

### A RAINY DAY ACCOUNT
If you want to save regularly for vacations, celebrations or large bills, get a savings account with a bank, but remember these accounts often have notice periods for withdrawals.

### CHECK YOUR HOME
Don't wait until your appliances and household items break before replacing or repairing them. Check them regularly and watch sales and offers so you don't have to panic buy.

### GET UP SOON
If you do fall and aren't too badly hurt, get up as soon as you can because a lot of the problems people experience after falls are from lying on the ground for too long and getting cold. Pull or push yourself up if possible.

## over-eighties

### KEEP MOVING
Studies have shown that 'exercise deficiency syndrome' is the biggest risk to older people. Regular exercise prevents high blood pressure, heart disease, stroke, poor circulation, depression, obesity, and joint and bone problems.

### BE A SOCIALITE
Having a strong network of family and friends and a range of activities is vital to the health of your mind and body, not only because it makes you feel happier, but because mental stimulation is important to stay alert and engaged with life.

### SEEK HELP
Don't put up with health problems on the grounds of "age" or assume that old age means nothing can be done. Age is not neccessarily a cause of illness or reason for poor healthcare.

### STAY HYDRATED
Remember that alcohol and caffeine-containing drinks, such as tea, are diuretics. You should try to balance them with clear fluids. Make it a rule of thumb to carry a bottle of water with you everywhere in the summer, so you make absolutely sure you don't get dehydrated.

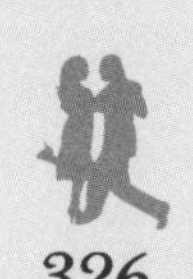



## LITTLE AND OFTEN

People who regularly drink small amounts of alcohol tend to live longer than people who don't drink at all because alcohol helps prevent coronary heart disease. The maximum benefit is achieved by drinking between one and two units of alcohol a day.

## THINK POSITIVE

Spend 20 minutes a day focused on a positive thought or memory – you will feel better and it will boost your immune system. Be positive – studies show that longevity appears to be linked to a determination to stay in control.

## MENTAL AGILITY

Research shows that cognitive functions can be kept agile by doing regular mental gymnastics. Crosswords, Sudoku and puzzles are excellent mental gyms, as are discussion groups and many kinds of voluntary work.

## BE ASPIRING

Talk to your doctor about taking aspirin regularly. There is some evidence that it can help to prevent coronary thrombosis, cancer of the colon and possibly cataracts. Not everyone can tolerate aspirin so it's important to check with your doctor, especially if you have gastric problems.

## COVER UP TO STAY WARM

Putting on an extra layer or wrapping up under a blanket can keep you warm if your home is cold, especially at night. Keep a blanket near your bed for the early hours and wear layers that are easier to adjust than a heavy jumper (sweater).

## GET GREAT GUMS

Gum disease is often the cause of lost teeth, so brush your gums gently and see the dentist if they bleed. If you wear dentures, make sure they fit properly; dentures need to be changed from time to time as your jaw changes shape with age.

## BRUSH AWAY

Older adults are likely to take medications that can impact oral health. And as you get older, dental health is more important because loose and missing teeth can cause problems eating, which can lead to malnutrition. Brush twice a day and get regular check-ups from a dentist.

### THE EYES HAVE IT

Eating foods that are rich in lutein – such as sweetcorn, spinach, courgettes, green peppers, cucumbers, red grapes and kiwis – is thought to help protect against cataracts and macular degeneration.

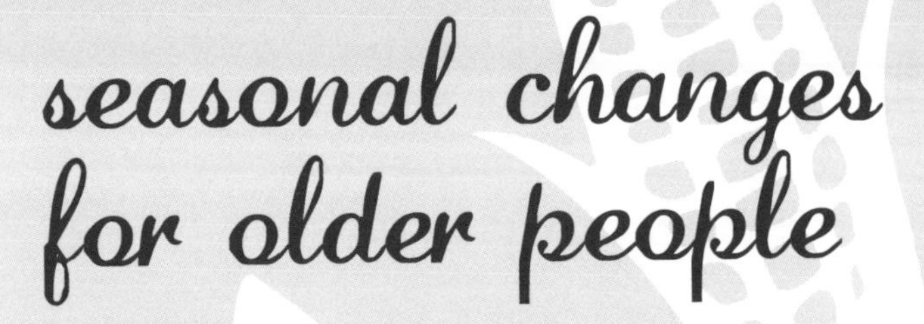


### GET A JAB

Everyone over 70 should get a flu jab every year to help protect them against the likely strains of flu, which can be dangerous in older people.

### MOVE FOR WARMTH

In the winter, many old people get dangerously cold because they don't move around. Even vacuuming or doing some gentle exercise in the home can help to get circulation moving again.

### TOP UP YOUR POTASSIUM

Fruit and vegetables are not only good to include in your diet because of their mineral and vitamin content, the potassium they contain is also thought to increase sodium (salt) excretion. Potassium is found in meat, bananas, dried fruits, potatoes and avocado.

### INSULATE IN THE SUMMER

Double glazing, loft and cavity wall insulation are good for summer as well as winter. Use draught-proofing strips and thick curtains in the winter.

### STAY IN AT MIDDAY

Avoid going out during the hottest part of the day in the summer, which is from about 11 am to about 3 pm. If you have to go out during this time, stay in the shade, wear a hat and loose-fitting clothes, and make sure your shoes are sensible. The idea is to stay as cool as possible, so natural fabrics are best.

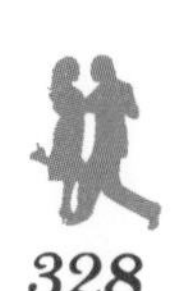



### KEEP WARM AT NIGHT

Keep your window closed, and help your health too – cold air on the head at night has been shown to raise blood pressure in older people, so stay warm if you can.

### START EARLY

If you want to spend some time in your garden in the summer, try to do it early in the morning or in the evening as the sun is going down, which means you'll be able to relax rather than overheat.

### EAT FOR TEMPERATURE

In the winter, two or three hot meals a day and regular hot drinks provide warmth and energy, and in the summer remember to drink lots of cool water and juices, and eat fruit and cold meals.

## *becoming a grandparent*

### SHARE EXPECTATIONS

You're bound to be excited about the prospect of becoming a grandparent, but don't assume your children will know what you want from it – talk to them about your expectations and theirs so you all know what to expect.

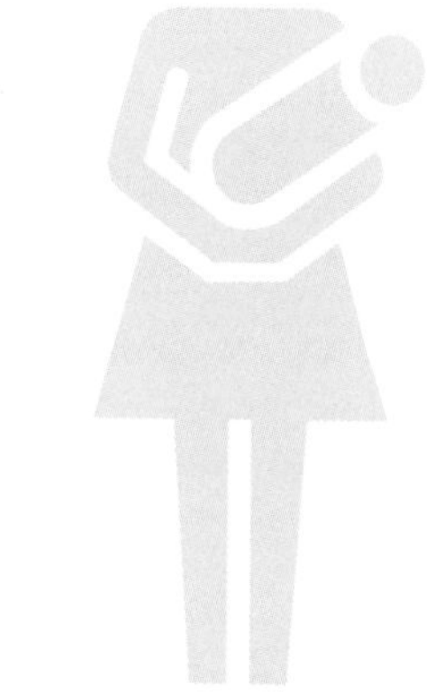

## HOLD BACK

There's nothing guaranteed to ruin the joy of being a new parent more than a grandparent interfering and constantly talking about how things used to be. Bite your tongue and let your children do it their way.

## BE PREPARED

Instead of relying on your children to fill you in on the dizzying array of new technology around childbirth, why not do some research yourself so you will know what to expect. The internet, doctors and libraries are all good sources.

## ASK QUESTIONS

Don't be afraid to ask your children whether they are planning a family of their own. If you are open to their answers and not judgemental, they will relish the chance to talk about their decisions.

## TAKE A CLASS

Many hospitals and groups run classes for grandparents-to-be, helping fill you in on the nitty-gritty of what to expect as well as explaining the methods and techniques that have changed since your day.

## OFFER SUPPORT

Remember that your job as a grandparent is not only to support your new grandchild but also your children – they are likely to need you a lot more after the birth than they have for several years.

## START EARLY

Don't assume your job starts when the baby is born – the last few months of a pregnancy are a great time to start bonding and laying the foundations for a good relationship.

## BE ADAPTABLE

It's good to start talking as early as possible about what your input as a grandparent will be – will it be daycare, babysitting or maybe financial? But don't set anything in stone; all of you may change your mind once the baby comes along.

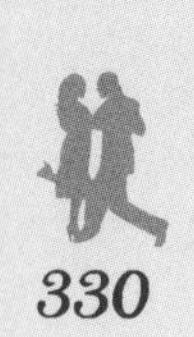



### WAIT TILL YOU'RE ASKED

Your children know you have lots of advice and experience to give, but don't risk ruining your relationship by offering it unless they ask. Try to express doubts or worries in non-threatening ways and always be ready to listen – your children may need someone to unload their worries to but that doesn't mean they will necessarily take any advice you offer.

### STAY YOUNG

Being a grandparent should be fun – free of responsibility and full of laughter – all the benefits without the burdens. If you find your 'job' of caring for your grand-children is making you feel older rather than younger, maybe it's time to put limits in place.

### ENJOY THE SPOILS

Many grandparents look forward to spoiling their grandchildren, but make sure this means lots of love and time rather than disregarding their parents' rules or giving them everything they ask for.

## age discrimination

### OMIT DATES

When applying for a new job, leave out any dates that will age you from your covering letter and CV (résumé). Put the focus on your recent job experience and keep it to the last 10–15 years and to relevant jobs.

### GAIN NEW SKILLS

If you're looking for a new job, try spending some time updating your skills. Employers respond well to people who adapt to change, and learning new skills is a great way to demonstrate flexibility.

### POSITIVE ATTITUDE

Don't go about looking for work thinking people don't want you because you're older. Negativity is catching, so work at projecting a positive image which is bright, neat and alert, and concentrate on what you can offer TODAY, in addition to your wealth of experience.

### EMBRACE CHANGE

Be adaptable in your approach to finding new work and embrace new opportunities and responsibilities. If you are forward-thinking enough, prospective employers won't notice your age.

## being a student

### HEAD DOWN

Studying at home can be tough, as the rest of the family often don't understand how to help, or want to. Try to talk to them reasonably about what would help you in the run-up to exams and ask them what you could do for them in return when your exams are over.

### BE SURE TO ASK

Often, a cause of people failing at school is not understanding what's needed when it comes to homework or assignments. Talk to your teacher or lecturer and make sure you know exactly what's required.

### KEEP IT VARIED

University is an opportunity to learn about life as well as your chosen subject so make sure you don't just stick to the course. Check out public noticeboards for groups or clubs and join a few to further your interests.

### EAT BREAKFAST

Even if you're getting up halfway through the day, eating breakfast is an essential way to start your day. When it comes to keeping your energy high for studying, it's even more important.

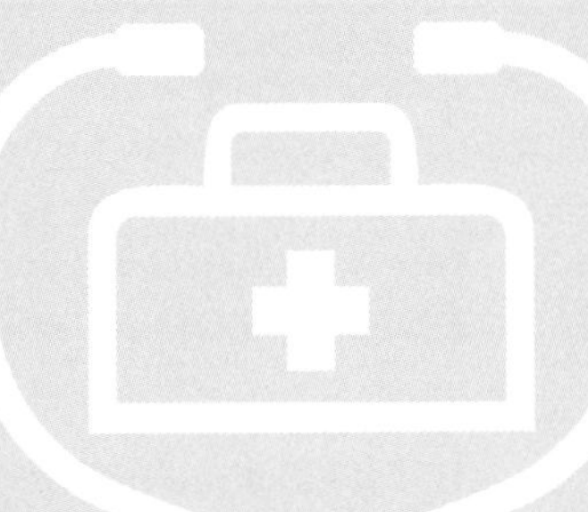

### GET REGISTERED

It's important to make sure you register with a local doctor or clinic as soon if you have travelled to study in a new town so that you can seek help quickly and easily if you become ill.

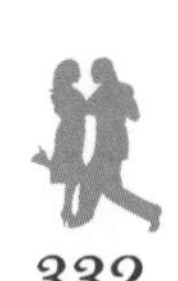



## PLAN THE REST

In the run-up to exams, try to give your memory a break by writing down to-do lists and work plans, both for revision and after the exam period, rather than keeping them in your head. It will help focus your time-keeping as well.

## TAKE AN HOUR

For one hour a day, do something that has nothing to do with your course. Watching TV or doing an exercise class can help clear your mind, or simply have a coffee break or take a walk with your friends.

## DO IT HOURLY

Split each hour you spend studying into work time and break time to make sure you're working most effectively. Work for 45–50 minutes and then take a 10–15 minute break, which will leave you refreshed for the next stint. Working without breaks is non-productive.

## KEEP YOUR FRIENDS

Even if your course is ultra-demanding, make sure you don't isolate yourself at university or college. Making time for your friends is really important, as they will help reduce your stress.

## HAVE FUN

Studying can be a lonely business. Make a point to schedule some fun into your day. For instance, make a rule that you won't work after 9.30 pm and get out of the house to meet some friends.

## SEEK ADVICE

If you become ill while you are away from home and need to get some rest, make sure someone knows, so they can check on you in case you worsen or get dehydrated.

## GET PHYSICAL

Take care of your physical health by exercising at least three times a week. You may never have as many opportunities to join sports teams and clubs again, so there's no excuse. A tennis match or a few laps in the pool are great ways to relieve tension too.

## KEEP UP-TO-DATE

Medical experts suggest that before you embark on your university or college career you make sure your vaccinations are up to date, especially for meningitis C, which is more common among students.

## TAKE A BREAK

When it comes to the breaks from college or university, lots of students need to work, but make sure you give yourself at least a few weeks a year when you take time out to relax and recharge.

## GET A ROUTINE

Try to timetable your studying so you sit down in the same place at the same time each day. This will give your brain and body a chance to get used to studying and make you more efficient.

## SET YOURSELF LIMITS

When it comes to exams, there will always be more to do than you can achieve, so don't get bogged down. Write your list in order of priority and set time limits for each item.

## DON'T OVERDO IT

It's tempting to join in with everything you can when you first start college or university, but try to be realistic about what you can handle. Working and playing too hard and not getting enough rest can lead to anxiety and depression, so stay sensible.

## MAKE A STUDY DATE

Don't always study alone when it comes to exam revision. Study with a friend but don't just stick to the same ones. For each subject, choose people of the same ability and who are compatible with your way of learning and form separate groups.

## STAY AWAY

Resist the urge to go home every weekend. Leaving home for the first time can be a difficult adjustment, but you're likely to cope with it better and stop feeling homesick quicker if you throw yourself into your new surroundings and don't leave every week. It will also give you the opportunity to develop new friends, which can take time.

## EAT REGULARLY

Skipping meals has been shown to lead to snacking on high-fat, high-calorie, sugary foods, which are not nutritious. Also, it has been scientifically proven that meal skippers accomplish less work, are physically unsteady and slower at making decisions. Avoid empty calories and feed your body and brain nutritiously on a regular basis.

## GET A THIRD STARCH

For best energy levels, aim to make a third of your food starchy – for example, bread, pasta and rice. A great way of doing it is to mentally divide your plate into three and make sure a third is filled with starchy stuff.

## SAY NO TO SUGAR

When you're studying until the early hours, snack on foods like cereal or sandwiches rather than high-sugar foods or drinks which can actually reduce concentration. Bear in mind that a can of coke contains 8 rounded teaspoons of sugar, a pack of boiled sweets (hard candy) 24 teaspoons and a typical chocolate bar 9.

## FIVE-A-DAY

Make sure you take in at least five portions of fruit and vegetables a day, especially if you are hitting the town, to help make up for lack of sleep and increased alcohol intake. For student cooking, frozen vegetables are great choices.

## BE COMPLEMENTARY

For vegetarians, the best way to ensure you're getting enough protein is to eat foods in the right mixtures, like cereal foods with dairy or pulses, and pulses with seeds or nuts.

## FEED YOUR BRAIN

Keep the brain well nourished with a diet rich in fish oils (omega 3 and 6), B-complex vitamins (in cereals and grains), folic acid (in fresh vegetables and fruits), zinc (in cereals and nuts) and vitamin A (in dark green leafy vegetables and orange or yellow fruits).

## CARB HEAVY

If you're cooking on a budget, snack in between meals on starchy, simple foods such as cereal, toast or a baked potato, which will keep you going for a long time.

## GET LEAN

Instead of buying large amounts of fatty meat of which you will have to waste lots, try buying a small amount of leaner meat like chicken or lean steak. You will be able to use more of it and it will be healthier.

## FIND YOUR PULSE

Beans, peas and lentils are a cheap source of protein and are great for using to bulk up stews, soups and casseroles with, or instead of, meat. One-pot meals like casseroles are great because they can be used for more than one meal – and save on washing up!

## COMMUNAL COOKING

If you live in a student house, instead of everyone cooking for themselves every night, create a cooking club where you take turns to cook for each other a few nights a week. It will give you a rest and help you socialize. It will also save you money in ingredients.

## MARKET SAVVY

Instead of buying fruit and vegetables at a supermarket where they can be expensive and high on packaging, why not visit a market? Most towns and cities have one and students usually have some time off in the day to shop, so are well placed to find healthy bargains.

## CAN IT

If you can't afford fresh fruit and vegetables, particularly if it's out of season, buy them canned in natural juice or water, which keep well.

## CLUB TOGETHER

Instead of each buying your own meat source if you live in student accommodation, why not club together for a joint of meat to share and add your own accompaniments. Cheap joints like shoulders of lamb are great choices.

### STOCK UP A STORE

At the beginning of term, buy store-cupboard essentials like lentils, beans, dry pasta, packet soups, peanut butter, canned fruit and vegetables. These will help to see you through when money gets tight.

### REHEAT WELL

When reheating food leftovers make sure everything is piping hot throughout, particularly if you're using a microwave, which can heat irregularly. Do it within 48 hours and don't reheat more than once.

# *pregnancy*

### PUT YOUR FEET UP

Feet and ankles can often get sore and swollen in pregnancy because of fluid retention and the added weight you're carrying around. Whenever you can, rest with your feet elevated to help fluid drainage.

### GET COMFY

Sleeping on your left side with your knees slightly raised is often considered the best position for you and your baby because it is said to help relieve nausea as well as increase blood flow to the foetus and decrease swelling. Put a pillow between your legs for extra comfort.

### CONNECT WITH YOURSELF

Antenatal yoga is a great choice during pregnancy because it not only helps you stretch and relax hard-working muscles but it will also help you connect with the changes in your body.

### STRETCH OUT CRAMPS

If you suffer from leg cramps during the night you should gently stretch the muscle and massage the area until the pain has subsided. Stretching out your calf muscles before bed may help to reduce their incidence, as will making sure you're properly hydrated – lack of fluids is one of the main causes of cramping.

## BE POSITIVE

Being pregnant involves a lot of tests and information about things that could go wrong but bear in mind that most pregnancies are fine and try to focus on the positive.

## JOIN A GROUP

Wherever you can, join groups that will help you meet women who are going through the same experience as you. Not only will making pregnant friends help you now, they'll be invaluable when your kids come along.

## SPLASH ABOUT

Swimming is ideal exercise during pregnancy as your body is weightless, so reducing pressure on joints and muscles. The breaststroke and backstroke are the best strokes to use during pregnancy.

## BODY AWARE

Skin, hair and nail growth often changes during pregnancy so make sure you alter the products you buy accordingly. Use a good moisturizer on your stomach and breasts to avoid stretch marks. Taking care of your body will make you feel nurtured.

## SLEEP IT OUT

Night-time toilet visits become a frequent occurrence throughout pregnancy but to minimize them, avoid caffeinated foods and drinks, reduce the amount of fluids you consume in the hours before bedtime and take a trip to the toilet before you settle for the night.

## DREAM EASY

Many women suffer from vivid dreams or nightmares during pregnancy, and the broken sleep patterns make it more likely you'll remember them. Try not to worry about dreams, but do talk to your partner or a friend if they are making you anxious.

## ENJOY SOME ADULT TIME

Pregnancy is the last chance you'll have for a while to enjoy some time with your partner and friends, so make the most of it. Try to go on a date with your partner every few weeks to just enjoy being together and alone.

### TRAVEL SAFELY

If you're flying during pregnancy, make sure you wear support stockings. When you're pregnant your fluid levels increase and you're more prone to swollen feet and ankles.

### SAY NO TO SPICE

To avoid night-time indigestions, avoid eating heavy or spicy meals before bed. Instead, snack on plain food such as a banana, toast or crackers, and drink milk or herbal tea.

## parenting

### ENCOURAGE PERSISTENCE

Don't teach children to be perfect; teach them to be persistent because that is what is more likely to bring them success in life. Going after perfection brings with it a fear of failure, which won't help their future.

### A POSITIVE OUTLOOK

One of the biggest indicators of happiness in adults is how positive their outlook is and parents can help their children grow up positive by concentrating on the good – "well done for cleaning your room"; "don't forget to put your socks in the drawer" rather than, "you haven't done it properly, your socks are still out".

### HELP THEM FOCUS

It's important to instil a sense of achievement into your children so they understand that effort and hard work are linked to praise and pleasure – adults who don't make this connection end up not achieving things.

### MAKE SUNDAY SPECIAL

It has been shown that families who spend time together at weekends (or any other specified day if weekends are difficult) develop closer links and are less likely to suffer depression.

## WRITE A LIST

If your child is resistant to go to school, get them to write a list of everything they like and don't like about school and work with them to reduce the 'don't like' list. Enlist the help of their teacher if necessary.

## LOOK AFTER YOURSELF

Research shows that the number-one worry for children is the health of a loved one. Children count on their families so make sure you give the right message by showing them you look after your health.

## TALK IT THROUGH

Talk to your children rather than shouting at them. If they have done something wrong, explain what it was rather than expecting them to read your mind. Keep your thoughts positive and it will rub off on them.

## TEACH THEM WELL

Remember that today's children are tomorrow's adults, and it falls to you to help them develop the capacity for happiness. Each day when you put them to bed, remind them of all the positive things they have seen and done that day.

## GROW GRATITUDE

Help your family see the half-full glass (instead of the half-empty one) by making a habit of being grateful for at least one thing a day. Even if it's something as simple as 'I'm grateful the sun was shining', it will help them develop a positive outlook.

## HELP THEM OPEN UP

Studies say that only about a quarter of kids discuss their worries with their friends. About the same number talk to their parents, but the majority try to deal with problems alone. Talk to your children often and help them open up to you. Kids in families who talk openly are more likely to turn to a parent first if faced with a crisis.

### KEEP IT CHEAP

Don't worry if you haven't got lots of money to take your children on expensive outings. Research has shown that children are just as happy having a picnic in the park or simply hanging out at home with their parents – what they really need is for you to spend quality time with them.

## taming teens

### TOO MANY NOS

Before you bite back with a "no" to all your teenager's requests, examine why you want to say no and be open to discussion. If your teenager feels you are compromising, they will be more inclined to do the same.

### GIVE PRAISE

You might assume your teenager doesn't now need or want your approval, but in fact they probably need it more than ever. Make sure they know you are proud of them.

### KEEP RULES FLEXIBLE

Instead of setting out rigid rules with strict boundaries, try to keep them flexible so your teenager feels they have some say in the rule making and is more likely to obey.

### ENJOY THE JOURNEY

Parents who give their teenagers their love, time,boundaries and encouragement to think for themselves may find that they actually enjoy this period in their kids' lives.

## special needs

### DON'T LAY BLAME

Many parents who have children with special needs feel anger or the desire to blame somebody (or themselves) for their child's condition. Understand that this is a very difficult time of adjustment and the acceptance process will take time.

## REMEMBER YOUR OTHER KIDS

If you have a child with special needs, the temptation can be to give them lots of attention instead of your other children. Try to get some help organized so you can build in a morning or afternoon alone with each of your other children so they don't feel neglected.

## BE A COUPLE

Having a child with special needs can put a lot of strain on marriages and partnerships and it's important to remember your relationship needs time too. Try to get out together once a month and find time to talk.

## DO YOUR RESEARCH

There's a wealth of information available on the internet about most conditions and arming yourself with knowledge about your child's needs will put you in a stronger position to fight red tape and indifference.

## CHANGE DOCTORS

If you don't feel your doctor or healthcare team is taking your child's problems seriously, don't be afraid to change to a different doctor. Set out your case clearly and avoid emotion.

## BE A PUSHY PARENT

Parents of children with special needs have to speak out on their children's behalf even more than other parents. Often, being the best parent you can for your child means being pushy and asking questions.

## GET SOME HELP

If you are the sole carer for a child or adult with special needs, make sure you take advantage of schemes available to give you a break. You'll be a better carer.

## SEEK ADVICE

If you're concerned that your child may have special needs or you're worried about a specific condition, seek help as soon as possible. Many problems respond better to help when addressed at an earlier age.

### DON'T TAKE NO FOR AN ANSWER

If there's something you think your child needs or would benefit from, fight for it and don't take no for an answer. Engage people to help you with your battles and give your child the best care you can.

## menopause

### KEEP A THERMOS

To help with night sweating, keep a thermos flask of ice water or an ice pack alongside your bed which you can use to help you cool down if you get hot in the night. At the onset of a hot flush, drink a glass of iced water or diluted fruit juice, which will help cool your body from the inside.

### KNOW YOUR TRIGGERS

If you have hot flushes, mood swings, palpitations, panic attacks or other symptoms, take a pen and paper and write down what you were doing, thinking, feeling, who you were with and what you ate or drank just before so you can identify patterns.

### KEEP DOING KEGELS

Menopause is a really important time to keep doing your Kegel exercises (clenching and relaxing the pelvic floor muscles) to stop future urinary incontinence and uterine prolapse. Tighten, hold for a few seconds then slowly release. Work up to holding for 10 seconds at a time and performing a set of 10 at least three times a day.

### ONE A DAY

Because your body systems change after menopause, it can make you more susceptible to clotting problems such as stroke and heart attack. Taking an aspirin a day (under doctor's supervision) could help reduce your risk.

### JUNK THE JUNK

Processed foods, nicotine, caffeine and artificial sweeteners are no-nos for menopausal women as they can exacerbate symptoms like flushing and mood swings. Try to keep your blood sugar levels as constant as possible.

## BE SWEET ENOUGH

Try cutting out the artificial sweetener aspartame, which is found in many low-fat products, cordials and other sweetened foods, and which some believe can make menopausal symptoms worse.

## NATURAL FIBRES

To help reduce the intensity of hot flushes and let your skin breathe, make sure you use cotton sheets at night and try to choose natural fibres for the clothes you sleep in, lingerie and clothing that will touch your skin.

## BE A MAG LADY

If you suffer menopausal palpitations, try taking 500 mg of magnesium, which is thought to help stop muscle flutters and spasms. Magnesium is also thought to help reduce migraines if taken early.

## TURN OFF THE NEWS

Studies have shown that watching the local news is actually a contributor to high stress levels, which can make mood swings more likely. Do something relaxing instead.

## DON'T GET ANGRY

Many women going through menopause report having uncontrollable anger and rage. Try to avoid situations that set you off and take lots of vitamin B to help tranquillize moods.

## SPRINKLE CINNAMON

Adding cinnamon and ground flaxseed to your morning cereal can help your heart stay healthy, keep cholesterol low and reduce blood pressure, all of which are increased risks after menopause.

## EDUCATE YOURSELF

One of the best ways to help yourself cope with the changes associated with menopause is to find out as much as you can about it and what to expect, which will help cut down anxiety. Research on the Internet and talk to friends and family who have already gone through the process.

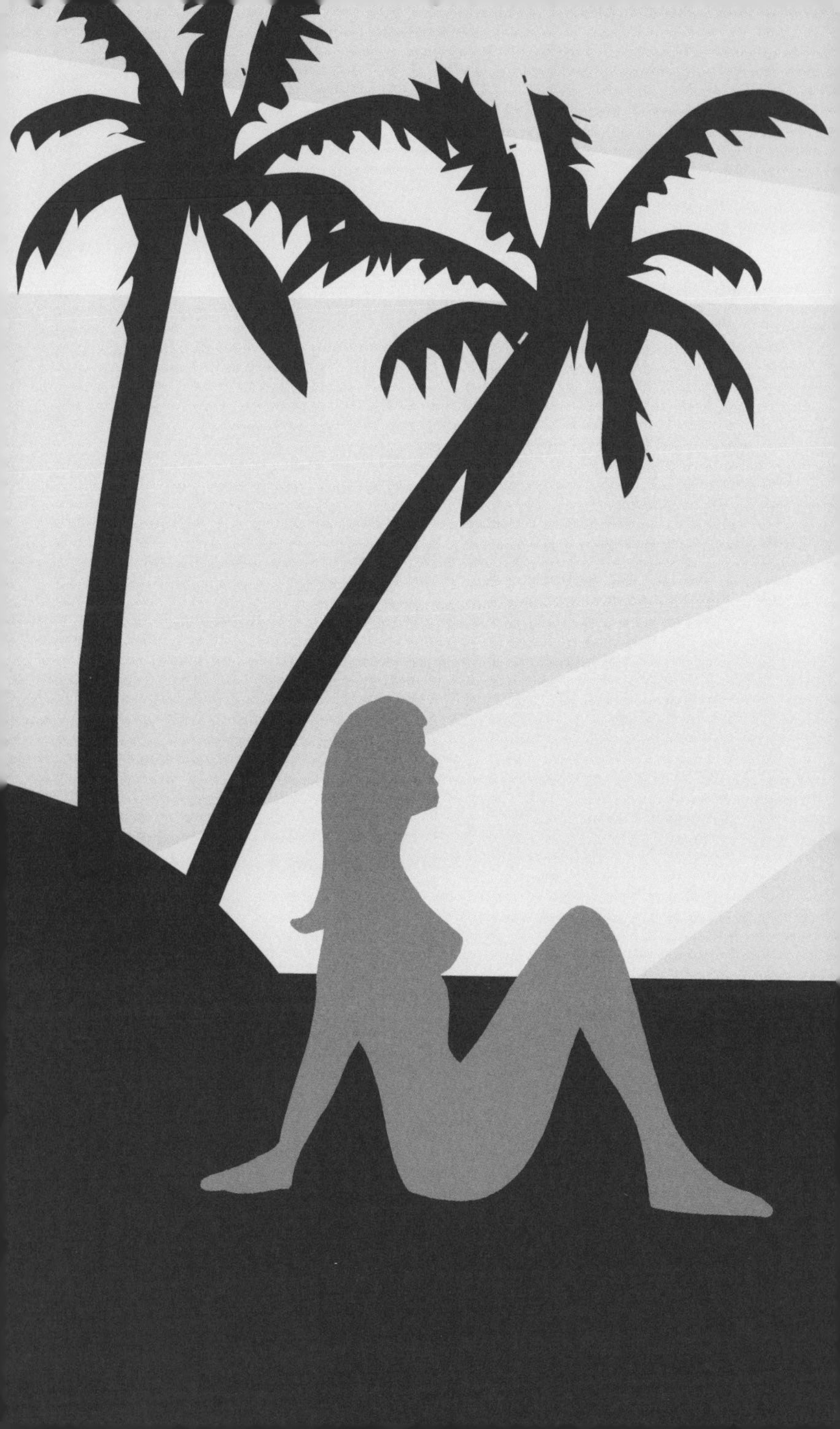

# Mind & Body

Addressing problems such as stress, insomnia, negative thinking and anger management, as well as mental health issues, this chapter includes astonishingly simple changes that can help you break bad habits and maximize your potential for happiness. Advice is also given on therapies that can help your mind, body and spirit, such as meditation, massage, feng shui, reflexology and neuro-linguistic programming.

# depression

## DON'T PUT YOURSELF DOWN

Although it's important to be able to recognize your weak areas, instead of just thinking about your weaknesses, match them with strengths to help keep confidence levels high. For instance, if you're impatient, chances are you are also good at adapting quickly to change.

## WATCH YOUR WEIGHT

A change of more than 5% in your bodyweight in a month, especially if accompanied by sleep changes or feelings of exhaustion, could be a sign you're suffering from depression. Seek help if you're worried.

## DON'T RUSH IT

If you're being treated for depression, remember it takes time for antidepressants to work. So although you may start to feel better within a couple of weeks, the full effect may not be seen for several weeks or months. Be patient.

## GET A MASSAGE

It might sound obvious, but it's amazing how many people never get a massage. A treatment doesn't need to cost a lot and having someone take care of you for an hour can make you feel happier and more whole.

## CHOOSE YOUR COUNSEL

When you first call a health professional, spend a few minutes asking them questions about their philosophy and approach. Interview several and choose the one you feel most comfortable with.

## FIND THE RIGHT ONE

If you're having therapy, don't stay with the therapist if you feel the treatment isn't working for you. Review progress regularly and don't be afraid to point out areas you feel could be improved.

## STRETCH AWAY TOXINS

During the winter, don't neglect exercise. Walking, yoga and pilates are all great ways to keep body's circulation going and alleviate the winter blues.

## TRIP THE LIGHT FANTASTIC

Winter is the most important time to make sure you get some natural light. A walk at lunchtime is a great way of boosting your sunlight levels. However, if you suffer from seasonal affective disorder (SAD), you may need to buy or hire a light box for regular exposure to light during dark months. You need 30 minutes a day at a light level that you'd get on a clear spring morning, which is five times brighter than a well-lit office.

## FIND A PROJECT

Take up a project or hobby that is something you used to enjoy before you started feeling down – such as art, politics or volunteer work. Dedicating yourself to a goal means you don't have time to think about being sad.

## KEEP TAKING THE PILLS

Don't be tempted to take yourself off antidepressants if you start feeling better without talking to your doctor first. Continued use under medical supervision has been shown to lower chances of future bouts of depression.

## KNOW YOUR SYMPTOMS

Depression isn't just about crying a lot or feeling sad. Other symptoms are loss of interest in doing things, changes in appetite and trouble concentrating, sleeping or eating. Seek help if you feel you might be depressed or are suffering from chronic anxiety.

## TAKE A CLASS

If you find it difficult to meditate, breathe deeply or concentrate on one thing at a time, consider taking classes in meditation, which could help give you a valuable life tool for relaxation.

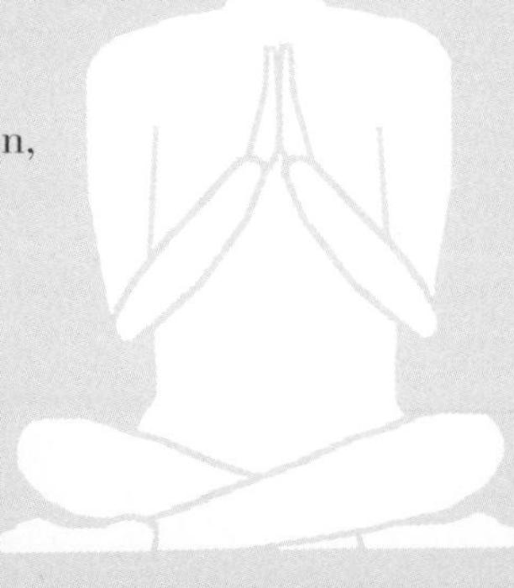

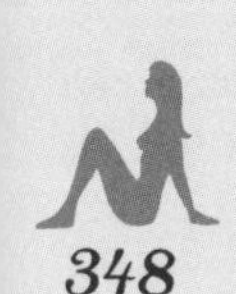

# relaxation



### HAVE A TEA PARTY

Simply going through the motions of making a cup of tea can reduce stress; added to this, each of the four main types of tea (oolong, black, green and white) have their own specific health-giving benefit.

### TAKE IT WITH YOU

If you're on the move all the time, take a home sanctuary with you. Use a portable basket or case to carry around your candles, oils, reading materials and music so you can create your relaxation area wherever you go.

### BREW UP SOME RELAXATION

Chamomile, sage, lemon balm and mint can all be used as relaxing infusions. Add two teaspoons of dried herbs to a cup of boiling water and let it brew for a few minutes.

### GET SOME SPACE

Try to ensure that everyone in the family has their own space, which they can make their own. A bedroom is ideal, but it could also be a corner of a room, a chair or even a shelf if space is tight.

### RETREAT TO THE SPARE ROOM

If you have a spare room, why not turn it into a sanctuary where you can retreat for a few hours to get away from it all. All you need is a CD player, some candles or incense and maybe even a DVD player, so you can chill out alone.

### BIG AIR

If you're using candles to help you relax, make sure the room is well ventilated with fresh air circulating so the air doesn't get stale or deprived of oxygen.

### GET SIDELIGHTS

Light your home to create a sense of comfort and intimacy and think about using different bulbs to provide different moods. Red can help warm up a cold-looking space, and blue can be extra soothing at bedtime.

## MAKE IT MOODY

Put on a favourite piece of music. It can be something that reminds you of a pleasant memory like a happy holiday or your first romance. Then sit back in a comfortable chair, dim the lights and just listen. The memories you associate with the music will help you relax. Music is also said to appeal to directly to the primal part of the brain to calm and soothe.

## BE A GUEST IN YOUR OWN HOME

For one night a week, treat yourself like a guest in your own home and lift your spirits with small touches – buy yourself some flowers, change the sheets so they're fresh and use luxurious towels, blankets and toiletries.

## DO IT ROOM BY ROOM

If you live alone or with a person who shares your interest in relaxation, turn a small area of every room into a relaxation space with a shelf of art objects, floating flowers or some candles. Then you will be reminded of calm wherever you go.

## THE CHIMES OF FREEDOM

Gentle sounds, such as chimes, can aid relaxation and act as a reminder to make your life more peaceful. According to feng shui, wind chimes can counteract the negative affects of unnatural sounds, such as noise from cars and building works.

## BE BEAUTIFUL

Fill your home with those things that give you pleasure. Don't worry about conforming to others' perception of beauty; simply choose things that appeal to you.

## SING ALOUD

Singing not only helps you relax because it feels good, it also helps to regulate your breathing, which itself reduces stress. So next time you take a shower, let rip.

## NURTURE YOUR FRIENDSHIPS

Every couple of months have a night out with one or two of your closest friends. It doesn't have to be expensive – just having a take-away meal at home is a great way to spend some quality time.

### OPEN A BOOK

Reading is a great way to escape the stresses of your day, because having the mind focused visually on the words makes it difficult to think of other things. Once a week, turn off the TV and make it a reading night.

### MAKE THAT CALL

Make one evening a week your phone-a-friend night and really take time to talk to your friends. Sharing your worries and triumphs with friends is important.

### BATHE AWAY STRESS

Treat yourself to a whole evening of pampering at home. Use a face pack or hair mask in your bath, wrap yourself in warm towels afterwards, do your hair and nails and you'll emerge feeling great.

### EAT LIKE A KING

Treat yourself to a meal of your favourite food and make it special – set the table with your best cutlery and crockery, dim the lights and really enjoy it. Even if you're on your own you'll feel pampered.

### AN ORANGE A DAY KEEPS STRESS AWAY

Research shows that vitamin C helps combat anxiety and lower stress hormones. Just one orange provides the RDA of 60 mg and makes a refreshing mid-morning snack. Choose whole oranges rather than juice as they are higher in fibre.

## de-stressing

### LOOK AROUND YOU

For a quick-fix relaxation exercise, if you're out and about, look straight ahead at a wall opposite and just above eye level. Keeping your eyes on that point, begin to broaden your vision so you notice more and more of what's around it. Gradually bringing your attention to the present like this will help your body relax.

## STRIP OFF

Did you know that nakedness has been shown to help combat stress? Close the curtains, turn up the heating and have some naked time at home to help you feel really free.

## BAG AWAY ANXIETY

Get a small brown paper bag, squash the top together as if you were going to pop it and breathe in and out through it as slowly as you can for 30 seconds to a minute. Stop if you feel light-headed. It's a great remedy for anxiety, panic attacks and general stress.

## WHAT A SCREAM

If you feel the stress building up inside you and don't know what to do about it, take yourself off to a quiet corner and scream it out. Primal screaming has been shown to lower blood pressure and unleash stress and deep-held feelings, so make it as loud and heartfelt as you like.

## DIVE INTO CALM

Many people believe water has spiritual qualities for healing, so a gentle swim is a good choice after an argument or to wind down after a stressful day at work. Swimming is also a particularly good form of exercise because you're weightless in the water, which has positive physical and emotional effects.

## BUBBLICIOUS ENERGY

Imagine you have a bubble of energy projecting from your central point and surrounding you, like a force field. Give it a colour if you want, and use it to shield you from stress and tension. This is especially good on public transport.

## FLOAT ABOVE

In emotional situations, it can be useful to be able to step outside yourself, so let your imagination do just that. Imagine you are floating above your body, higher and higher, until you reach a comfortable point. Then use your new perspective to help you deal with the situation better.

### AN INVISIBLE FRIEND
Imagine you had an invisible friend who told you all the negative things you tell yourself during the day. Would you take that kind of abuse? Make your own voice your best friend by striving to be positive. Practise the empty chair technique, where you sit with an empty chair or cushion opposite you, imagine yourself facing you and speak positively to yourself about concerns.

### DESK MATE
If you often get irate or stressed at your desk, give your hands something to do to help relieve the irritation. Keep a ball or other "fiddling" toy to hand and use it when you feel stressed, remembering to breathe slowly and relax.

### GET TO YOUR CORE
To reduce anxiety, concentrate your attention on a point a few inches below your navel and halfway between your front and back. Let your body relax and make sure your knees and jaw are soft.

## boosting energy

### PEDAL PUSHERS
Cycling to work is not only good for the environment, it will help you start the day feeling fresh and revived. Exercising in the morning is a great way to boost your system – just don't forget to fuel up with a power breakfast first.

### DITCH THE CAFFEINE
Give up caffeine – it's a temporary fix and can actually make your brain and body more sluggish and less alert in the long run. Instead, choose water, herbal tea, diluted fruit juice or decaffeinated alternatives to your usual drink.

### BRAIN FREEZE
If you have a shower in the morning, finish with a two-minute cold burst to boost your circulation and get your scalp tingling. Not only will this wake up your body, it will give your brain a boost of adrenaline to help wake you up naturally, without caffeine.

### GET WALKING
Walking uses virtually every muscle group in the body and can burn up 520 calories an hour. Not only that, a brisk walk has been shown to flood the body with feel-good endorphins, helping to beat depression and boost mood.

### BREAK YOUR FAST
Avoid carbohydrates for breakfast and plump for proteins instead to boost your brain's levels of dopamine and increase alertness, as well as keeping your blood sugar steady. Choose eggs, mushrooms, tomatoes or yogurt sprinkled with nuts and seeds.

### WATER YOUR ENERGY
If you suffer from a late-afternoon slump in energy and concentration levels and have eaten a healthy non-fast-food lunch you are probably dehydrated. Aim to drink around eight glasses of water steadily throughout the day and avoid tea, coffee and fizzy drinks which can add to dehydration.

## sleeping soundly

### GET PASSIONATE
If you suffer from sleepless nights, try an extract of passionflower in tea, extract or capsule form. It has been proven to have a mild sedative effect and alleviates nervous symptoms and cramps that can interfere with sleep patterns.

### FREEDOM FROM CLUTTER
If you want to get the most benefit from your night's sleep, make sure you always sleep in a room that you find calm and restful. For most people that means keeping the bedroom free of clutter, dust, pets, electronic equipment, books, TVs and telephones.

### WRITE IT DOWN
Keep a pen and paper by your bedside. It can help you in two ways: first, write a list of things you need to tackle the next day; second, write down (and therefore let go) anything that's playing on your mind and that you might find hard to stop thinking about.

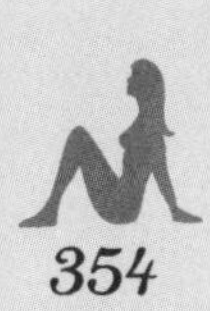



## DO SOMETHING

If you really can't sleep, don't waste time lying there worrying about it. Get up and do something you find relaxing (like reading or watching TV) until you feel sleepy again. You might find going into another room reduces your anxiety about not falling asleep.

## STAY COOL

Research has shown that people who have fresh air circulating in their bedrooms and who keep the temperature at 18–22°C (65–70°F) have a better night's sleep.

## SSSSSHHHHHHH!

One of the worst culprits for sleep deprivation is a noisy bedroom. If you live near a road, street or railway make sure your windows are double glazed or well insulated to help reduce noise.

## DAYLIGHT HELPS

Studies have shown that people who get a good dose of natural daylight every day sleep better at night. Try to get at least 20 minutes outside every day.

## DITCH THE BOOZE

A small nightcap might help you drift off to sleep more easily, but drinking heavily during the evening is likely to lead to waking in the early hours as your body copes with metabolizing it.

## GET FRESH FOR SLEEP

Sex is a great way of winding down because it helps relax the body and releases endorphins, which make you feel good and reduce stress.

## KEEP IT MODERATE

Scientists believe that people who exercise regularly have less sleep troubles, but be careful of exercising late at night. If you must exert yourself close to bedtime, choose moderate exercise like yoga.

## KEEP IT REGULAR

Many people who have trouble sleeping have erratic time schedules. Aim to go to bed and get up at roughly the same time every day, which will help train your body's rhythms into a daily schedule. Taking time to prepare for bed will also help aid a good night's sleep by bringing you towards a state of relaxation.

## DON'T DRINK COFFEE

Avoid stimulating drinks like coffee, tea, cola and other drinks containing caffeine during the evening because they can prevent deep sleep from occurring.

## LOWER YOUR SUGAR

Some experts believe that eating foods high in sugar in the evening can cause waking during the night as your body's systems deal with the subsequent sugar crash that follows. Aim for low-GI foods for your evening meal.

## DIM THE LIGHTS

You naturally come into a light sleep several times during the night. To help you sleep smoothly through them, make your room as dark as possible so the light won't encourage you to wake up.

## HAVE A HERBAL

Although it's best to steer clear of coffee and tea before bed, herbal teas like chamomile and peppermint can relax your system and help you settle down more easily.

## DITCH THE FAGS

Smoking is bad for sleep because nicotine is a stimulant. Smokers take longer to fall asleep, wake more often and have more sleep disruption than nonsmokers.

## B A SLEEPYHEAD

Eating foods that contain lots of vitamin B, such as bananas and avocados, is supposed to help relieve sleep problems caused by adrenal stress. Alternatively, take a B-complex vitamin or the Chinese herb astragalus, which enhances the body's immune function.

## MAKE IT MILKY

Milky drinks help you sleep because they line your stomach and have a variety of slow-release sugars. Drink them warm for greatest effect but avoid hot chocolate as it contains caffeine.

## MUSIC ON YOUR PILLOW

Try spending 5 minutes before you go to sleep listening to music as you lie in bed. Helping relax your mind and body in this way will help you drift off to sleep more easily. Nature sounds, such as birdsong, cascading water or wind through the trees, are particularly relaxing.

## BE A LAVENDER GIRL

Sprinkling a few drops of lavender oil on your pillow, or on a handkerchief near your bed, will help you sleep as the herb is linked to restfulness and helps your body feel calm and sleepy.

## BEDTIME BREATHING

Spend a few minutes every night before you turn out the lights doing deep breathing while visualizing any areas of tension in your body and releasing them.

## PLAY A MIND GAME

Counting sheep is the most popular mind game, but anything repetitive will help, like repeating the word "sleep" over and over again, or imagining walking slowly around a room that is covered in black velvet.

## CARE WITH PILLS

Be cautious about sleeping pills because although they might help you go to sleep, they do not give you a natural sleep and there is a risk of dependency. If you do use them, it should be for the short term only.

## BATH BEFORE BED

A warm bath will gently warm and relax you, and not only that, the corresponding reduction in body temperature about 15 minutes after your bath is a great way to mimic your body's natural sleep rhythms.

### TRY TRYPTOPHAN
Foods containing the amino acid tryptophan are thought to help sleep by boosting the brain's natural sleepy chemicals. Turkey, bananas and wholemeal bread are all good tryptophan trips.

# take a deep breath

### BREATHE YOURSELF HAPPY
When you breathe deeply and allow your body to relax, levels of stress hormones reduce in the bloodstream; the more you practise the better your body gets at it. Aim for 10 minutes a day to rejuvenate.

### FOCUS ON THE BREATH
The best relaxation tip is also the simplest – just close your eyes and focus on your breathing. If your attention wanders, bring it back to your breathing and if you have tension in any part of your body help it relax by breathing into that part.

### TAKE CONTROL
Changing your breathing is one of the quickest and easiest ways to take control of how you feel. The rapid, shallow breathing we do when we feel fear or anxiety not only makes us more stressed but also lowers immunity and increases susceptibility to heart problems. Concentrate on allowing your breathing to become deeper and calmer.

### FOLLOW THE SIGHS
For a quick anxiety releaser if you find yourself getting wound up, force yourself to STOP. Breathe in through your nose and then very slowly breathe out. Relax the muscles in your jaw, neck and shoulders as you do so. It only takes a few seconds but can have great benefits.

### DON'T PANIC
Instead of letting your feelings of anxiety, panic or stress overwhelm you, take control by concentrating on using breathing to help you stay calm. Breathe in and out slowly and you'll feel you're doing something to help yourself.

# anger management

## LET'S PRETEND

A great way to control your anger if you need help is to pretend you're calm. Projecting an outward vision of calmness will actually help you feel more calm and less angry inside.

## WALK AWAY

If you are in a situation that is making you angry, leave the room for a while or take a walk. It's easier to think of solutions to problems when you have calmed down.

## EXPRESS YOURSELF

Next time you feel your temper might get the better of you, try to explain your feelings to yourself to get at the root of your anger. Aim to be assertive but not aggressive in your dealings with others.

## SPOT THOSE TRIGGERS

If you feel your anger is out of control, wait until you're feeling positive and try to think about the things that trigger loss of temper. Then, work out how you could avoid those triggers.

## PLAY MUSIC TO AVOID ROAD RAGE

Instead of sitting in a silent car with nothing but the sounds of traffic to spark off road rage, listen to your favourite music or the radio to distract your anger.

## RELAX AWAY RAGE

Gripping the wheel, slouching and arching your back while driving all cause muscles to become tense. Take a moment when you're driving to consciously relax tense muscles and help you remain calm.

## TAKE A BREATH

When you get angry a big surge of adrenaline goes through your body and your heart rate and blood pressure go up. This causes the reasoning part of your brain to shut off for a short while. Taking a deep breath short circuits this system to help you regain control.

## SUPPRESS ANGER

If you have anger problems, instead of allowing yourself to fly off the handle the next time you feel angry, make a deliberate effort to quash your feelings. Then, when you have calmed down, you can take that energy and put it to positive use.

## ALLOW MORE TIME

If you find yourself getting angry when you're driving on particular journeys, allow more time and avoid travelling at high traffic periods. The same applies when you're not driving – always leave plenty of time to allow for delays. One of the most stressful aspects of modern living is being under time pressure.

## BE REASONABLE

Use words to describe your anger and help you decide if it's appropriate or not. For instance, if someone causes you pain it's reasonable to feel angry, but if they simply get in your way or slow you down it's not.

## CONFUSED EMOTIONS

Don't confuse anger with jealousy. It's not reasonable to feel angry with someone simply because they have something you don't or are better than you at something.

## DEFINE YOUR ANGER

Learn to define your problem and face it head-on rather than let it build up. Passively allowing circumstances you are unhappy with to continue will lead to suppressing your anger, which can stop you being able to act to real and serious threats to your wellbeing.

## ACT, DON'T REACT

Stop reacting to what others say or do, and act positively instead. Changing the situation through deeds, rather than words, is less inflammatory and requires thinking it through.

# think positive

## KEEP A DIARY

Every day for a month, write down ten things for which you are thankful. Choose an attractive bound journal or cover a plain book in photos you love. Not only is it a great way to become a more thankful person, but it's good to read through in your low moments.

## MAKE ONE GOOD DECISION

Make a decision – today – to change one thing and one thing only. Make the change, then when you've achieved it, think about making another. If you can't face the big changes like stopping smoking, start small by making an extra 10 minutes for your family each day, or limiting your intake of junk food to once a week.

## BOX UP POSITIVITY

Make a collection of quotes, statements, and compliments about being positive or thankful and keep them in a box. Once in a while, get the box out and read through the quotes to help you feel better.

## SAY THANK YOU

When people give you gifts, however small, send a thank you note. It can be an email or text if you're really pushed for time, but saying thank you makes you stop and think about being grateful, which, in turn, helps you feel more positive.

## VOLUNTEER

One of the best ways of helping you get a positive outlook on your own life is to volunteer to help those less fortunate than you. Helping out at special needs groups, shelters or hospitals is a good start. Check the local press or the internet for details of voluntary groups.

## ADMIRE YOUR REFLECTION

Make time each week to reflect on the decisions you have made and how they have affected your life positively or negatively. Then make a promise to yourself to learn from your successes and failures.

### TIME ALONE
Don't be afraid to let your family and friends know if you feel you need some time alone, especially during holidays and festivities. Be honest and say, 'I could really do with an hour alone,' then come back feeling refreshed.

### LEARN FROM ANOTHER
Find a story about someone who has less opportunity than you who is nonetheless achieving satisfaction with life. Use their story to help you stay positive about your life and the opportunities you have.

### GET CLOSE
Close relationships are important for preventing depression and boosting wellbeing. Most people have around six really close friends who can help them in times of stress, so if you have only one or two make an effort to enlarge your circle.

### DON'T LOSE TOUCH
When people are at their busiest and most stressed is often the time they let friendships drop in order to get things done, but it's a false economy. Keep a good balance by making time for your friends, however busy you are.

### EMBRACE CHALLENGES
It's all too easy to be grateful for things like your house, family and loved ones, but remember to be grateful for life's challenges too. Often, it's facing challenges that helps uncover hidden strengths.

## harnessing happiness

### KNOW YOURSELF
It might sound strange, but spending some time really getting to know yourself could pay huge wellbeing dividends. Identify what it is that makes you really happy and try to make sure every aspect of your life is working towards it.

## USE YOUR WORDS

Next time you feel emotional or overwhelmed by feelings, think about what exactly it is you're feeling. Instead of using words like "angry" or "upset", try to think of the reasons behind your feelings, like "jealous" or "frustrated". Knowing your triggers can help you control moods.

## SAY WELL DONE

Research has shown that people who are enthusiastic and demonstrative with their congratulations when their partner does well at something have stronger and longer relationships, so don't be afraid to let your close ones know when you're proud of what they've done.

## BE GRATEFUL

Spend some time each day being grateful for what you do have rather than focusing on what you don't have or what has gone wrong. First thing in the morning or last thing at night is often best to help you get your day in perspective.

## GET ACTIVE

Studies show that people feel less anxious while they are exercising and for the several hours following. It doesn't need to be for long – you only need to exercise for 20 minutes for this natural tranquillizer to kick in. A brisk walk or even some gardening or housework will work.

## LEARN TO ASK

The times when people feel overwhelmed and really need help are often the hardest moments of life to ask for help. Instead of cutting yourself off and pretending things are fine, allow yourself to ask for, and accept, help and let your friends and family do something useful for you.

## TAKE TEN

Try this exercise if you're feeling low or depressed, or if you've got a specific problem you need to solve. Set an alarm for 10 minutes and for that time write or draw continuously about the issue to help you to release hidden insights.

## LOVE BEFORE MONEY

Research repeatedly shows that loving relationships rather than money lead to people being happier for longer. Don't neglect the people you love in order to make money and be a success. Spend time with your partner, children, parents and friends, making sure they know they are important to you.

## THE PAST IS PAST

Don't let bad experiences in the past put you off trusting friends or partners again. It is better to risk the occasional let-down than to live a life without trusting others, which is seldom happy.

## LOSE YOURSELF

Think about an activity in which you lose yourself but emerge fulfilled and feeling that you have done well. Try to work out what it is you do right at that time and how you could channel it to other tasks.

## FIND OTHERS

If you've got a problem you're not sure how to handle and you don't want to share it with friends or family, join a support group. Talking with people who have undergone similar problems can be really helpful.

## DON'T MISTAKE FINANCIAL SECURITY FOR HAPPINESS

Try to see people's lives and your own as a whole. For instance, your friend might have lots of money, but would you rather swap her single life for your relationship?

## TRY A REMEDY

If you tend to dwell on emotional hurt from the past that you feel may be holding you back, try the homeopathic remedy natrum mur, which could help you to look forward.

## DITCH THE GREEN MONSTER

Jealousy is a negative emotion and often a hidden one, but it can be very damaging to relationships. Try not to listen to what outsiders say and trust your own instincts. The Bach flower remedy of holly is said to be good for general jealousy and chicory is thought to be helpful if you are jealous of another's possessions.

### FIGHT THE FEAR

If you're a naturally anxious and fearful person, the tendency is to think that everyone else is fearless. To get perspective, ask your friends about what they worry about most and what they are afraid of – remember everyone has something they fear even if they don't show it.

### START A DISCUSSION

Discuss problems with your partner or friends when things are good between you. It's at these times that misunderstandings are less likely to occur, and you're more likely to sort out problems if neither of you is angry or upset. You are also more likely to see the other's point of view or simply to agree to disagree.

### STAY TRUE TO YOURSELF

Trying to be – or pretending to be – someone you're not will only lead to anxiety and tension, and people will see through the false exterior. Don't be afraid to be yourself – everyone likes a genuine person more than a wannabe.

## embracing change

### ONE AT A TIME

Don't try to change more than one bad habit at a time, and instead of concentrating on what you haven't done, look at what you have done. Try to replace each negative behaviour with a positive one.

### THE OCCASIONAL SLIP IS OK

If you're committed to changing a bad habit, don't worry if you slip every now and again – but make sure you don't get lax and allow too much slippage, or allow yourself to let slips be a reason to give up.

### COME UP WITH A SLOGAN

Using a positive slogan can help you harness the power of habit because repetition of a phrase hardwires it into your brain. Create a slogan such as 'stay on track' or 'one step at a time' and repeat it ten times a day to burn the thought into your brain.

## ASK ADVICE

Talk with your partner or a close friend about how to reward your good behaviour if you quit a bad habit – keep the reward reasonable and achievable and stick to it.

## THE RIGHT SUPPORT

Before you discuss making a life change with someone, make sure you are choosing someone who will be supportive. Don't ask a smoker for support on giving up, for instance!

## GIVE YOURSELF A CHANCE

If it was easy to kick bad habits nobody would have any, so accept you may be in it for the long haul. Chart your progress so that you can see how things develop over time and look back to motivate yourself.

## MOVE YOUR NOTES

Posting motivational notes around the house to remind yourself to be positive is a great idea, but keep in mind that after a few days your brain will "background it" unless you move it to a new place.

## KEEP THE CHANGE

To help you form a positive new habit, put ten coins in your left pocket and each time you remember to do your chosen thing, move one to the right pocket. When you have moved all ten several days in a row, the habit is formed.

## DO IT FOR THIRTY

Focus on one change only for 30 days and during that time concentrate solely on that one thing and don't try to change anything else about your life. After 30 days, move on to the next change, or take a break from change for a while. Trying to focus on several things is difficult and makes it more likely you'll give up on all of them.

## PULL THE TRIGGER

Come up with a trigger, which is a short ritual you link with a change to condition new patterns of behaviour. Examples include snapping your fingers every time you want a cigarette if you're trying to quit, or jumping out of bed as soon as the alarm starts if you're used to sleeping in.

## KICK BUT

Use the word "but" to help you change negative thought cycles. If you find your inner voice telling you you're bad at something, use "but" to make it positive like, "I'm crap at this ... but if I keep practising I'll get better".

## PRINT YOUR PROMISES

If you've made a commitment to yourself to change, don't keep it in your head where it could become warped or forgotten. Writing down promises makes them harder to break.

## KEEP SCHTUM

Studies have shown that people who talk about things to exhaustion before they do them are less likely to follow through. By all means discuss your chosen course of action, but don't let words take over from actions.

## BET ON IT

Motivate yourself to make a habit change by having a wager with a friend. Making a public commitment and promising to give up something you will miss is a great motivator for the low times.

## BE CONSISTENT

Make sure your habit is as consistent as possible and doesn't require thought or attention. Keeping it consistent will allow the habit to be drilled into your subconscious instead of you having to remind yourself.

## REPLACE LOST NEEDS

If you're trying to give up a habit that gives you something, like comfort eating or watching television to relax, bear in mind that the feeling you're giving up will need to be replaced with an alternative behaviour.

## STAGGER YOUR REWARDS

If you're trying to reinforce behaviour, plan to reward yourself as often as possible the first week, then every week for a month and then every month for three months.

### DO THE CAN CAN

Be vigilant in your hunt for negative thoughts, like "I can't do it", and keep squashing them and replacing them with positives like "I can do it; I am doing it". If you think positive, you will succeed.

### KEEP IT SIMPLE

Don't let your behaviour change become too complicated. Keep it to a few rules to help form habits and avoid confusion. Exercising every day for half an hour is easier to remember than a complicated weekly regime, for example.

### MAKE LINKS

Try to link your rewards to your behaviour change. If you're replacing smoking with exercise, for example, use the money you would have spent on cigarettes to buy yourself new exercise gear, a gym membership, or a sports massage.

## being a better you

### SAVOUR THE SMALL STUFF

Allow yourself to enjoy small pleasures each day. Take a walk, sing in the car, have a glass of wine, read your favourite magazine or do whatever it is that relieves stress and leaves a smile on your face.

### TRAIN THE BRAIN

There are many books, puzzles and even computer games on the market that can help keep your brain active with brain training. Or simply aim to learn a new thing every week to keep your grey cells working effectively.

### BE POSITIVE

For every negative thing you hear yourself say, try to think of three positives. For example, if you hear yourself complaining about the rain, remember how important rain is for modern life as well as nature, and how it makes you appreciate the sunshine even more.

## MAKE A CHANGE

People who are concerned about their stress levels are less likely to exercise and more likely to be smokers than those who don't smoke and lead active lives. Instead of worrying about your bad habits and the problems they cause, make some positive lifestyle changes.

## GET A GOAL

Set yourself a goal – be it with relationships, work or home – and make a list of the steps you'll need to take to achieve it. Anything is do-able if you break it down into small enough steps and take each one at a time.

## MAKE UP YOUR MIND

Unresolved decisions are very stressful. Most decisions are reversible, but getting back time you waste by not making a decision isn't, so be decisive and help reduce stress.

## FIND A PLACE

Locate a place near to your home which you can use as a relaxing getaway. Whether it's a museum, riverbank, café or the beach, it's good to have somewhere you can take yourself to think things through.

## TAKE RESPONSIBILITY

Don't plead helplessness when it comes to your life not being perfect. Acknowledge that it's partly down to you and the choices you have made and are making and then do what you can to change them.

## BE DECISIVE

What's holding you back? Are you waiting for someone to hold your hand, the children to grow up, a lottery win? Being decisive means doing something to enhance your life now, not hanging on for a dream future.

## AVOID COMFORT EATING

One in four people is thought to turn to food to help alleviate stress or deal with problems, but it rarely works – comfort eaters report higher levels of stress, fatigue and sleeping problems. Try something else instead.

### DON'T GRAB AND GO

Stress levels are higher among frequent fast-food eaters than those who eat more natural foods. Make time to cook your own meals and eat them at home.

### KNOW THE DIFFERENCE

Women dealing with stress report nervousness, wanting to cry or lack of energy while men talk about trouble sleeping or feeling irritable or angry. Understand the differences to help support your partner in times of stress.

### SHARE THE BURDEN

Stress is higher for the family's health-care decision-maker, which in 75% of families is the mother. Try to share decisions with your partner to avoid piling on the stress.

## brainpower

### DRINK UP TO THINK UP

The brain weighs about 1.3kg (3lb), the equivalent of a medium-sized chicken! Three-quarters of this is water, so letting yourself become dehydrated really will sap your brainpower. Aim for 1.5–2 litres (2½–3½ pints) a day.

### EAT A BRAINY BREAKFAST

The best food to boost your brainpower at breakfast is high-fibre, carbohydrate-rich food that releases energy slowly, such as wholegrain breads and cereals, porridge or fresh fruit, plus some protein from milk, bacon, eggs or peanut butter.

### WHIZZ UP SOME QUICK-FIX IQ FOOD

If you're feeling sluggish, whizz up a quick-fix brain boost, like a thought-boosting fruit smoothie with oats or apple purée and honey, which will keep your brain firing faster for longer.

### BANANAS ON THE BRAIN

The glucose released into the bloodstream from carbohydrates is the brain's favourite food, and the slower and steadier it's released, the better. Bananas, apples, porridge and stoneground bread are all good snacks.

## BREATHE DEEP TO CLEAR YOUR HEAD

The brain is the body's second largest organ and uses 20% of the total oxygen pumping around your body. Make sure you feed it well with daily deep breathing exercises to boost oxygen circulation.

## DO SOME OLIVE GOOD THINKING

Both memory and concentration are better in people whose diets include high levels of monounsaturated fats, such as those that are to be found in olive and flaxseed oils. This is because of the beneficial effect these healthy fats have on the structure of brain-cell membranes.

## GET CREATIVE WITH CREATINE

Studies have shown that the dietary supplement creatine, used for building body muscle, could increase brainpower by maintaining a high energy flow to the brain.

## BE A MUSICAL GENIUS

Babies who listen to classical music have been shown to be cleverer than their peers who don't, and there is some evidence that music can help adults think clearly, too – but it's Mozart, not Motown, that brings out the brilliance!

## BE A DOUBLE-SIDER

Try using your other hand (your left hand if you're right-handed or your right if you're left-handed) for activities such as writing, eating and sports. Experts say that this will stimulate parts of your brain that routine habits cannot reach.

## EAT MORE CHOCOLATE

No, seriously! Studies have shown that dark chocolate has a protective effect on the brain. Combine this with trying new activities or hobbies – for example, bake your own chocolate recipes for extra mental stimulation.

## SHUN FAT TO STAY SHARP

High intakes of saturated fat could put people at greater risk of cognitive impairment. The healthiest diets for sharp brains are those containing oily fish like salmon and mackerel, which not only prevent degeneration of mental faculties but actually boost brainpower too.

## IRON OUT MEMORY PROBLEMS

A deficiency of iron in the body will impair learning and memory skills along with cell growth in the rest of the body. To counter this, stock up on leafy green vegetables, figs, raisins, peas and meat, which contain high levels of the mineral.

## BE A PILLOW LOVER

Sleep allows your brain to regenerate, keeping you clear-headed and bright throughout the following day. Experts think that between seven and eight hours a night is best for optimal brainpower.

## GET FIT TO THINK

Approximately 750ml (1¼ pints) of blood pumps through your brain every minute of the day and night, and you can boost your potential brainpower simply by increasing the efficiency of your heart by introducing a 30-minute exercise programme into your routine three times a week.

## BREAKFAST LIKE A KING

People who have a proper meal at breakfast tend to have better reaction times, problem-solving abilities and a more acute memory than people who skip, skimp on or rush through their first meal of the day. So make time to breakfast royally.

## BE AN ALL-DAY GRAZER

The brain needs nourishment 24 hours a day as it cannot store significant reserves of energy to keep it working. Missing a meal is detrimental to your thought processes, so aim to eat little and often to keep the brain's energy levels topped up.

## GIVE YOUR BRAIN A WORKOUT

Each day, pick an object and study it for several minutes, then shut your eyes and recreate the image. Remember as much as you can, then open your eyes and see how much you missed. Repeat with different objects daily to boost concentration.

## BE A PROTEIN PRO

Proteins are essential building blocks for the brain to make neurotransmitters, which are crucial for all thought processes. Optimize feelings of alertness by eating meat, fish, peas, beans, lentils, soya beans and soya bean products, eggs or a range of dairy products.

## BE BERRY CLEVER

A cup of blueberries a day could improve short-term memory by protecting against age-related mental decline.

## SANDWICH SOME REST TIME

Carbohydrate foods, including starchy vegetables, pasta, potato, cereals and bread, stimulate the release of the relaxation chemical serotonin in the brain, which enables your brain to wind down after a long day.

## GO MENTAL WITH MINERALS

Both sodium and potassium are vital ingredients when it comes to the optimal functioning of the brain, enhancing connections between neurons. Bananas are a tasty snack and high in potassium, while sodium is readily found in salt, meat and many other foods.

## GET A MEATY REMINDER

Foods that are rich in protein, such as meat, fish, cheese, soya products and nuts, help the brain create dopamine, which is an essential chemical for quick thinking. Eating 75g–125g (3oz–4oz) of protein should help make you more alert and energized.

## FISH FOR MEMORIES

Shellfish contain zinc, which boosts short-term memory and recall as well as enhances verbal and visual memory. Zinc is also found in beans, dark turkey meat and peas.

## GET A BEANY BRAIN

Beans, peas, apples and pears contain high levels of boron, which helps enhance alertness and memory power.

## NIBBLE NUTS FOR MEMORY

Nuts – particularly walnuts and brazil nuts – are full of the memory-boosting substance magnesium, which can improve brain function and alertness.

## GO SLOW FOR QUICK THINKING

Low-density carbohydrate vegetables such as broccoli, spinach and pak choi, fresh herbs and low-glycaemic fruits like berries and melons release sugars slowly and help the brain work hard all day.

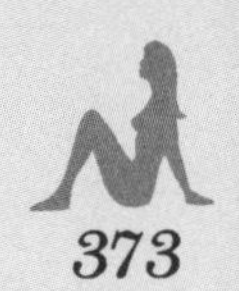



## MAKE MINE AN ESPRESSO

Caffeine may improve memory by making existing brain cells swell and new ones grow, but too much can cause attention problems, so stick to espresso, which has less caffeine per serving than other coffees.

## CHOOSE CHEESE FOR A CHAMPION BRAIN

Cheese can help to increase levels of the neurotransmitter acetylcholine in the brain, which assists general functioning. Other foods you can eat that do the same job include liver, fish, milk, broccoli, cabbage and cauliflower.

## DRINK YOURSELF CLEVER

Your brain circuitry needs to be fully hydrated in order to function at its optimum levels, so drinking eight glasses of water a day is an essential requirement for concentration and mental alertness.

## EAT SMALL FOR BIG SUCCESS

After a big meal, most of the body's oxygen is taken up by the intestines as they deal with the process of digestion, which means the brain gets less. This is why you often feel sleepy after a blow-out business lunch. If you want to stay alert to clinch that deal, eat light at lunch.

## ADDRESS STRESS TO GET AHEAD

Stress hormones like cortisol destroy brain cells, which means the more stressed you are, the fuzzier your head will be. Allowing yourself to relax will help you concentrate.

## BECOME SOYA CLEVER

Soya and soya products contain high levels of lecithin, which is essential for forming the structures of the brain, so make sure you include them in your diet.

## RISE TO THE CHALLENGE

Challenging normal routines occasionally, like enrolling on a new course or feeling your way around your bedroom with your eyes shut, improves reaction times by forcing the brain to work harder.

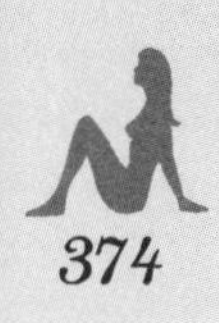



## TAKE A BREAK TO GET A BRAINWAVE

Concentrating on something for long periods of time might not be the best way to solve problems. Instead, give yourself a break to allow ideas to incubate.

## STIMULATE YOUR SENSES

By stimulating more than one sense at once in unusual ways – for example, by sniffing vanilla essence while listening to orchestral music – you can force your brain to create new connections, thus building up your thinking potential.

## DON'T SAY NO

Your brain does not understand negatives, so telling yourself not to think about something simply will not work. Instead, distract yourself by concentrating fully on something else and you will find that the worrying thought disappears.

## GIVE YOURSELF A VEGETARIAN BRAIN BOOST

Vegetarians needing a brain boost could get instant benefits by upping the levels of protein (from nuts and soya) in their food or by taking a protein supplement, both of which will help stimulate the flow of blood to the brain.

## DITCH THE CALCULATOR

Using a calculator to save time could be a false economy. It's much more beneficial for your brain if you do the maths in your head instead.

## REMEMBER TO ADD GARLIC

Garlic has been shown to improve spatial memory and to help protect against age-related memory loss. Use it in sauces, Italian-style meals and stir fries.

## MAKE AN ENTRANCE

First impressions do count, so every time you walk into a room, hold your head up and your shoulders down and back. This will make you appear more confident – and if you look more confident, you will be more confident.

## SALUTE THE SUN

Sunlight boosts the body's natural levels of mood-boosting serotonin, so if you're feeling low on confidence a breath of fresh air could be just what you need.

## BE YOUR OWN HERO

If you feel your confidence slipping at a business meeting or in a social situation, just think of someone you respect and admire and spend a few minutes acting like them. Eventually it will become second nature and their self-assurance will become part of your own.

## STAND UP TO FEEL OUTSTANDING

Standing up straight encourages you to breathe more deeply, which will in turn reduce anxiety levels and help you feel more confident.

## CALM DOWN WITH VALERIAN

The herb valerian has been shown to help more than two-thirds of people with anxiety. Make tea infusions from roots or take supplements when you feel low.

## LEARN TO LOVE YOURSELF

Make a list of at least five to ten things you like about yourself and carry the list around with you so you can refer to it when your self-image is low.

## CURTAIL THE CAFFEINE

Caffeine increases heart rate, which can increase nervousness and anxiety. If you want to feel cool, calm and collected, opt for water or herbal tea instead.

## NEGATE NERVES WITH A SNACK

If you feel sick with nerves, it could be because your stomach is empty. Confidence levels drop when we're in need of food, so have a healthy snack even if you think you're not hungry.

## ACCENTUATE THE POSITIVE

The next time you catch yourself having a negative thought, however small, make an effort to turn it into a positive one. Negative thinking is a bad habit that needs to be broken, and conquering the small negatives is the best way to do it.

## LEARN TO TAKE A COMPLIMENT

People with low self-confidence often find it difficult to accept a compliment, so the next time someone says something nice about you, make an effort to listen and then thank them.

### BE GENEROUS WITH PRAISE

Learn to pay others compliments. Giving a genuine compliment not only makes someone else feel better but can bolster your self-esteem. Look for the good in someone and tell them what you've found.

### PAY IT FORWARD

Doing something nice for someone else has been shown to make people feel more confident, probably because it stops them thinking about themselves and focuses their attention on the positive.

## motivation

### THINK HAPPY FOR HEALTH

People who are happy and relaxed find it much easier to summon up motivation for things they don't want to do. Try to plan a time to do boring jobs and reward yourself when you finish – that way they won't take over your life.

### GIVE YOURSELF GOALS

Setting yourself achievable goals to aim for throughout the day will help your body enter a natural cycle of effort and reward. Remember to reward yourself by allowing yourself a few minutes off every time you achieve something, rather than rushing on to the next task.

### DO IT IN INTERVALS

If you struggle mentally to keep going during your workout, you might want to switch to interval training instead. Using this method, your brain may respond better to short bursts of activity, so enabling you to work harder for longer.

### DRINK UP ENERGY

Fatigue during exercise could be mostly due to dehydration, which causes the body to slow down in order to preserve essential fluids. Make sure you sip regularly to stay well hydrated.

## SEE YOURSELF SUCCEEDING

Visualizing yourself achieving something you want could actually help you achieve it. This is because you are moving the thought patterns in your brain away from negative thoughts towards positive, productive action.

## TREAT YOURSELF

You can train yourself to be motivated in the same way that you train a dog or teach a child – by using rewards. Allow yourself treats when you achieve something and you'll soon race through that "to do" list.

## BUDDY UP TO WORK HARDER

Finding a friend or gym buddy to work out with could increase your productivity by up to a third. Gym buddies help each other by making workouts fun and diverting attention away from the fact that exercise routines are often boring and repetitive.

## MIX IT UP

No one said you had to walk the exact same route each morning or cycle the same roads day in, day out. Keep things varied and don't get stuck in a routine. You'll find that you'll look forward to the changes in scenery and varieties of activity.

## SET REALISTIC GOALS

Set goals you know you can follow through with. Choose activities you know you can do and do well. If you find yourself constantly frustrated with your workout, for example, it could be that it's time to rework your strategy and find a better fit.

## DRESSED FOR SUCCESS

If you look good, the chances are that you'll feel good, too. If you're feeling low, make an effort to dress up and make yourself look good, then look in the mirror and smile. You'll be amazed how much better you feel.

## PUT IT IN WRITING

Keeping a log – of whatever it is you're trying to improve on – will help you see how well you're doing and guide you in setting new goals. If you feel you're "stuck in a rut", set a new challenge and track your progress. Having some 'homework' could make you more diligent.

### GIVE THE GYM A BREAK

Being active still counts as exercise, even if it's not strictly a proper workout. If you're bored with the regime at the gym, take a break. Designate an 'active' day when you don't go to the gym but make a conscious effort to exert energy in other ways. You will feel good for being active, and will have given yourself a break from your normal routine.

### BOOGIE ON DOWN

Playing your favourite music or a selection of uplifting, inspiring songs while you work out or do unpleasant tasks has been shown in studies to increase enjoyment and motivation. Grab that broom and don't be afraid to dance around the kitchen while you clean!

## negative thoughts

### THINK POSITIVE TO STAY PAIN-FREE

Negative thoughts not only make you feel bad but also increase the perception of pain. People who are inclined to think negatively about things perceive more pain than those with a tendency towards a more positive frame of mind.

### LOCK AWAY NEGATIVITY

Start keeping a negative notebook in which to lock away destructive thoughts. Every time you think negatively, write the thought down in the notebook and leave it there so the notebook gets filled up, instead of your brain.

### ATTEND TO THE DETAILS

People who are in the habit of over-generalizing are more likely to have negative thoughts than those who pay attention to the details. So the next time you feel low, instead of just accepting it, think about why you feel bad and try to do something about it.

### BE A CONTROL FREAK

Instead of worrying about things you can't change, concentrate on the things you can change and control – that way you'll feel you're achieving something.

## A THOUGHT FOR THE DAY

Start every day with a positive thought about yourself. It could be something you like or enjoy doing, or something you feel – just as long as it's positive.

## BREATHE DEEPLY TO STOP THE DOWNWARD SPIRAL

If you feel negative thoughts beginning to overwhelm you, stop and take a deep breath. The idea here is that negative thinking is linked to the stress response, which can be halted by a series of long, slow, deep breaths.

## LISTEN FOR THE GOOD THINGS

The next time you feel defensive about something someone has said, think about the comment again before you react. Then, instead of taking it as criticism, try to extract positives from it.

## DON'T SPEAK OUT OF TURN

Listen to the way you say things, particularly to those you love the most. Do you say what you mean or do the words come out in a critical way? Often people can seem to be criticizing without meaning to. Think positively about other people, and make sure they know it.

## MAKE A THOUGHT CHAIN

Carry around a pocketful of paperclips and every time you have a negative thought about yourself, simply hook another paperclip onto the chain. At the end of the day, you might well be amazed to discover just how negative you are. Once you've identified your negative triggers, work at transforming them into positive ones.

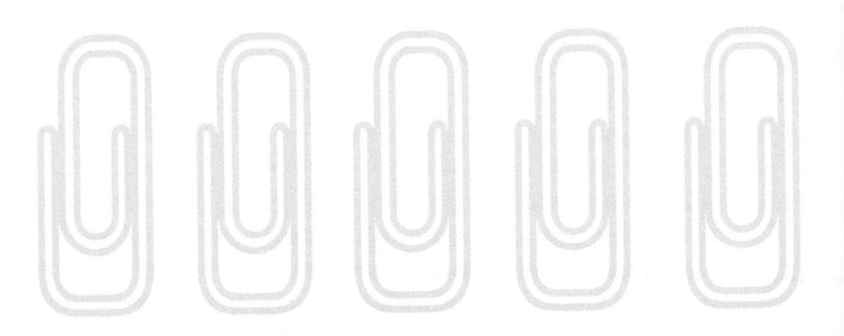

# seasonal affective disorder

## WATCH OUT FOR WINTER BLUES

Seasonal affective disorder (SAD) can manifest itself in feeling low, anxiety, fatigue, weight gain, carbohydrate craving, lack of energy and difficulty concentrating during dark winter months. Slight depression isn't the same thing.

## FLY OFF TO FREEDOM

Taking a holiday abroad at the darkest time of the year could be the key to alleviating SAD. Just a week of sunlight can stave off symptoms for up to a month afterwards.

## CHOOSE PROTEIN TO BOOST YOUR MOOD

To avoid blood sugar surges, which can affect mood, stick to protein-rich foods that release sugar slowly – such as turkey, chicken, salmon, kidney beans or lentils – or slow-release complex carbohydrates like wholemeal bread and brown rice.

## RELAX TO STAY HAPPY

Relaxation therapies, such as Tai Chi, meditation, yoga and massage have been shown to reduce the symptoms of SAD. So next time you feel like you are suffering, get yourself to a class – a deep relaxation treat and being around others may help.

## WALK IT OUT

Getting outside for a 15-minute walk every day can help relieve SAD because sunlight enables the body to produce vitamin D, raising mood-boosting brain chemicals and aiding circulation.

## HAPPINESS IN A BOX

Exposure to light boxes has been found to help sufferers of SAD by safely mimicking the effects of summer sun.

## HERBAL HIGH

The mood-boosting effects of the herb St John's Wort were marked in almost half of those who took it in one study. It can have side effects, so check with your doctor before taking it.

### D FOR DEPRESSION

In a trial, SAD sufferers who took 400 IU (international units) of vitamin D a day during the winter felt more enthusiastic, inspired and alert, probably because the vitamin raises levels of the mood-lifting brain chemical serotonin.

### TIME OF THE MONTH?

If you find your PMS (PMT) symptoms get worse during the winter months, it could be a sign of SAD. Exercise and spending more time outside in the natural light should help alleviate symptoms.

### PARTY ON

If you're suffering from SAD, the last thing you want to do is go out and party the night away, but it could really be the best thing for you. Studies have shown that people who make themselves socialize when they're low feel happier sooner than stay-at-home hermits.

### GET ON YOUR BIKE

Regular exercise – inside or outside – could be almost as effective as light therapy for sufferers of the winter blues, probably because of the mood-boosting endorphins that are released into the body following any type of strenuous exercise.

## acupuncture & acupressure

### POP A PLACEBO

The placebo effect is powerful – it often works even when we know it's a placebo. Even if you don't totally buy into alternative remedies, they can still work for you, so don't be afraid to try something you're sceptical of.

### DON'T BE LATE

Many complimentary therapies, including acupuncture, are most effective if you are calm and unstressed. To help achieve an unstressed state, arrive ten minutes early so you have time to relax before treatment.

## NOSTRIL RELEASE

To release nasal 'stuffiness', push down directly below the outer border of each nostril, on either side of the base of your nose. Feel for a small indentation (flaring and relaxing your nostrils can accentuate the point) and press into the point equally on each side for five minutes.

## GET STUCK IN

Research shows that acupuncture can help a range of conditions, including pain, premenstrual tension, stress and insomnia as well as anxiety and depression. It works by balancing flow of chi (the 'life force') through the body. But make sure you see a trained and licensed professional.

## BE UPFRONT

To get the most out of your acupuncture treatment, it's important to start off on the right foot. Tell the acupuncturist about any medical conditions, drugs or problems you have and if you are, or could be, pregnant.

## MAKE YOUR POINT

Choose your acupuncturist carefully – make sure they belong to your country's professional register and that you feel comfortable with them. Don't be embarrassed about asking questions, especially if you have specific conditions you want them to treat.

## TREAT ADDICTIONS

There is increasing evidence to show that visiting an acupuncturist could help to overcome addictions like alcohol and smoking by reducing cravings and instilling a sense of wellbeing.

## GET SOME YANG

One of the telltale signs of stress is also an acupressure trick for reducing it – massage your temples in slow, circular motions with flattened fingers. Breathing deeply and closing your eyes can help accentuate the result.

## STICK YOUR TONGUE OUT

Drinking and eating before an acupuncture appointment could affect the natural coating of your tongue, which is often used to help diagnosis. Similarly, don't brush your teeth or use a tongue scraper beforehand either.

## WHEEZE AWAY WITH PRESSURE
To help reduce wheezing for asthmatics, cross your hands over your chest and using your fingers to press down on the middle point between neck and end of shoulder for a few minutes (don't do this if you're pregnant).

## KEEP IT LOOSE
If you're going to see an acupuncturist, make sure you wear loose clothing that you'll feel comfortable lying down in. This will also help you feel comforted afterwards.

## DON'T FILL UP
Before you have acupuncture you should avoid large meals, alcohol, coffee and smoking, which may change the "pulses" your acupuncturist will need to feel for in order to choose the right treatment.

## BE QUIET
After you've visited an acupuncturist, it's sensible to build in 20 minutes or so of quiet time to allow yourself to 'come back' to your normal life pace. Many clinics have rooms where you can do this.

## PINCH YOURSELF
If you start to feel light-headed or tired, pinch yourself on the very centre of the tip of your nose. Hook your index finger over the 'bulb' of your nose to anchor it, then dig your thumbnail in firmly.

## HEAL YOUR SCARS
Promote healing with moxibustion, the therapy of burning herbs at acupressure points, often used in conjunction with acupuncture. For recent scars (allow eight weeks of initial healing) wave a lit moxa stick (available from Chinese therapists) a few inches above the scar site to warm the area and restore good chi flow.

## PRESS IT OUT
If you're performing self-acupressure and your fingers get tired, use the rubber (eraser) end of a pencil or the thick end of a chopstick instead.

### MASSAGE AWAY JAW PAIN

To help relieve jaw pain and toothache, use your thumb to massage small circles into your acupressure point in the base of the fleshy valley where your other thumb meets the fingers (do not do this if pregnant).

### PRESS AWAY INSOMNIA

When you can't get to sleep or you're restless, massage underneath the bony ridge around the back of your head, working your thumbs under the ridge line from the ears to the centre above your neck. You can also apply steady pressure for three minutes, using several fingers, to the point on the inside of the wrist crease, in line with the little finger.

## massage & self-massage

### TOUCH BASE

To relieve a tense neck and shoulders, try this self-massage tip: make small circular movements with your fingertips, on either side of your spine, working up the neck and around the base of the skull to ease away spasms in muscles.

### A TIGHT SQUEEZE

One of the most effective ways to reduce tension and spasm in muscles is to go for the squeeze. Apply pressure to the muscle – your shoulder, say – and hold for several seconds, then let go. Work around a whole area.

### CIRCULATION POUND

A great circulation booster if you've been sitting at your desk too long is to use a loosely clenched fist to gently work the muscles of your opposite shoulder. Keep the wrist flexible and avoid applying too much pressure.

## GET YOUR FOOT IN

Resting one foot on the opposite leg, put one hand on the top of the foot and the other on the sole and gently work your fingers into the muscles to relieve tension. Better still, get your partner to do it for you.

## A LEG UP

Knowing how to massage your own legs is really useful for athletes to help post-exercise recovery. It also boosts lymphatic drainage and is thought to help reduce cellulite. Work from ankle to thigh.

## DEAL WITH CRAMPS

If you are prone to night cramps, giving your legs a massage before bed to boost circulation may help. Stroke the whole leg from ankle to thigh three to five times and knead gently into the thigh and calf.

## STROKE AWAY NECK PAIN

To help a stiff neck, stroke your right shoulder with your left hand, starting at the base of your skull and ending at the elbow. Repeat three times then do the other side.

## GET AN AROMA DURING MASSAGE

It might sound like a 'lightweight' therapy, but when you consider that it takes around 20 kg (45 lb) of rose petals to create just a single teaspoon of essential oil, it's worth giving aromatherapy a try, particularly for stress release treatments. Aromatherapy diffusers release the oils into the air, enabling you to breathe them in during a massage.

## STRETCH IT OUT

Most of the things we do with our hands – particularly at keyboards – are contractions, so make sure you take time to stretch them out as well. Spread out your fingers and open the palms as far as possible to stretch them out.

## FEEL THE PRESSURE

Pressure points in your skull can help relax your whole body. To work them, put two tennis balls in a sock and tie the end. Lie on your back on the floor with the sock behind your upper neck so that each ball touches the part of the skull directly above the hollow spot. Relax for at least 5 minutes, preferably 15 to 20.

### EAR WE GO

A great tension reliever if you only have a few minutes is to use your ears to help relax your face and jaw muscles. Pull the sides of your ears outwards, then up and down, then use your index finger to press behind the earlobe where it attaches to the head. Hold for several seconds and release.

### FACE UP TO IT

Don't forget your face when it comes to self-massage. Our faces hold much of the tension of our bodies so make sure you gently work your fingers and palms over it to bring warmth and relaxation.

### RUB YOUR KIDNEYS

Give yourself a quick energy boost if you're feeling low by rubbing the area above your kidneys – push your fists gently into your back either side of your spine at waist level and rub in a circular motion.

### NATURAL PAINKILLER

Massage is a great choice for pain relief because it is thought to interfere with the brain's pain signals as well as causing the body to release endorphins, its natural painkillers.

### THE HEALING TOUCH

Research shows that even a touch from someone else lasting a single second can help people feel better. Ask a friend or partner to help you if you feel you need another's touch.

### KNUCKLE FOOT PAIN

If your feet are painful at the end of the day and muscles feel fatigued and tense, use a loose fist to make knuckling movements all over the sole of your foot, which helps muscles relax.

## *meditation*

### SAY THANK YOU

Get into the habit of feeling grateful for the opportunity to do a meditative practice and your mind's ability to focus. Spending a few minutes being grateful at the end of a session will help reinforce the positive effects of meditation.

## KEEP GOALS IN MIND

The goal of meditation is to create mental space so that your subconscious mind can come to the surface, and to promote a positive outlook and feelings of happiness. Remember this while you practise and the meditation will be more fulfilling.

## PICTURE HAPPINESS

Your safe place doesn't have to be real; you can create a safe haven for meditation in your mind by picturing a happy place where you feel comfortable and "going" there when you feel stressed.

## KEEP PRACTISING

Meditation is a skill and, like any other skill, practise makes perfect. Don't expect to be able to do it straight away, but practise regularly and soon it will be second nature.

## BE ACTIVE

It's easy for beginners to think meditation is the same as going to sleep, but it is an active process. The art of focusing on a single thing takes a lot of hard work and practice, and requires great commitment.

## DON'T ALLOW FRUSTRATION

If you're just starting to learn meditation, frustration is common as thoughts crowd in and threaten to overwhelm the desire for quiet. Focus on the breath if this happens, which helps link body and mind.

## TAKE IT WITH YOU

If you're just beginning to learn meditation, try it throughout the day by generating small moments of awareness (at your desk, walking through the park, and so on) to strengthen the mind and promote calm.

## LIGHT A CANDLE

Meditating with your eyes closed can be difficult, as thoughts can crowd in. To strengthen your concentration, try lighting a candle and using it as your point of focus.

## BRING A FRIEND

Meditating with someone can have many wonderful benefits and can help you both improve your practice. Make sure you set rules before you begin so you both know what to expect.

## BE AN EARLY BIRD

A great time to meditate is in the early morning when it is naturally quiet and the body is well rested. Ideally you should get up half an hour early and do a few stretches before beginning your practice.

## STRETCH IT OUT

Stretching loosens the muscles and tendons, allowing you to sit more comfortably, so gentle stretching or yoga is a great pre-meditation choice, as is a brisk walk or swim.

## LEAVE THOUGHT BEHIND

The goal of meditation is to go beyond the mind – it can't be done by thinking alone, we have to help our minds become quiet before they can really relax. Do this by acknowledging thoughts but not allowing them in – picture yourself turning them away from your "quiet space".

## NOTICE YOUR BODY

A great practice for beginners is to take notice of the body when a meditative state starts to take hold. Put all your attention to the feet and then slowly move your way up the body, becoming aware of each part in turn.

# laughter

## CUT THE NEGATIVES

If you've got friends who always leave you feeling low or depressed, try to spend less time with them and more time with someone who makes you laugh and feel good about yourself. If a negative friend always has that effect on you, you may need to reevaluate the friendship.

## FEED YOUR HUMOUR

Instead of watching heavy dramas that leave you feeling wrung out, spend at least one night a week watching or listening to a comedy programme, sitcom or stand-up.

## CREATE A FUNNY BOX

Take a box (an old shoe box will do) and use it to store things you find funny, like old cards and cut-outs from magazines, or even DVDs or audio comedy. Dip into it when you feel in need of a boost.

## HAVE A LAUGH

A recent study by the University of Maryland Medical Center found that people with heart disease were 40% less likely to laugh, and watching a funny movie boosts the flow of blood to the heart in the same way aerobic exercise does. Every day, make a conscious effort to read or watch something funny.

# feng shui

## SOOTHE YOURSELF

Use colours to help create a feng shui sanctuary in your bedroom. Opt for colours which mimic the natural human skin – from pale pinky white to rich chocolate brown.

## CLOSE YOUR DOORS

Keeping bedroom doors closed at night – including those to en suite bathrooms and walk-in closets – will allow for the most nourishing flow of feng shui energy.

## BLACK AND BLUE

The feng shui colours of water are black and blue. They are used to help create abundance, including good health. Use them in the north, east and southeast areas of your home.

## GET FRESH

Open your bedroom windows often or use an air purifier to keep your bedroom fresh and full of oxygen. Plants are good for air quality but try not too have them too near the bed.

## THE BEDROOM YOU DESIRE

Everyone has different tastes when it comes to décor, but keep in mind two keywords when you are creating your bedroom: pleasure and dreaming. Everything you put in your bedroom should reflect the desire for love, relaxation and healing sleep.

## CREATE SOME BED SPACE

The best place to have your bed according to feng shui is where it is approachable from both sides, with bedside tables on each side to balance and declutter. Do not position the bed directly in line with the door. A firm mattress, solid headboard and sheets made with natural fibres are all good for creating harmony.

## GO EAST

To boost health with feng shui, try to incorporate wood or water features in the east of your space (concentrate on your main living area and your bedroom in particular). If you don't want wood or water, choose art that depicts them.

## ROOM WITH A VIEW

According to feng shui, the most important views to concentrate on are the view from your bed and the first view you see when you walk in the door. Make sure these are attractive and clutter free.

## BE FRESH

When you're using feng shui techniques to help harmonize your home, the important elements are fresh air, light and a lack of clutter. Concentrate on these three before you embark on specific changes.

## BE METALLIC

If you want to boost your clarity and precision, try to incorporate some of the feng shui metal elements to the north and west areas of your space. Use metal or grey and white colours.

## DIM THINGS DOWN

A great way to make your bedroom feel relaxing is to use a dimmer or have lots of different levels of lighting. Candles are great but they're not always appropriate, so other means of low-level lighting are useful.

## GET A GOOD IMAGE

Make sure the paintings and prints you choose for your bedroom reflect what you want to see happening in your life. Avoid colours that clash or anything violent or too bright. Nature scenes such as landscapes are calming and relaxing.

# yoga

## GET TOASTY

If you're meditating at the end of a yoga or pilates session, make sure you keep yourself warm with a blanket or shawl. Being still and reducing heart rate with deep breathing after exertion can cause the body temperature to drop, and that will reduce your ability to relax.

## MAKE A CHOICE

Read up on different types of yoga before you pick one that is right for you. For most complete beginners, a Hatha or Vinyasa class will be most appropriate as they are least demanding physically.

## EAT LIGHT

Don't have a big meal before a yoga class as this could affect your energy levels and give you a cramp. Aim to eat a light meal a few hours before the class is due to start and drink water to stay hydrated.

## GO BARE

It's best to take off socks and shoes and to practise yoga in bare feet, as many of the postures involve your feet being aligned properly and being aware of the ground. If your feet get cold you can wear socks during relaxation, though.

## GO AT YOUR OWN PACE

Whenever you're doing exercises at home like stretching, pilates or yoga, pay attention to pain. Do things at your own pace and never be tempted to push yourself too far to keep up with someone else.

## DO LIKE A DOG

The Downward Dog yoga position (with hands flat on the floor, feet flat or heels pressing down towards the floor and bottom in the air to form a triangle) is great for clearing your head of stressful thoughts. It helps reduce blockages in the neck and shoulders and allows blood flow to the brain.

## SPEAK OUT

The first time you attend a yoga class make sure you tell the teacher and, if possible, choose a place near to them so that they can keep an eye on you.

## HOT TO TROT

Bikram yoga is a series of exercises practised in a heated room. As you can imagine, a vigorous yoga session at high temperatures promotes profuse sweating and loosening of muscles. It is said to be cleansing and to rid the body of toxins but it is not for beginners. Make sure you drink plenty of water before and after the class and don't eat for two hours beforehand.

## DRINK UP BEFORE

Because yoga is designed to have beneficial effects to your internal organs as well as the muscles and bones of your body, it's a good idea not to drink water during class – but make sure you top up before and after.

## YOGA FOR LIFE

A holistic therapy, yoga heals the mind, body and spirit. Yoga means "yoke" or "union" in Sanskrit and its aim is to integrate all the various aspects of your life so that your mind and body work together.

## GET INTENSE

If you're an active person who enjoys exercise, Ashtanga yoga might be the right choice as it is an intense style based on constant movement, or flow, from one pose to the next. Attend a beginner's class first.

## HOLD THE POSE

If you are a naturally precise person, you will probably enjoy Iyengar yoga, which is a style based on postural alignment that concentrates on holding poses for a long time.

## STAY UNSTIMULATED

If you're new to yoga, the effects can be fairly dramatic. Avoid energizing and stimulating postures like the Sun Salutation and standing Warrior poses in the evening. Try practising slow forward bends and the prone Corpse pose, which creates a deep state of relaxation.

## DON'T PUSH IT

While it's natural – and often helpful – to look around you in a yoga class to see what everyone else is doing, don't worry if they seem to be able to do more than you. Everyone's bodies are naturally different and it's dangerous to try and push yourself. You'll feel the benefit whatever your level.

## ALL OR NOTHING

If you are the type to throw yourself into something wholeheartedly, choose Sivananda yoga, a form of Hatha, which is based upon the five principles of proper exercise, breathing, relaxation, a vegetarian diet and meditation.

## KEEP AT IT

You will probably feel a bit stiff or sore after your first yoga class, especially if you don't take regular exercise, but stick at it for a few weeks before you decide not to go back – you'll be amazed at how quickly your body adapts.

## HAVE A HATHA

If you're a naturally relaxed person who likes taking things slowly, a Hatha yoga class is probably for you as it's likely to have a slow pace and provide a good introduction to basic poses and breathing exercises.

## HANG LOOSE

If you're practising yoga at home, even if you're a beginner, be sure to wear clothes that allow for freedom of movement but which are not so baggy that they could restrict flow. Lycra and cottons work well.

## STAY BALANCED

If you're trying yoga poses that involve balance, put a "focus" object a few metres (yards) away from you to fix your gaze on as you balance. A painting or photo at eye level is best, but a plant or even a pile of clothes will do.

## RUNNING ON EMPTY

Dedicated yogis will only perform exercises on an empty stomach, but there's no real evidence that this makes it easier or gives greater benefits. As with any form of exercise, however, it's sensible to avoid doing anything strenuous straight after a large meal.

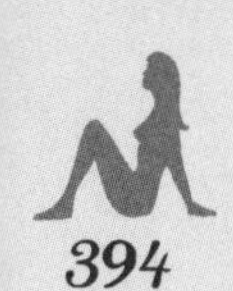



# reflexology

## HOLD YOUR HEELS

For a home reflexology treatment to help problems in the pelvic area, try massaging your heels or rolling them around on a soft ball. The heel of the foot is linked to the pelvic area so it's a great place to target if pregnant.

## EASE BREATHING

To help ease breathing problems, relieve stress and relax the chest and ribs, stand on or roll your foot over textured reflexology or massage balls (or golf or tennis balls if you don't have any to hand) in the centre of your foot at the toe end of the arch.

## TOE THE LINE

The bottom of the big toe in reflexology is thought to link to the hormone-controlling pituitary gland, so if you're feeling low and think it might be hormonal, or if you're premenstrual, give it a rub.

## PAD IT OUT

If you're having problems with your lungs, chest area and breathing, give yourself a reflexology treatment by massaging the pad of the foot, under the toes as far down as the beginning of the arch.

## PULL YOUR FINGER OUT

For some hand reflexology, grasp each finger or thumb at its base and tug firmly. Allow your grip to loosen slightly and let your finger gradually slide out of its grasp.

## CENTRE YOURSELF

If you're feeling low or out of sorts, sit cross-legged or with knees dropped to the side on the floor with your thumbs gently pressing into the soles of your feet. This will help redress energy imbalance.

## PINCH AN INCH

For headaches and stomach aches, pinch the webbing between the thumb and index finger and keep holding with the same pressure for a few minutes, when symptoms should start to disappear.

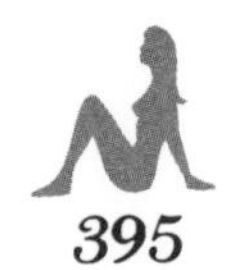



## HEAD, FINGERS AND TOES

If you suffer from headaches, massaging toes and fingers could help reduce symptoms. Massage all fingers in turn but concentrate on the thumb and big toe.

## REACH OUT

If you don't like your feet being touched but want to benefit from the relaxing effects of reflexology, try hand reflexology, which is based on the same principle but using hands instead of feet.

## GET BACK IN LINE

To help reduce back pain, apply pressure with your thumb along the inside of each foot, starting at the base of the big toe and ending at the heel. Do this about ten times and gently massage any tender spots.

## RUB IT OUT

To help relieve the symptoms of a cold, rub the balls of your feet with steady pressure. You can do the same to the pads under your fingers, but feet are more effective as there is more padding.

## BE IMMUNE

Encourage strong immunity by massaging the reflexology points on the top of the foot between the toe and ankle with gentle pressure from the fingertips.

## GIVE FINGERS A LIFT

For a quick hand boost, pinch the tops and bottoms of finger and thumb tips, then squeeze from side to side. They might feel a little uncomfortable, but you should never press if they are tender.

## PALM IT OFF

Rest the palm of your hand inside your other palm and use your thumb to massage the back of your hand, starting with the knuckles and areas in between the knuckles and ending up near the wrist.

## GO GOLFING

To help give your feet a complete reflexology boost that will kickstart sluggish internal systems, stand on golf balls. It might sound painful but in fact it will give you a great energy boost.

## PRESS YOUR PALM

For a quick reflexology trick to help you centre your energy, relieve stress and encourage your body to take a few moments out, close your eyes, breathe deeply and press your thumb into the centre of your opposite palm for 30 seconds to a minute. Afterwards, open your eyes and rotate wrists to bring back energy.

## SAY I LOVE YOU

If your child suffers from digestive complaints or constipation, give him or her an "I Love You" double foot massage by using a thumb to trace an I (from the heel to the middle of their right foot), an L (across the feet in a line) and a U (in a line over the outside of the left foot, ending at the heel).

## HEAL WITH REFLEXOLOGY

Although reflexology is not a substitute for a medical diagnosis, it can alleviate the symptoms of many health complaints, from migraines and PMS to back pain and poor digestion. It can kickstart the body into healing itself and strengthen immunity.

## HAVE A BALL

If your thumbs and fingers get tired from massaging your feet, or you find the position uncomfortable, invest in some foot balls which you can use while sitting down to target treatment areas more comfortably.

## GET SOME SOLE

A foot rub to the centre of the sole is a great way to help reduce the effects of a hangover, boost a detox or give you a lift if you're feeling down.

## TWIST YOUR WRIST

A great self-massage for anyone who uses a computer or writes a lot is to massage the inside of your wrist with the thumb of the opposite hand. Move the wrist and hand around during the massage for greater effect.

# neuro-linguistic programming (NLP)

## PICTURE ACTIVITY

Exercise is a key factor in losing weight but many of us don't enjoy it. Trick your mind into enjoyment by picturing the times in your life when you enjoyed an activity (like sex or dancing). After a while, your unconscious mind will connect the feeling of excitement and eagerness to the thought of exercising.

## FIGHT PHOBIAS

For phobias, NLP, which helps you 'rewire' your brain, can be a fantastic and relatively easy treatment. NLP claims to remove phobias in a couple of hours simply by altering your "self-talk", the inner voice inside, replacing negative messages with positive ones.

## VISUAL GOALS

Changes are implemented visually, auditorily and kinetically for greatest benefits in NLP, which means you need to see, hear and do them. Write down your goals and pin them to your fridge so you can see them, tell your family and friends what you're trying to do and put your plans into action.

## REDUCE APPETITE WITH NLP

One of the basic NLP premises is that the mind and the body are one system. If you make a change in your mind, there will also be a change in the body. NLP can help reduce your appetite by helping you understand your eating habits. Create a mental picture of the times you snack and replace it with one of drinking water, walking or doing something healthy. Many people believe water has spiritual qualities for healing, so a gentle swim is a good choice after an argument or to wind down after a stressful day at work. Swimming is also a particularly good form of exercise because you're weightless in the water, which has positive physical and emotional effects.

# index

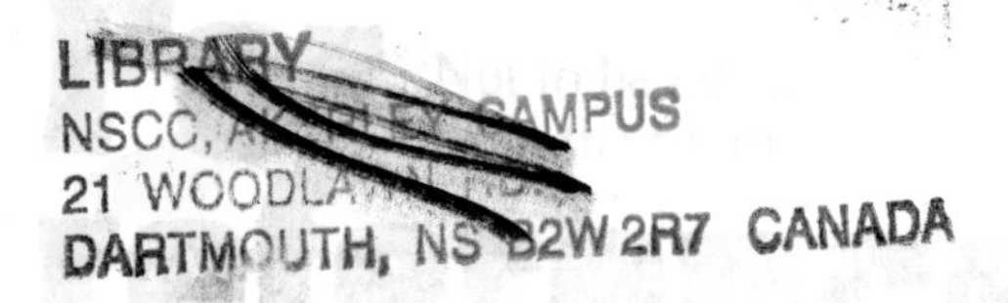
LIBRARY
NSCC, AKERLEY CAMPUS
21 WOODLAWN RD.
DARTMOUTH, NS B2W 2R7 CANADA



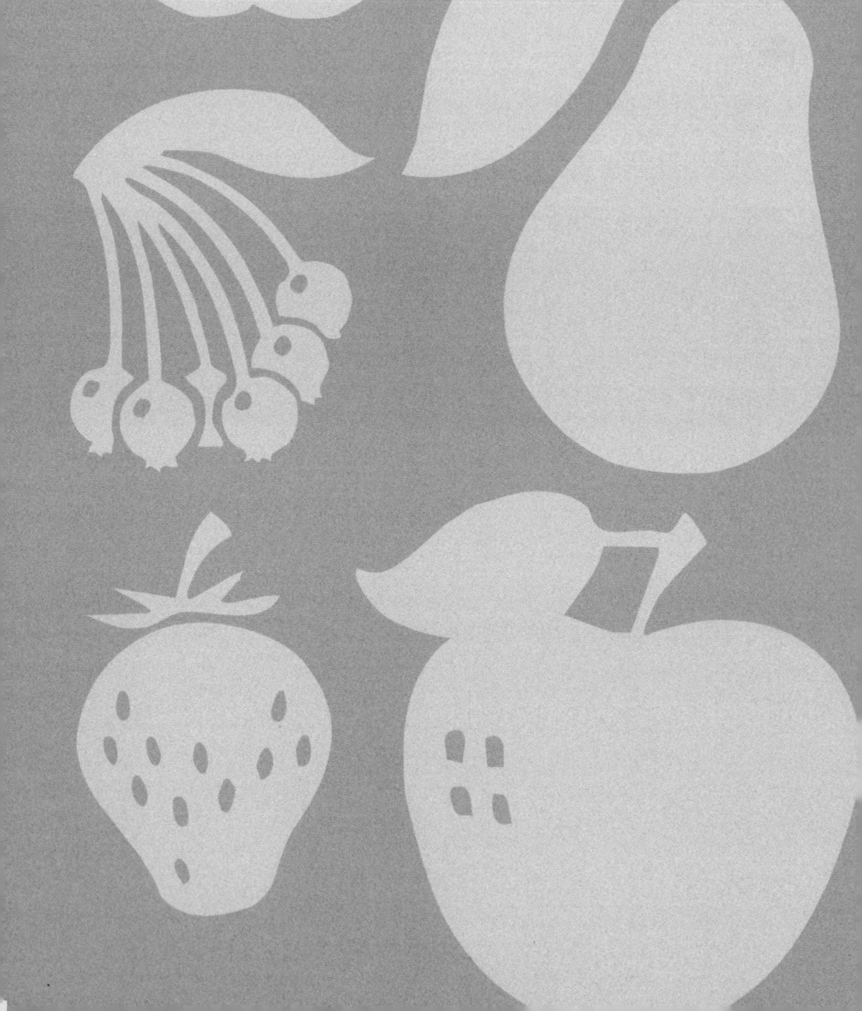